Arthroplasty - Advanced Techniques and Future Perspectives

Edited by Alessandro Zorzi,
Hechmi Toumi and Eric Lespessailles

Published in London, United Kingdom

Arthroplasty - Advanced Techniques and Future Perspectives
http://dx.doi.org/10.5772/intechopen.102234
Edited by Alessandro Zorzi, Hechmi Toumi and Eric Lespessailles

Contributors
Beakal Gezahegne, James M. Broderick, Tiarnán Ó Doinn, Jesua I. Law, Kunal Panwar, Brenden Cutter, Michael Holmboe, Ryan Card, William Pistel, Armin H. Paravlic, Andrew P. Kurmis, Rogério Teixeira de Carvalho, Jörg Lützner, Brigitte Altermann, Ana Laura Puente Reyna, Thomas M. Grupp, Atthakorn Jarusriwanna, Chaturong Pornrattanamaneewong, Leisheng Zhang, Zhihai Han, Zhongchao Han, Hui Cai, Tukaram Sambhaji Dudhamal, Alessandro Rozim Zorzi, Wander Edney de Brito, Gustavo Constantino de Campos, João Batista de Miranda , João B. Miranda

First published in London, United Kingdom, 2023 by IntechOpen
IntechOpen is the global imprint of INTECHOPEN LIMITED, registered in England and Wales, registration number: 11086078, 5 Princes Gate Court, London, SW7 2QJ, United Kingdom

British Library Cataloguing-in-Publication Data
A catalogue record for this book is available from the British Library

Additional hard and PDF copies can be obtained from orders@intechopen.com

Arthroplasty - Advanced Techniques and Future Perspectives
Edited by Alessandro Zorzi, Hechmi Toumi and Eric Lespessailles
p. cm.
Print ISBN 978-1-80356-401-2
Online ISBN 978-1-80356-402-9
eBook (PDF) ISBN 978-1-80356-403-6

For EU product safety concerns:
IN TECH d.o.o., Prolaz Marije Krucifikse Kozulić 3, 51000 Rijeka, Croatia,
info@intechopen.com or visit our website at intechopen.com.

Meet the editors

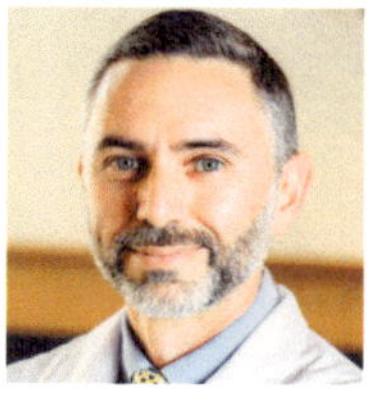

Prof. Alessandro Zorzi is a doctor with a specialization in orthopedic surgery. He received an MSc and Ph.D. in Surgical Sciences from Campinas State University (UNICAMP), Brazil. He obtained additional specialization in clinical research at Harvard Medical School and in research ethics at UNESCO. Currently, he is a researcher and undergraduate Professor of Medicine and Professor of Graduate Studies in Medical Sciences at São Leopoldo Mandic, Brazil, the clinical director of MedMandic Clinic, and coordinator of the Center for Rare Diseases, São Leopoldo Mandic. He is also a physician in the Department of Orthopedics and Rheumatology, UNICAMP, and a member of the Medical Assistance Group for Knee Surgery, Hospital Israelita Albert Einstein. He is the editor-in-chief of UNICAMP's science blog "Fêmur Distal." In 2022, Dr. Zorzi and his team received the Eric Wroclawski Award for the best scientific paper published in *Einstein*, the official scientific publication of the Instituto Israelita de Ensino e Pesquisa Albert Einstein, Brazil.

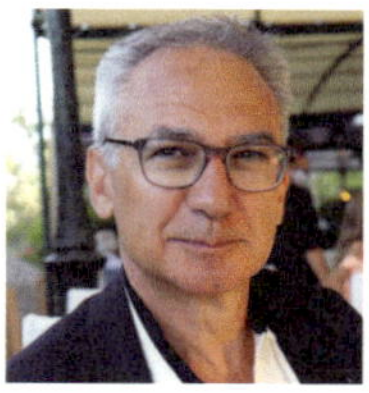

Dr. Eric Lespessailles is a doctor in the Rheumatology Department at the Regional Hospital of Orleans, France. He received his Ph.D. in Sciences and Techniques of Physical Activities and Sports at the University of Orleans. He obtained accreditation to supervise research and a qualification as a university professor in physiology. He is the medical director of the Translational Medicine Research Platform at the Regional Hospital of Orleans. He has published about 200 peer-reviewed manuscripts. His research focuses on osteoporosis, osteoarthritis, psoriatic arthritis, and musculoskeletal imaging.

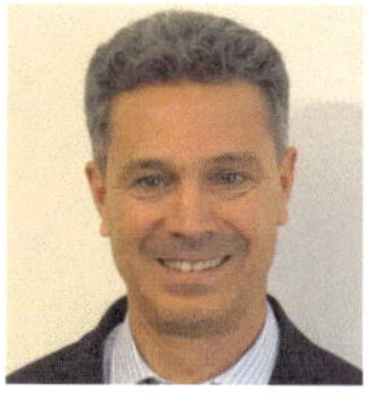

Professor Hechmi Toumi graduated from Blaise Pascal University, France. His primary research and teaching interests are musculoskeletal anatomy and pathologies, notably medical histology and imaging. He began his career as a research assistant at the University of Wisconsin, USA, and at Cardiff University, UK. He is a full professor at the University of Wales, UK. He was dean of the Faculty of Sciences at the University of Orleans from 2013 to 2020. Currently, Professor Toumi is the director of the translational medical research platform PRIMMO. He filed an international patent application for his invention on the use of algorithmic analyses to identify and quantify invisible detail in soft tissues using standard radiographs. Professor Toumi has lectured worldwide on the pathologies, treatment, and prevention of muscular-skeletal injuries. Currently, Professor Toumi is the acting consultant for healthcare development for Orleans Metropolitan.

Contents

Preface

Osteoarthritis is the most common cause of joint pain in adults. It is a growing problem due to population aging and the increasing prevalence of obesity in the world. Since the dawn of humanity, people have suffered from pain and difficulty walking caused by trauma, tumors, infections, inflammatory diseases, or genetic problems. Joint diseases culminate in the progressive destruction of the joints, a condition known as secondary osteoarthritis. This leads to enormous individual and family suffering, in addition to social overload. Only about 50 years ago did a successful surgical solution called replacement arthroplasty emerge for the treatment of the most serious and debilitating cases. This surgery is particularly effective for osteoarthritis in the hips. Although arthroplasty has made it possible to approach complex cases previously considered as contraindications, there is still a long way to go.

In this book, renowned international authors present their experiences, research results, and proposals for innovative solutions for the improvement and advancement of hip and knee arthroplasty. Chapters discuss non-surgical treatment of osteoarthritis as well.

I want to acknowledge the support and patience of Author Service Manager Miss Sara Tikel at IntechOpen for her assistance. I also thank my co-editors Dr. Hechmi Toumi and Dr. Eric Lespessailles. Finally, I thank the contributing authors for their excellent chapters. Without them, this book would not exist. Happy reading!

Alessandro Rozim Zorzi
Medical School,
São Leopoldo Mandic,
Campinas, Brazil

Hechmi Toumi and Eric Lespessailles
University of Orléans,
Orléans, France

Section 1

General Aspects

Chapter 1

Introductory Chapter: Past, Present, and Future of Joint Reconstructive Surgery

Alessandro Rozim Zorzi and João B. Miranda

1. Introduction

By 2030, the demand for primary total hip arthroplasty in the United States of America is estimated to grow by 174% and the demand for primary total knee arthroplasty is projected to grow by 673%. Overall, total hip and total knee revisions are projected to grow by 137% and 601%, respectively, between 2005 and 2030 [1]. This estimate demonstrates that joint problems, especially those correlated with population aging, are an important public health problem. The queues for performing arthroplasties in developing countries are among the longest in the health systems of countries such as Brazil. Governments around the world will need to take steps to ensure assistance with public policies aimed at increasing patients' access to treatment with surgery for joint reconstruction.

On the other hand, it is important to emphasize that arthroplasty is a very effective surgery, which resolves pain in most cases and restores mobility, functional independence, and quality of life for the patient. No wonder hip arthroplasty was elected the most important surgery of the twentieth century [2].

2. Definition

Arthroplasty is an orthopedic surgical procedure, where the articular surfaces of a synovial joint are removed, remodeled, or replaced, to restore function and relief pain. It is indicated in cases of advanced joint destruction caused by different etiologies (osteoarthritis, inflammatory arthritis, trauma, tumors, sequelae of osteoarticular infections, neurological injuries, among others), where three factors combine: severe and refractory pain, functional limitation, and poor quality of life.

3. Types of arthroplasty

Although nowadays the term "arthroplasty" is strongly associated with the placement of a "prosthesis", there are other forms of arthroplasty that are still practiced and need to be recognized by the specialist in joint reconstructions. Many of them have only historical value for the hip and knee joints, where the development and success of metallic prostheses, which follow Charnley's "low friction" concept, have made it the gold standard

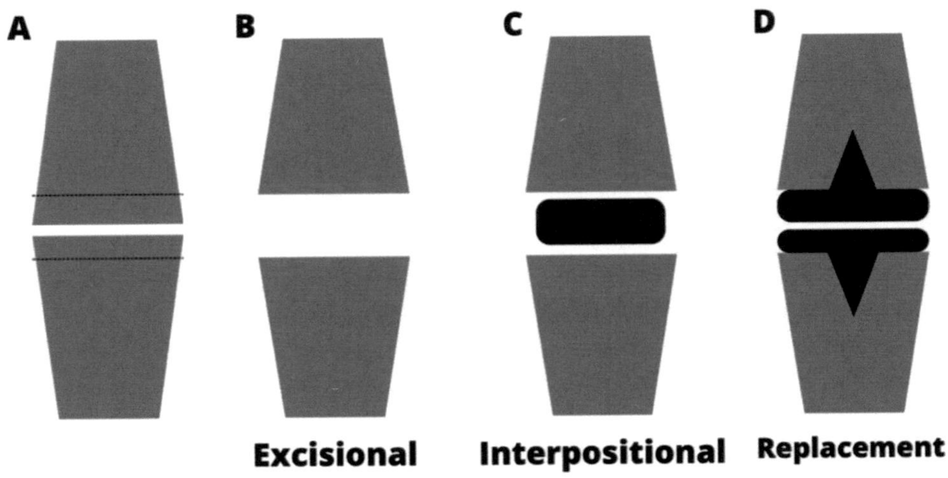

Figure 1.
Types of arthroplasty: A) severely damaged joint, with significant reduction of joint space. The dashed line shows the original joint space width; B) excisional, which consists of simple resection of joint surfaces; C) Interpositional, when, in addition to the resection, some biological tissue or synthetic material is interposed between the joint surfaces; D) replacement, when a prosthesis is implanted to restore joint geometry.

in the treatment of the vast majority of cases. But other joints, especially small joints and upper limbs can still benefit greatly from other forms of arthroplasty. **Figure 1** shows a schematic of the types of arthroplasty.

3.1 Excisional arthroplasties

Also known as resection arthroplasty, it consists of removing part of the joint. The space that is left fills in with scar tissue over time. Nowadays, its use is indicated most often for correction of deformities in the toes (hallux rigid, hammer toe, mallet toe), for the treatment of rhizarthrosis in the trapezio metacarpal joint of the hand, and for some elbow problems. In hemophiliac patients, for example, hypertrophy of the radial head causes pain and limitation of pronation-supination. Radial head resection promotes good results in these patients.

It can also be used as a salvage procedure in difficult cases of the shoulder (Jones surgery) or hip (Girdlestone surgery). The functional result in the knee is very poor and should be avoided. It may be rarely indicated in cases of refractory infection of the prosthesis, in elderly patients, or in patients with no gait prognosis, in which comorbidities would make the performance of an arthrodesis risky.

The problem with resection arthroplasty is that it generates instability, often so severe as to render the limb virtually nonfunctional. Therefore, its purpose is to relieve pain in patients with low functional demand and without surgical conditions for other forms of arthroplasty.

3.2 Interpositional arthroplasties

Interpositional arthroplasty consists of the resection of damaged joint surfaces, with the interposition of biological tissue or synthetic materials. Although it has presented poor results in the past, mainly in load-bearing joints of the lower limbs, it currently plays a role in the treatment of some specific pathologies.

In the small joints, an interposition arthroplasty is an option for surgical treatment of hallux rigidus, for elderly patients with low functional capacity. Also could be used to manage rizarthrosis, the so-called Eaton's arthroplasty with ligament interposition. Interpositional arthroplasty with temporalis fascia flap has been one of the most frequently performed procedures to treat temporomandibular joint ankylosis.

In large joints, it has been used frequently for elbow problems. It is considered a salvation option in young patients where conservative treatment has failed and total elbow arthroplasty is relatively contraindicated [3].

3.3 Replacement arthroplasties

The articular surface is partially or completely replaced by a prosthesis. The prosthesis protects the subchondral bone and restores joint geometry, returning normal tension to the ligaments and joint capsule. This is the most successful type of arthroplasty, the result of a long historical development, which led to the development of the prostheses currently in use. In joints such as the hip and knee, the superiority of replacement arthroplasty is indisputable, being considered the gold standard treatment in severe destruction. In the shoulder and ankle, promising results are beginning to be achieved.

4. The past: a brief history of replacement arthroplasties

Knowledge of the past is important to understand how we arrived at the present way of performing arthroplasty, in addition to making it possible to understand the directions of this surgery in the future. Although today, it is strongly linked to the activity of the implants and medical equipment industry, in the early days the first arthroplasties emerged thanks to the creativity and perseverance of important names in orthopedic surgery.

Modern days of replacement arthroplasty date back to the 1960s, with the development of "low friction arthroplasty," which reduced the wear sustained by artificial hip joints over time and provided more predictable outcomes. From the first femoral head attachments fashioned from ivory to current technologies, we can take this point in history as a milestone for the emergence of current models manufactured by the modern prosthetic industry (**Figure 2**).

However, without the first steps in any scientific endeavor, future steps are impossible. The nineteenth century brought three major technical advances that revolutionized surgery: Joseph Lister's aseptic technique, the discovery of anesthesia, and the discovery of X-Ray. Before the nineteenth century, people with severe joint problems and walking difficulties were called "cripples." There was not much to do, just the use of herbs to relieve pain and walking aids such as canes and crutches. In the eighteenth century, some surgeons dared to perform joint surgery to try to relieve the pain of these patients, but with poor results. Henry Park (1744–1831) in Liverpool, United Kingdom, was the first surgeon to report an operation with excision of the femoral head, basically performing an excisional arthroplasty. Later, in the 1940s, femoral head excision was popularized by Gathorne Robert Girdlestone (1881–1950) from Oxford in patients suffering from tuberculosis [4].

Later, surgeons began to consider using different types of materials or biological interposition tissues, developing the interposition arthroplasty without success.

It was only in the nineteenth century, with the use of aseptic surgery, anesthesia, and x-rays that the first attempts at joint reconstruction with prostheses began to become

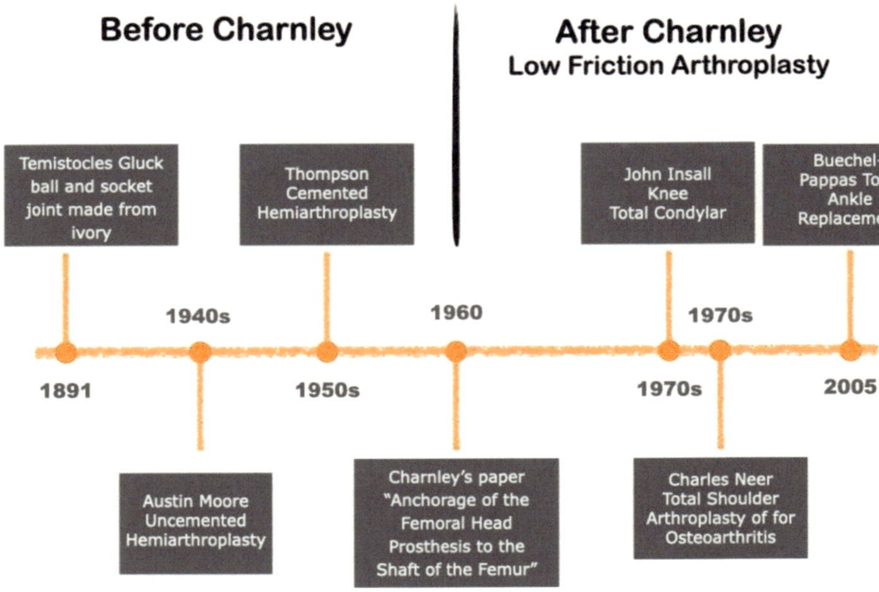

Figure 2.
Timeline of the evolution of arthroplasties.

viable. In 1891, Themistocles Gluck from Berlin developed a ball and socket joint made from ivory that was fixed to the bone with nickel-plated screws. French surgeon Pierre Delbet (1861–925) used a rubber prosthesis for replacing the femoral head in 1919. In 1927, the British surgeon Ernest W. Hey-Groves (1872–1944) used ivory. In 1948, the Judet brothers, Robert (1901–1980) and Jean (1905–1995) used an acrylic prosthesis.

In 1940, Austin Moore implanted the first Vitallium prosthesis to replace the proximal femur. Modifications were made to preserve the proper neck angle and the stem was fenestrated in subsequent years. In the 1950s, Thompson developed his hemi-arthroplasty for femoral neck fractures. Initially, it was operated without cement fixation, but with practice, it changed to a cemented procedure. This phase was marked by the pioneering spirit of great names in orthopedics at the time, who sought a solution to the problem of joint reconstruction. However, the results were still unsatisfactory. These were abandoned when Sir John Charnley defined modern hip arthroplasty [4, 5].

John Charnley developed the concept of "low friction arthroplasty" based on three principles: the idea of low friction torque arthroplasty, the use of acrylic cement and the introduction of high-density polyethylene as a bearing material. Low friction arthroplasty is the principle used until today, although with evolutions and small modifications, in all current prostheses. So we can say that Charnley's paper "Anchorage of the femoral head Prosthesis to the Shaft of the Femur", from 1960, was the birth of the current era of arthroplasties [4–7].

After Charnley, the realization of hip arthroplasties began to have promising clinical results, which led this surgery to become a routine practice and led to production on an industrial scale, contributing to the birth of the current implant industry. The success obtained in the hip encouraged other surgeons to seek similar solutions for other joints in the human body.

The evolution of knee arthroplasties follows a sequence very similar to that of the hip, with the first attempts to perform resection or interposition arthroplasties most of the time unsuccessful. The history of total knee arthroplasties made great progress with the application of the "low friction arthroplasty" principle and the launch of the "total Condylar" model created by John Insall in the 1970s. From then on, there were successful and replicable results, which made possible the flourishing of the modern knee implant industry [8].

In a similar way and practically at the same time, Charles Neer improved his model of hemiarthroplasty created in the 50s for the treatment of fractures of the proximal humerus and launched in the 70s a model of total prosthesis with a component for the glenoid, indicated for cases of shoulder osteoarthritis [9].

The ankle was the last joint in the lower limb where total joint replacement was attempted, and therefore, it is the least developed. The mobile bearing system for the ankle first used by Pappas and Buechel appears to have become widely accepted by orthopedic manufacturers as an accurate solution for replicating the biomechanics of the ankle.

5. The present: current results

Arthroplasties are currently among the most practiced surgeries in the world. Routinely, thousands of patients undergo this type of intervention daily in almost every country around the world. This is possible thanks to the effective and safe results obtained with the technique and the great impact on the recovery of people's quality of life.

The safety and effectiveness of the technique can be verified through data collected in large cohorts, called registries, available in many countries around the world. There are local, regional, and national registries. Four registries stand out as the main forces behind the effort to popularize the concept of evidence-based medicine: the Mayo Registry and the Harris registry are important institutional registries in the United States; while among national registries, both the Swedish Knee Registry and Hip Registry [10].

A total estimated 630,000 hip replacement procedures were performed in the United States in 2017. For total knee replacement, the increasing incidence of TKA is a universal phenomenon. In 2017, the United States had 911,000 total knee procedures performed [11].

6. Future perspectives

The arthroplasty surgery practiced today was developed about 50 years ago. It was created in the "analogical era." The rapid transformations that occurred with the fourth industrial revolution, accelerated by the COVID-19 pandemic, led us to live in the "digital age." In this scenario of intensive use of technology and computing in all sectors of human life, it is predictable that arthroplasty will undergo transformations. Some of them are already present, although still timidly, in clinical practice. We list below five technologies that are already available, although still timidly used, and that could lead to significant advances in the near future:

- Computer-assisted surgical navigation

Although there is still no consensus on what would be the ideal alignment of a limb with knee prosthesis, the traditional concept of neutral alignment have being questioned by concepts such as kinematic alignment, the quest for reliable and reproducible achievement of the intra-operative alignment goal has been the primary motivator for the development of Computer assisted surgical navigation (CASN). There are already a significant number of clinical studies showing that the use of CASN increases the accuracy of the planned alignment [12]. However, there is still a lack of clinical studies demonstrating that the long-term clinical outcome of using CASN is better than traditional alignment without the use of technology. Although the cost of using the equipment has been progressively decreasing over time and with greater use, it will be necessary for the future to improve the system to further reduce the cost of use and enable its use on a large scale. The reader is invited to explore the chapter in this book called "advanced, imageless navigation in contemporary THA: optimizing acetabular component placement" written by Prof Andrew Kurmis.

- Robotic-assisted surgery

As a natural evolution of the use of CASN, robotic systems with mechanical arms associated with the navigation system emerged. Companies such as Zimmer Biomet (Rosa), Stryker (Mako), Smith & Nephew (Cori), for example, already offer orthopedic surgeons the clinical use of robot-assisted prostheses. Current systems include robotic arms, robotic-guided cutting jigs, or robotic milling systems, with different navigation strategies using active, semiactive, or passive control systems [13–15]. One problem is that the robots used in arthroplasties are not very versatile. There are specific systems for hip or knee, some more recent systems already allow using the same robot for both hip and knee, but not for other joints. This greatly increases the cost for the hospital, making the technology even restricted to places with higher purchasing power. For a deeper understanding of the use of robots in arthroplasties, the reader is invited to read the chapter entitled "active robotic total knee arthroplasty" written by Prof. Andrei Gritsyuk.

- Augmented reality

However, in parallel with the development of navigation and robots, the recent digital technological advance (fourth industrial revolution caused by the emergence of the internet) already presents another type of innovative solution to assist the surgeon in the implantation of the prosthesis: the use of the augmented reality (AR). It is stated that AR could provide a more efficient and cost-effective solution than robotic surgery [16].

- Patient-specific implants

The development of new 3D printing technologies made it possible to design patient-specific implants and single-use instruments, which have also been proposed as an alternative technology to improve accuracy, while also improving efficiency and limiting the associated cost of arthroplasties. This technology has the potential of reducing operating room times over reusable sets, and benefit theater personnel ergonomically while presenting potential cost-saving benefits in terms of reduced sterilization costs and surgical times [17].

- Nanotechnology

The future also promises advances not only in systems to aid prosthesis implantation but also in the manufacture and composition of implants. The reader is invited to visit this book the chapters written by Mr. James Broderick on "Biomaterials in arthroplasty" and Prof. Jörg Lützner on "Modern Coatings in Knee arthroplasty."

Author details

Alessandro Rozim Zorzi[1,2*] and João B. Miranda[2]

1 São Leopoldo Mandic Medical School, Campinas, SP, Brazil

2 Department of Orthopedics, Rheumatology an Traumatology, University of Campinas (UNICAMP), Campinas, SP, Brazil

*Address all correspondence to: arzorzi@hc.unicamp.br

References

[1] Kurtz S, Ong K, Lau E, Mowat F, Halpern M. Projections of primary and revision hip and knee arthroplasty in the United States from 2005 to 2030. The Journal of Bone and Joint Surgery. American Volume. 2007;**89**(4):780-785. DOI: 10.2106/JBJS.F.00222

[2] Learmonth ID, Young C, Rorabeck C. The operation of the century: Total hip replacement. Lancet. 2007;**370**(9597): 1508-1519. DOI: 10.1016/S0140-6736(07)60457-7

[3] Almeida TBC, Reis EDS, Pascarelli L, Bongiovanni RR, Teodoro RL. Interposition arthroplasty of the elbow: Systematic review. Acta Ortopedica Brasileira. 2021;**29**(4):219-222. DOI: 10.1590/1413-785220212904238960

[4] Bota NC, Nistor DV, Caterev S, Todor A. Historical overview of hip arthroplasty: From humble beginnings to a high-tech future. Orthopedic Reviews (Pavia). 2021;**13**(1):8773. DOI: 10.4081/or.2021.8773

[5] Gomez PF, Morcuende JA. Early attempts at hip arthroplasty--1700s to 1950s. The Iowa Orthopaedic Journal. 2005;**25**:25-29

[6] Markatos K, Savvidou OD, Foteinou A, Kosmadaki S, Trikoupis I, Goumenos SD, et al. Hallmarks in the history and development of Total hip arthroplasty. Surgical Innovation. 2020;**27**(6):691-694. DOI: 10.1177/1553350620947209 [Epub 2020 Aug 3]

[7] Charnley J. Anchorage of the femoral head prosthesis to the shaft of the femur. Journal of Bone and Joint Surgery. British Volume (London). 1960;**42-B**:28-30. DOI: 10.1302/0301-620X.42B1.28

[8] Johal S, Nakano N, Baxter M, Hujazi I, Pandit H, Khanduja V. Unicompartmental knee arthroplasty: The past, current controversies, and future perspectives. The Journal of Knee Surgery. 2018;**31**(10):992-998. DOI: 10.1055/s-0038-1625961 [Epub 2018 Mar 7]

[9] Flatow EL, Harrison AK. A history of reverse total shoulder arthroplasty. Clinical Orthopaedics and Related Research. 2011;**469**(9):2432-2439. DOI: 10.1007/s11999-010-1733-6

[10] Malchau H, Garellick G, Berry D, Harris WH, Robertson O, Kärrlholm J, et al. Arthroplasty implant registries over the past five decades: Development, current, and future impact. Journal of Orthopaedic Research. 2018;**36**(9):2319-2330. DOI: 10.1002/jor.24014 [Epub 2018 May 24]

[11] Abdelaal MS, Restrepo C, Sharkey PF. Global perspectives on arthroplasty of hip and knee joints. The Orthopedic Clinics of North America. 2020;**51**(2):169-176. DOI: 10.1016/j.ocl.2019.11.003 [Epub 2020 Feb 6]

[12] Jones CW, Jerabek SA. Current role of computer navigation in Total knee arthroplasty. The Journal of Arthroplasty. 2018;**33**(7):1989-1993. DOI: 10.1016/j.arth.2018.01.027 [Epub 2018 Jan 31]

[13] Jacofsky DJ, Allen M. Robotics in arthroplasty: A comprehensive review. The Journal of Arthroplasty. 2016;**31**(10):2353-2363. DOI: 10.1016/j.arth.2016.05.026 [Epub 2016 May 18]

[14] Mancino F, Jones CW, Benazzo F, Singlitico A, Giuliani A, De Martino I. Where are we now and what are we hoping to achieve with robotic Total knee arthroplasty? A critical analysis of the current knowledge

and future perspectives. Orthopedic Research and Reviews. 2022;**14**:339-349. DOI: 10.2147/ORR.S294369

[15] Siddiqi A, Mont MA, Krebs VE, Piuzzi NS. Not all robotic-assisted Total knee arthroplasty are the same. The Journal of the American Academy of Orthopaedic Surgeons. 2021;**29**(2):45-59. DOI: 10.5435/JAAOS-D-20-00654

[16] Fucentese SF, Koch PP. A novel augmented reality-based surgical guidance system for total knee arthroplasty. Archives of Orthopaedic and Trauma Surgery. 2021;**141**(12):2227-2233. DOI: 10.1007/s00402-021-04204-4 [Epub 2021 Oct 26]

[17] Attard A, Tawy GF, Simons M, Riches P, Rowe P, Biant LC. Health costs and efficiencies of patient-specific and single-use instrumentation in total knee arthroplasty: A randomised controlled trial. BMJ Open Quality. 2019;**8**(2):e000493. DOI: 10.1136/bmjoq-2018-000493

Chapter 2

Biomaterials in Total Joint Arthroplasty

Tiarnán Ó Doinn and James M. Broderick

Abstract

Primary total hip and knee arthroplasty (THA, TKA) are among the most common procedures performed in the United States. The volume of revision TKAs and THAs are also exponentially rising each year. Paramount to the success of total joint arthroplasty (TJA) is the correct choice of biomaterials which are used to reconstruct a particular joint. This chapter explores the history of common arthroplasty biomaterials, their biomechanical properties and current applications. This chapter also discusses modern strategies of improving biomaterial mechanical properties, survivability and sterilisation methods. The contents of this chapter will form an essential resource for practicing orthopaedic surgeons, orthopaedic trainees, researchers and engineers interested in tribology and biomechanics of biomaterials in adult reconstruction.

Keywords: primary hip arthroplasty, primary knee arthroplasty, biomaterials, alloy, polymer, ceramic, sterilisation

1. Introduction

Primary total hip and knee arthroplasty (THA, TKA) are among the top 5 most common procedures and among the top 5 fastest growing procedures performed across all surgical specialties in the United States [1]. Compared to the available 2014 National Inpatient Sampling figures, the estimated total annual United States use for primary TKA and THA is expected to increase in 2030 and 2040 by 182% and 401% for primary TKA and 129% and 285% for primary THA, respectively [2]. Similarly, projections for revision TKA (rTKA) and THA (rTHA) are estimated to increase from 2014 to 2030 by between 43% and 70% for rTHA and 78% and 182% for rTKAs [3]. Paramount to the success of total joint arthroplasty (TJA) is the correct choice of biomaterials which are used to reconstruct a particular joint.

Biomaterials are defined by the European Society for Biomaterials as "a material that interacts with the biological system to evaluate, treat, reinforce or replace a tissue, organ or function of the organism [4]." In THA and TKA these materials should exhibit a yield stress greater than physiological loading of the joint, while also preventing stress shielding of adjacent bone. These materials should also have an endurance limit which reduces the number of revisions required over a patient's lifetime, particularly as TJA procedures are increasingly being performed among younger patients [5]. Biomaterials can be considered as being either bioinert, biotolerant or

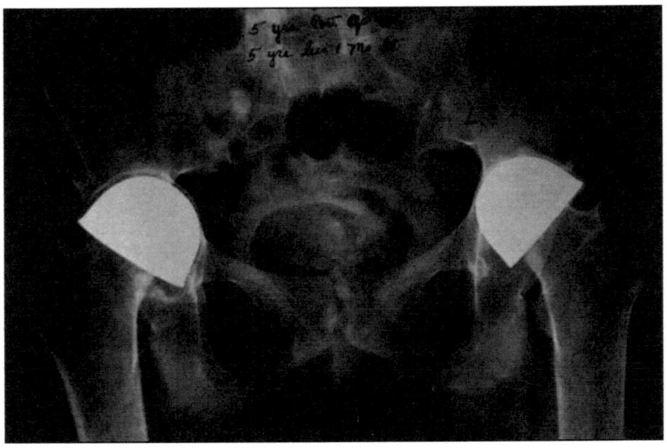

Figure 1.
Smith- Petersen acrylic Mould arthroplasty [9].

bioactive. Bioinert materials such as ceramics and titanium, do not illicit a biological response from surrounding tissues. Biotolerant materials, such as stainless steel, result in the formation of a fibrous layer due to irritation of surrounding tissues. Bioactive materials, such as hydroxyapatite coatings, result in direct bone on-growth, bonding prosthesis to bone.

The development of orthopaedic biomaterials closely follows the evolution of arthroplasty. Glück used ivory secured with nickel plated screws to replace femoral heads destroyed by tuberculosis in 1891 [6]. Ivory heads were also adapted by Hey-Groves several years later [7]. Delbet developed rubber prosthetic femoral heads in 1919 [8]. Smith-Petersen, in 1932 developed the first mould arthroplasty (**Figure 1**), which consisted of a hollow glass hemisphere which was fitted over the femoral head to provide a new articular surface [9, 10]. This design was subsequently revised to a Vitallium cup, a cobalt-chromium-molybdenum alloy. Subsequently, during the 1940s and 1950s a plethora of stemmed prosthesis were popularised in an effort to achieve a more anatomic design. Attempts to enhance fixation of these stemmed prostheses resulted in the adoption of dental acrylic cement by both McKee and Haboush in 1953 [11, 12]. Another significant advancement in the field of THA came in the form of articulating prostheses. Wiles popularised the first metal-on-metal THA in 1938, which was among the earliest articulating designs, with both prosthetic femoral and acetabular components [13]. However, poor component stability led to high failure rates, which were later modified by McKee and Ring using varying metal-on-metal prostheses with more reliable fixation methods.

Ultimately, these early designs gave way to the Charnley era in the 1950's which laid the foundation for modern THA design. Charnley made three major contributions to THA including 1) low friction torque arthroplasty 2) use of polymethylmethacrylate to reliably fix components to bone and 3) the use of high-density polyethylene as a bearing material [6, 14].

A core understanding of the biomaterials used in joint arthroplasty is key to selecting the most appropriate materials for a specific task, patient and type of prosthesis. This chapter provides a practical general overview of modern arthroplasty materials (metal alloys, ceramics, polyethylene and polymethylmethacrylate) rather than an exhaustive description which can be found elsewhere.

2. Metal alloys

The use of metal implants in orthopaedics dates as far back as 1775 with the use of brass wire for fracture osteosynthesis [15]. All metal alloys consist of metals constituted from metallic and non-metallic elements which form a highly organised repeating microstructure. The solvent metal determines the name of the alloy and is considered the base or primary metal. Non-metallic alloying components or solutes, such as oxygen, carbon or nitrogen are added to the base metal, which alters its properties. In their pure form metals tend to have one of three crystalline arrangements. This can be body-centred cubic, face-centred cubic and hexagonal close packed. In the FCC arrangement each atom is in contact with 8 other atoms. Whereas in the BCC and HCP arrangement each atom is in contact with 12 other atoms. During alloy formation, when a molten mixture undergoes solidification, the alloying components substitute for atoms of the base metal in the crystalline arrangement. The size of the non-metallic alloying elements relative to the size of the metallic elements determine the alloy crystal arrangement. If the non-metallic and metallic atoms are of similar size a substitutional alloy is formed, whereby non-metallic elements substitute for metallic elements in the crystalline arrangement, such as brass. If the non-metallic atoms are smaller than the metallic atoms on the other hand then an interstitial alloy is formed, whereby non-metallic atoms occupy spaces in the crystalline structure, such as stainless steel.

The above metallic alloy crystals, group together to form clusters of crystals termed grains. Grains are imperfectly aligned with each other creating gaps between adjacent grains, termed grain boundaries. Microstructure defects such as grain boundaries as well as dislocations and vacancies can all act to increase the propensity for alloy failure. Macrostructure defects, such as scratches and voids can also be a focus for stress and precipitating failure. Several processing methods have been introduced to address these defects including cold and hot working, powder metallurgy techniques to reduce grain size, precipitation hardening and thermomechanical processing.

Metals are susceptible to chemical wear, which is typically the result of corrosion from reactions with the surrounding aqueous physiologic environment [16]. Corrosion is the undesirable dissolution of metal in a solution. This occurs through the formation of an anode and cathode, resulting in metal cation ejection. Typically, passivity through the formation of a thin oxide film on certain metals serves as a kinetic protective barrier. In arthroplasty implant modularity, which results in relative motion between two materials can disrupt the passive oxide layer, resulting in dissolution of metal particles, which is termed fretting corrosion. This has resulted in modular components falling out of favour in primary THRs. Other types of mechanically assisted corrosion such as pitting and crevice corrosion, result in the formation of localised defects and the formation of a stress riser. While implant longevity is a concern, the local and systemic effects of corrosion must also be considered. Therefore, knowledge of the relative corrosion resistance of various metal alloys is essential in TJA, to ensure that they are employed correctly.

Metal alloys with relevance to TJA fall into three main groups 1) stainless steel 2) alloys based on the Cobalt-Chrome (Co-Cr) system and 3) Titanium and its alloys, which will be discussed in this section.

2.1 Stainless steel

Stainless steel was first used in orthopaedic implants in 1926 [17]. Later, Charnley and the Exeter group employed stainless steel for their femoral stems (**Figure 2**). An iron-based alloy, the stainless steel used in orthopaedic implants is austenitic American Iron and Steel Institute (AISI) 316 L. The number 300 indicates that it is a member of the 300 series of austenitic steel. Austenite steel denotes an FCC crystalline arrangement, with a solid solution of carbon in a nonmagnetic form of iron, which is stable at high temperatures. The FFC structure increases susceptibility to plastic deformation. The alloy includes 3% molybdenum, which increases resistance to pitting and 16% nickel which stabilises the austenitic structure, improving ductility and reducing the alloy's yield stress. The letter 'L' refers to the low carbon content of <0.03% which improves corrosion resistance by reducing sensitisation, a process which results in carbide formation in grain boundaries.

Furthermore, the addition of chromium to stainless steel results in the formation of a thin chromium oxide layer (Cr_2O_3), a process termed passivation which shields the alloy from corrosion. Despite these properties, stainless steel remains susceptible to stress and crevice corrosion. Stress corrosion occurs as a result of exposure to chloride- rich environments whereas crevice corrosion results from the disruption of the passive oxide layer which occurs with undulating deformation.

3. Titanium based alloys

Titanium and titanium-based alloys have been available since the 18th century and are widely used today as biomaterials. They were first applied as a biomaterial in the 1940s in dentistry. However, their mechanical properties and excellent biocompatibility led to

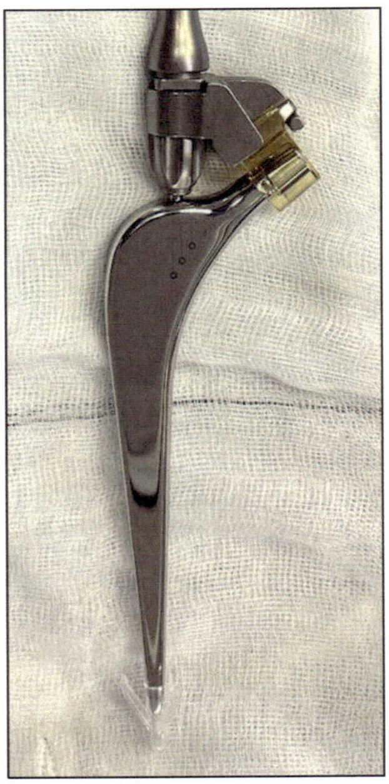

Figure 2.
Exeter V40 stainless steel femoral stem.

them becoming a desirable orthopaedic alloy. Titanium has a low density, high tensile strength and is highly corrosion resistant. The presence of chromium in titanium results in the in vivo formation of a passive oxide layer producing good corrosion resistance. Pure titanium is available in various grades, with the relative oxygen content determining the degree of impurity. Titanium alloy exists as a biphasic structure. As it precipitates from its molten state, an alpha phase results in a HCP arrangement and the beta phase produces a BCC arrangement. This biphasic precipitate results in improved fatigue resistance.

Titanium is commonly alloyed with aluminium, vanadium, niobium, zirconium and tantalum. The most common titanium alloy used in orthopaedics is Ti-6AL-4 V, often termed Titanium 64 due to the 6% aluminium and 4% vanadium concentrations. This alloy possesses a higher ultimate tensile strength than pure titanium and a modulus of elasticity closer to that of bone compared to stainless steel, preventing stress shielding. Additionally, newer generation titanium alloys (TiMoFe, TiMoNbZr and TiNbZrTaSiFe) demonstrate increased elasticity which may improve this capability further [18–20]. Another, distinct advantage of titanium alloys is MRI compatibility, given that it is non-dielectric and does not rise in temperature when placed in a magnetic field. These properties make titanium an ideal material as an orthopaedic implant. The main disadvantage of titanium, however, is titanium's poor abrasion resistance and notch sensitivity. Accordingly, titanium is not suitable as a bearing material and should be handled meticulously intraoperatively.

3.1 Cobalt chrome alloy

Cobalt-Chrome (Co-Cr) alloy was introduced into total joint arthroplasty in the early 1900s, as a modification of Vitallium, a common alloy which was in use in dentistry at the time [21]. Most Co-Cr orthopaedic implants contain Cobalt (62–68%), Chromium (27–30%), Molybdenum (5–7%), and Nickel (<2.5%). The alloy was initially used by Smith-Petersen in 1939 in mould arthroplasty and later in the Charnley femoral stem following a move from stainless- steel [9, 22]. Co-Cr possesses several properties which make it a highly suitable alloy for use in arthroplasty. The presence of Cr, as with other alloys, results in the formation of a passive oxide layer providing protection against corrosion, and as a result excellent biocompatibility. Co-Cr alloy has among the highest modulus of elasticity among all commonly used arthroplasty materials. It also possesses a high ultimate tensile strength and has excellent wear resistance.

Modern techniques for implant production use powder metallurgy to reduce the carbon content and thus limit carbide phases which negatively impacts Co-Cr mechanical characteristics. Previous techniques involved cast-wrought production which resulted in increased carbide formation. In contrast, powder metallurgy, involves sieving a fine powder alloy, heating it to a temperature just below melting point before compressing the alloy components in a die cast of the final component shape. Compared to cast-wrought production this method reduces grain size and carbide formation, improving its strength and corrosion resistance.

4. Orthopaedic polymers

4.1 Polyethylene

One of Charnley's legacy to modern arthroplasty is the introduction of polyethylene as a bearing material for THA [14]. Polyethylene is a linear homopolymer, composed of hydrogen and carbon, represented by the formula ~(CH2-CH2)~. Charnley originally used polytetrafluorethylene, termed Fluron G1 and Fluron G2 manufactured by Imperial Chemical Industries (London, England) as a bearing material for THA due to its low coefficient of friction and biocompatibility [23]. However, poor abrasive characteristics lead to failure of Charnley's polytetrafluorethylene acetabular cups within 2 years, due to low resistance to creep deformation. Fortuitously, Charnley's technician, Craven tested a material termed high-molecular- weight polyethylene (HMWPE) which was given to him by a plastic gear salesman. This material was first implanted in 1962 by Charnley when a HMWPE cup was used in combination with acrylic bone cement which was compressed into a reamed acetabulum (**Figure 3**) [24].

Ultra HMWPE (UHMWPE) is composed of long chains of polymerised alkene, ethylene. It is a semicrystalline polymer, having both a crystalline and amorphous phase. UHMWPE contains a set of ordered crystalline lamellae, with tightly packed randomly orientated macromolecules, embedded in a disordered amorphous phase. UHMWPE consists of up to 200,000 monomers per molecule and a molecular weight ranging from 2 to 6 10^6 g/mol. Increased molecular weight and degree of cross-bond

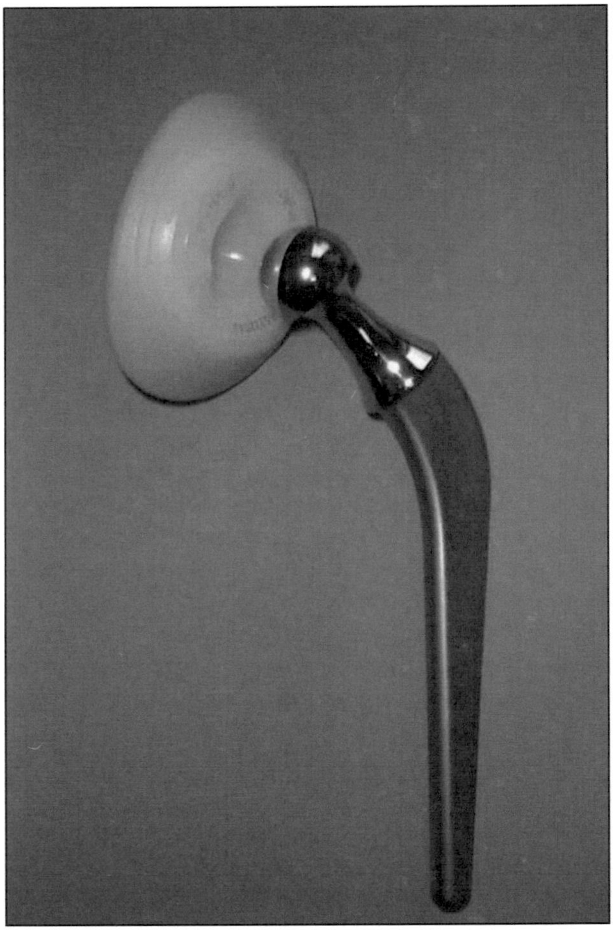

Figure 3.
Charnley hip consisting of HMWPE cup with a Moore stem [25].

formation between chains increases the strength and wear resistance of UHMWPE. These properties combined with a low coefficient of friction, resistance to abrasive wear and corrosion, with a high impact strength and toughness have made UHMWPE the arthroplasty bearing material of choice. Comparatively high-density polyethylene has a lower molecular weight (0.05–0.25 10^6 g/mol) and higher density which results in inferior mechanical properties.

4.1.1 UHMWPE processing

Historically there have been 3 modes of UHMWPE production for orthopaedic implants. Direct moulding involves placing polyethylene powder into a mould of the final configuration of the implant. The powder is then placed under pressure and heated to consolidate it into its final shape. Ram extrusion involves a similar process; however, the powder is fashioned into a cylindrical bar stock which is later machined into the desired final shape of the implant. The final method involves moulding large sheets of polyethylene in which implants are later machined from. A more modern technique has recently been pioneered by Zimmer Biomet termed Hot Isostatic pressing. This process uses high temperature and pressure with argon gas and compression moulding. The process is then completed by a machining operation. These fabrication methods do not significantly alter the physical, chemical or structural properties of the original polymer other than the crystallinity. As the original polyethylene is heated to above melting point, its crystallinity is irreversibly decreased, decreasing fatigue strength. As a result, all polyethylene components possess their original properties prior to sterilisation.

4.1.2 Sterilisation

Polyethylene sterilisation presents a challenge as it cannot be carried out using traditional heating methods due it's low melting point. The main sterilisation methods used today include high energy radiation (gamma irradiation or electron beam irradiation) or surface treatment. Gamma irradiation is emitted from the decay of a ^{60}Co unstable nucleus whereas electron beam is produced by heating a tungsten filament. Both radiation methods have the advantage of sterilising PE but also causing cross-linking of polymer chains which enhances fatigue strength and wear resistance [26]. However, electron beam irradiation can be performed in a shorter period of time (seconds) and with lower doses of radiation required to achieve a similar degree of crosslinking.

The main disadvantage of high energy radiation is oxidative degradation of the implant through radiolytic bond scission and free- radical generation [27]. Irradiation results in scission of chemical bonds of UHMWPE resulting in free radical formation. Environmental oxygen binds with free radicals permanently breaking the carbon-carbon bonds, a process termed oxidative degradation. This process results in reduced molecular weight and a final component with inferior wear resistance and increased wear debris generation. Macroscopically, oxidative degradation can be seen in retrieved and new components as appearing as a white band or crown effect, which results in severe failure, through delamination and fracture.

Several methods have been employed to reduce the effect of oxidative degradation during irradiation. Manufactures have trialled irradiating PE components in an inert gas such as argon or in a vacuum. Similarly, more sophisticated packaging methods have also become available with particle barrier material, preventing ambient oxygen exposure. Packaging has also been designed to allow the penetration of select gases when chemically sterilised. During the 1990's, post-irradiation thermal stabilisation melting was also introduced as a means to reduce oxidative degradation by quenching residual free-radicals, allowing them to recombine, improving oxidative resistance. This was initially demonstrated to maintain mechanical property performance standards, but remelting decreased crystallinity, reducing PE fatigue strength.

Subsequently in 2007, UHMWPE stabilisation with antioxidant Vitamin E-diffusion was introduced in the United States [28]. Vitamin E diffusion, limited the need for post-irradiation melting, maintaining PE crystallinity. Synthetic α- tocopherol, the vitamin E used during implant processing, decreases the macro alkyl radicals available to interact with oxygen, inhibiting the ensuing oxidative cascade. Vitamin E can be incorporated into UHMWPE either by post-irradiation vitamin E diffusion or by mixing vitamin E with UHMWPE powder prior to pressurisation. Post-irradiation vitamin E diffusion has the benefit of avoiding the effect of Vitamin E on reducing the number of alkyl radicals available for cross linking but places the cross-linked PE at increased risk of oxidation prior to Vitamin E stabilisation. Mixing Vitamin E with UHMWPE powder has the converse effect.

4.2 Polymethylmethacrylate

The earliest use of acrylic bone cement was by Glück in 1891, for use with an ivory hip prosthesis [6]. However, in 1901 a German chemist, Otto Röhm developed polymethylmethacrylate (PMMA), which is the earliest form of the bone cement which is in widespread use today in orthopaedics [29]. The Judet Brothers developed acrylic femoral hemiarthroplasties prosthesis as a treatment for hip arthritis [30]. However, it was Haboush who was the first to use PMMA as a grout to fix implant to bone [31]. Subsequently, Charnley pioneered to modern use of self-curing PMMA to achieve an implant- bone- cement construct for femoral and acetabular components, in the 1950s and 1960s. Charnley proposed that PMMA, creates an interface between prosthesis and bone to allow for distribution of contact forces and rigid fixation [14, 32]. PMMA acts as a grout which interdigitates with cancellous bone, enhancing interface shear strength. Cement may also act as a shock absorbing layer between elastic bone and a stiff implant with a Young's modulus (2400 MPa in tension) between cortical and cancellous bone. Cement therefore acts as an elastic interlayer between 2 stiff layers facilitating a more gradual transfer of stress from implant to bone. Currently, cement has a number of orthopaedic applications including; prosthesis fixation, percutaneous vertebroplasty, antibiotic delivery and as an interpositional material for bone defects.

PMMA ($C_5H_8O_2$) is packaged as 2 separate components; a powdered polymer and a liquid monomer in a 2:1 ratio [33]. The liquid component is supplied as 20mls of fluid, in a brown vial to avoid the deleterious effects of direct sunlight. The liquid monomer contains methyl methacrylate monomer, consisting of microspheres of variable diameter with the size of particles determining the viscosity of the cement. Additionally, heat stable antibiotics may also be added such as gentamicin or vancomycin. Other compounds contained in the liquid component include N,N dimethyl- p toludine (DMPT), hydroquinone, and a colouring agent (e.g green chlorophyl or cobalt blue). The powdered polymers is typically packaged as 40 g of powder containing pre-synthesised PMMA, barium sulphate or zirconium oxide and benzoyl peroxide.

Addition polymerisation of PMMA occurs via an exothermic reaction when the liquid and powdered components are mixed together. Benzoyl peroxide, in the powder component, acts as a catalyst, initiating polymerisation by interacting with DMPT in the liquid component [33]. This interaction liberates free radicals, breaking carbon-carbon bonds within MMA, allowing MMA monomers to couple with the growing polymer chain. Hydroquinone stabilises this reaction, preventing premature polymerisation. The radio-opacifier (barium sulphate or zirconium oxide) and colouring agent (cobalt blue or green chlorophyl) allow for identification of cement, radiologically and intra-operatively.

This chemical reaction is characterised by 4 distinct phases. The mixing phase or sandy stage (phase 1) occurs when powder and liquid components are mixed together (lasting roughly 30s). The waiting phase or sticky phase (phase 2), lasts approximately 1 to 3 minutes (depending on cement viscosity) and ends when the cement will easily separate from a gloved finger. The working phase (phase 3) occurs when the cement can be easily handled and signals when implants can be inserted, lasting approximately 5 minutes for high viscosity cement. The setting or hardening phase (phase 4) lasts approximately 1 minute 30 seconds to 2 minutes for high viscosity cements. These phases are influenced by a number of endogenous and exogenous factors. Increasing environmental temperatures and humidity decreases cement working time. Other factors such as a decreased powder liquid ratio increases setting time. The final biomechanical performance of cement can also be influenced by a number of exogenous factors such as mixing technique, sterilisation methods, antibiotics additives and choice of radio-opacifier.

5. Ceramics

Ceramics were popularised in the 1970's as bearing materials. Ceramics consist of metallic elements such as aluminium, zirconium and silicon covalently and or ionically bound with non-metallic elements. The main advantage of ceramic bearings is the reduction of wear debris in the periprosthetic space, which can precipitate the osteolysis cascade and aseptic loosening [34] associated with metal-on-metal and metal-on-PE bearing couples. Oxide ceramics used in total joint arthroplasty (TJA) are chemically inert after binding to oxygen, resulting in excellent biocompatibility. Ceramics also possess a low surface roughness and high hardness, possessing the highest modulus of elasticity of any other biomaterial used in TJA.

Unfortunately, the trade-off of high hardness is ceramic bearing brittleness and subsequent catastrophic failure. The first ceramic bearings used in THAs in 1971 were marred by catastrophic failure due to acute debonding at the implant-cement interface of cemented ceramic sockets resulting in aseptic loosening and implant fracture. In more modern systems this has been corrected with the addition of metal backed acetabular shells to ceramic liners [35]. The primary mode of failure, in more modern systems is now edge loading due to implant mispositioning, resulting in stripe wear. This process disrupts the oxide layer, reducing fracture toughness and increasing surface roughness. Microscopic flaws, introduced during the manufacturing process or machining such as notches, pores and scratches can also result in stress concentration, propagation of cracks and subsequent abrupt failure [34].

Ceramics are fabricated by mixing fine ceramic powder and water together and compressing the mixture into casts of the desired final shape. The mixture is then sintered in a kiln to bond the particles together and to increase density before being polished. The resulting organised crystalline microstructure and mechanical characteristics are subsequently determined by the grain size, porosity, crystallinity and density together with the implant design. Ceramics can be classified as non-oxides, oxides and composites, with oxide ceramics the material of choice in THA.

With the increased uptake of ceramic-on-ceramic bearings globally, audible squeaking arose as a new complication, with an incidence between 0 and 24.6% [36]. There have been a number of purported mechanisms described accounting for this complication. Suggested risk factors for COC squeak have included increased stripe wear and disruption of film-fluid lubrication, edge loading due to malposition of the acetabular cup, increased body mass index and femoral stem design geometry, among many others [37].

5.1 Aluminium oxide

Aluminium oxide (Al_2O_3) was developed as a biomaterial in the 1960's, making it a well characterised biomaterial. Modern alumina is processed using hot isostatic pressing, a process which reduces inclusions, grain size and grain boundaries, increasing hardness and increasing scratch resistance. Alumina also possesses a very low coefficient of friction due to a low surface roughness, resulting from its low grain size. This excellent tribological performance is further compounded by alumina' s high wettability and resulting film-fluid lubrication, which reduces in vitro wear. Retrieval studies have demonstrated alumina-on-alumina wear rates of a few micros per year [38]. Biologically the typical response to alumina wear debris is fibrocytic with no giant cell formation and little induction of macrophages, reducing osteolysis [35]. The estimated lifetime risk of catastrophic failure of alumina femoral heads is estimated to be 0.004% [38].

5.2 Oxidised zirconium (zirconia)

Oxidised zirconium (ZrO_2) is a ceramic composite bearing which was introduced as a means to reduce the catastrophic failure rates associated with alumina heads, while still also retaining the desirable wear characteristics of smaller femoral heads on polyethylene [34]. Pure zirconia is not used as a bearing material as it undergoes phase transformation between its three crystalline arrangements (monoclinic, cubic, tetragonal). This can result in volume and shape changes that increase the susceptibility to fracture. As a result, pure zirconia, requires stabilisation through a process known as transformation toughening. Zirconia can be stabilised with CaO, Y_2O_3 or MgO which controls phase transformations.

Zirconia toughened alumina (ZTA), is a composite which consists of zirconia dispersed in an alumina matrix (**Figure 4**). This modification resulted in the improved strength, fracture toughness and tensile strength compared to aluminium oxide [34]. ZTA can be strengthened further by the addition of Cr_2O_3 and SrO, which prevents crack propagation.

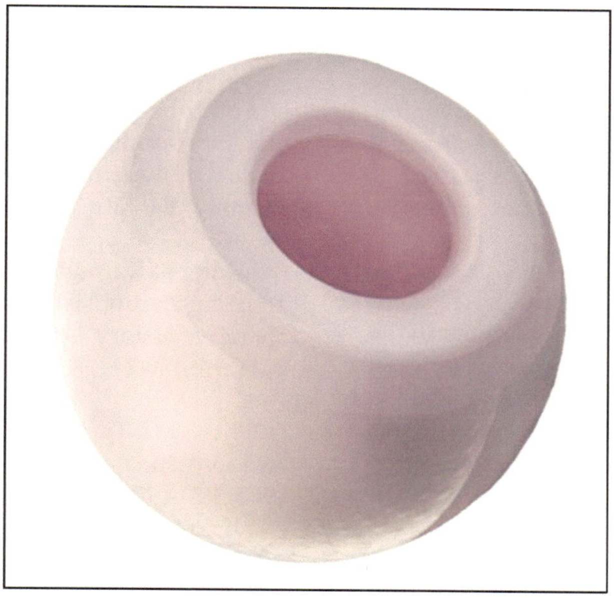

Figure 4.
BIOLOX Delta composite ceramic femoral head containing Aluminium oxide, zirconia and strontium oxide [39].

6. Summary

The responsibility of choosing the correct biomaterial in TJA lies solely with the operating surgeon. Surgeons should have a good working knowledge of the properties of commonly implanted biomaterials and should regularly scrutinise joint registry data when determining the most suitable biomaterial according to its intended use, in order to optimise patient outcomes.

Author details

Tiarnán Ó Doinn* and James M. Broderick
Department of Trauma and Orthopaedics, St. Vincent's University Hospital, Elm Park, Dublin, Ireland

*Address all correspondence to: tiarnanodoinn@rcsi.ie

References

[1] McDermott KW, Freeman WJ, Elixhauser A. Overview of operating room procedures during inpatient stays in US hospitals, 2014: statistical brief# 233. 2018

[2] Singh JA, Yu S, Chen L, Cleveland JD. Rates of total joint replacement in the United States: Future projections to 2020-2040 using the national inpatient sample. The Journal of Rheumatology. 2019;**46**(9):1134-1140

[3] Schwartz AM, Farley KX, Guild GN, Bradbury TL Jr. Projections and epidemiology of revision hip and knee arthroplasty in the United States to 2030. The Journal of Arthroplasty. 2020;**35**(6):S79-S85

[4] Williams DF. Definitions in Biomaterials: Proceedings of a Consensus Conference of the European Society for Biomaterials. Chester, England: Elsevier Science Limited; 1986. p. 1987

[5] Ravi B, Croxford R, Reichmann WM, Losina E, Katz JN, Hawker GA. The changing demographics of total joint arthroplasty recipients in the United States and Ontario from 2001 to 2007. Best Practice & Research Clinical Rheumatology. 2012;**26**(5):637-647

[6] Learmonth ID, Young C, Rorabeck C. The operation of the century: Total hip replacement. The Lancet. 2007;**370**(9597):1508-1519

[7] Groves EWH. Some contributions to the reconstructive surgery of the hip. Journal of British Surgery. 1927;**14**(55):486-517

[8] Gomez PF, Morcuende JA. Early attempts at hip arthroplasty: 1700s to 1950s. The Iowa Orthopaedic Journal. 2005;**25**:25

[9] Smith-Petersen M. Evolution of mould arthroplasty of the hip joint. The Journal of Bone and Joint Surgery British Volume. 1948;**30**(1):59-75

[10] Knight SR, Aujla R, Biswas SP. Total hip arthroplasty-over 100 years of operative history. Orthopedic Reviews. 2011;**3**(2):72-74

[11] McKee G. Total hip replacement—Past, present and future. Biomaterials. 1982;**3**(3):130-135

[12] McKee G, Watson-Farrar J. Replacement of arthritic hips by the McKee-Farrar prosthesis. The Journal of Bone and Joint Surgery British Volume. 1966;**48**(2):245-259

[13] Wiles P. The surgery of the osteo-arthritic hip. British Journal of Surgery. 1958;**45**(193):488-497

[14] Charnley J. Arthroplasty of the hip: A new operation. Clinical Orthopaedics and Related Research®. 1973;**95**:4-8

[15] Hernigou P, Pariat J. History of internal fixation (part 1): Early developments with wires and plates before world war II. International Orthopaedics. 2017;**41**(6):1273-1283

[16] Jacobs JJ, Gilbert JL, Urban RM. Current concepts review-corrosion of metal orthopaedic implants. JBJS. 1998;**80**(2):268-282

[17] Li B, Webster T. Orthopedic Biomaterials: Progress in Biology, Manufacturing, and Industry Perspectives: Springer; 2018. pp. 175-195

[18] Abdelrhman Y, Gepreel MA-H, Kobayashi S, Okano S, Okamoto T. Biocompatibility of new low-cost (α+ β)-

type Ti-Mo-Fe alloys for long-term implantation. Materials Science and Engineering: C. 2019;**99**:552-562

[19] Nnamchi PS, Obayi C, Todd I, Rainforth M. Mechanical and electrochemical characterisation of new Ti–Mo–Nb–Zr alloys for biomedical applications. Journal of the Mechanical Behavior of Biomedical Materials. 2016;**60**:68-77

[20] Kopova I, Stráský J, Harcuba P, Landa M, Janeček M, Bačákova L. Newly developed Ti–Nb–Zr–Ta–Si–Fe biomedical beta titanium alloys with increased strength and enhanced biocompatibility. Materials Science and Engineering: C. 2016;**60**:230-238

[21] Callaghan JJ, Rosenberg AG, Rubash HE, Clohisy JC, Beaulé PE, Della Valle CJ. The Adult Hip: Hip Arthroplasty Surgery. United States: Wolters Kluwer Health Adis (ESP); 2015

[22] Smith-Petersen M, Larson CB, Aufranc OE, Law WA. Complications of old fractures of the neck of the femur results of treatment by vitallium-mold arthroplasty. JBJS. 1947;**29**(1):41-46

[23] Li S, Burstein AH. Ultra-high molecular weight polyethylene. The material and its use in total joint implants. JBJS. 1994;**76**(7):1080-1090

[24] Charnley J. The long-term results of low-friction arthroplasty of the hip performed as a primary intervention. The Journal of Bone and Joint Surgery British volume. 1972;**54**(1):61-76

[25] Jackson J. Father of the modern hip replacement: Professor sir John Charnley (1911-82). Journal of Medical Biography. 2011;**19**(4):151-156

[26] Grobbelaar C, Du Plessis T, Marais F. The radiation improvement of polyethylene prostheses. A preliminary study. The Journal of Bone and Joint Surgery British volume. 1978;**60**(3):370-374

[27] Sobieraj M, Rimnac C. Ultra high molecular weight polyethylene: Mechanics, morphology, and clinical behavior. Journal of the Mechanical Behavior of Biomedical Materials. 2009;**2**(5):433-443

[28] Oral E, Wannomae KK, Rowell SL, Muratoglu OK. Diffusion of vitamin E in ultra-high molecular weight polyethylene. Biomaterials. 2007;**28**(35):5225-5237

[29] Rohm O. On the Polymerization Products of Acrylic Acid. Chemistry (dissertation). Tubingen: University of Tubingen; 1901

[30] Judet J, Judet R. The use of an artificial femoral head for arthroplasty of the hip joint. The Journal of bone and joint surgery British volume. 1950;**32**(2):166-173

[31] Haboush E. A new operation for arthroplasty of the hip based on biomechanics, photoelasticity, fast-setting dental acrylic and other considerations. Bulletin of the Hospital for Diseases Orthopaedic Institute. 1953;**14**:242-277

[32] Charnley J, Charnley J. Acrylic Cement in Orthopedic Surgery Baltimore. Philadelphia, PA, USA: The Williams and Wilkins Co; 1970. p. 36

[33] Jaeblon T. Polymethylmethacrylate: Properties and contemporary uses in orthopaedics. JAAOS-Journal of the American Academy of Orthopaedic Surgeons. 2010;**18**(5):297-305

[34] Bal B, Garino J, Ries M, Rahaman M. A review of ceramic bearing materials in total joint arthroplasty. Hip International. 2007;**17**(1):21-30

[35] Hannouche D, Hamadouche M, Nizard R, Bizot P, Meunier A, Sedel L. Ceramics in total hip replacement. Clinical Orthopaedics and Related Research®. 2005;**430**:62-71

[36] Owen D, Russell N, Smith P, Walter W. An estimation of the incidence of squeaking and revision surgery for squeaking in ceramic-on-ceramic total hip replacement: A meta-analysis and report from the Australian Orthopaedic Association National Joint Registry. The Bone & Joint Journal. 2014;**96**(2):181-187

[37] Currier JH, Anderson DE, Van Citters DW. A proposed mechanism for squeaking of ceramic-on-ceramic hips. Wear. 2010;**269**(11-12):782-789

[38] Willmann G. Ceramic femoral head retrieval data. Clinical Orthopaedics and Related Research®. 2000;**379**:22-28

[39] Exactech Inc. BIOLOX Delta Ceramic Femoral Head | Total Hip Arthroplasty. 2022. Available from: www.exac.com

Section 2

Hip Arthroplasty

Chapter 3

Hemiarthroplasty

Beakal Gezahegn

Abstract

Hemiarthrroplasty is a procedure in which the head and neck of femur are only replaced with prosthesis. Currently, almost exclusively used now for displaced intracapsular femur neck fracture in older adults and is the surgery of choice for hip fracture in patients who minimally ambulate or do not function at a very high level. This surgical procedure(arthroplasty) eliminates the risk of non-union, fixation failure, and reoperation in the treatment of femur neck fracture. There are two forms of HA: unipolar and bipolar, as well as conventional and dual-mobility THA. Both HA types have comparable results in terms of stability, but there is a danger of acetabular wear that may eventually need conversion to THA. HA is indicated in patients whose self-sufficiency and physical activity are limited. A unipolar implant should be used, as no evidence exist that bipolar implants provide additional benefits. THA is associated with better functional outcomes and a lower risk of revision surgery in self-sufficient, physically active patients. Instability is the leading complication of conventional THA and occurs with a higher incidence compared to HA. Because of the potential for instability, the posterior approach should be avoided while doing HA. In the hands of a skilled surgeon employing a dual-mobility cup, the posterior route is a solid alternative for THA. Cement fixation of the stem is advised to reduce the possibility of peri-prosthetic fracture.

Keywords: hemiarthroplasty, femur neck, internal fixation, total hip replacement, bipolar hemiarthroplasty, unipolar hemiartroplasty, cemented, uncemented hemiartroplasty

1. Introduction

Hip arthroplasty is a surgical procedure where the entire or part of the hip joint is replaced with a prosthetic implant. Hip arthroplasty comes in a wide range of variations. There are two types of procedures involving femoral head replacement: total hip arthroplasty and hemiarthroplasty. The femoral head is replaced with a prosthesis while the native acetabulum and acetabular cartilage are kept in hemiarthroplasty. The acetabulum, as well as the femoral head, are both replaced during total hip replacement.

A hip or proximal femoral fracture in an elderly patient is the most common reason for hemiarthroplasty. The displaced intracapsular fracture is the most common type of hip fracture treated with arthroplasty. The majority of extracapsular fractures are treated with fracture internal fixation. There is still debate about the best treatment for displaced intracapsular fractures in the elderly. Internal fixation reduces operative trauma, but complications such as fracture displacement, nonunion, and avascular necrosis may necessitate revision. Although internal fixation is still preferred in some countries, most surgeons now treat this fracture with arthroplasty.

The Moore prosthesis (1952) and the FR Thompson Hip Prosthesis (1954) are the most well-known early hemiarthroplasty designs (1954). Both of these implants are monoblocks that were designed prior to the development of poly (methyl methacrylate) bone cement, so they were initially inserted as a "press fit." The Moore prosthesis has a fenestrated femoral stem as well as a square stem with a shoulder to allow for stability within the femur and to resist rotation within the femoral canal. It is commonly used without cement, and bone in-growth into the fenestrations can occur over time. Thompson prostheses have a smaller stem with no fenestrations and are frequently used in conjunction with cement. There are numerous other designs of unipolar hemiarthroplasties that are based on stems used for total hip replacements [1].

In bipolar prostheses, there is an articulation in the femoral head component itself. In this type of prosthesis, there is a spherical inner metal head with a size of between 22 and 36 millimeters in diameter. This fits into a polyethylene shell, which in turn is enclosed by a metal cap. The objective of these condjoints is to reduce acetabular wear by promoting movement at the interprosthetic articulation rather than with the native acetabulum. There are a number of different types of prostheses with different stem designs. Examples of bipolar prostheses are the Charnley-Hastings, Bateman, Giliberty, and Monk prostheses, but many other types with different stem designs exist [1].

The femoral stem can be fixed during hip arthroplasty using cement or by bone growth into a porous-coated implant, depending on the surgeon's inclination. In elective total hip arthroplasty for osteoarthritis, some orthopedic surgeons now use uncemented femoral components, whereas some prefer cemented stems [2].

Hemiarthroplasty requires different considerations than complete hip arthroplasty. In the latter, clear exposure of both the femur and the acetabulum is essential, necessitating a very long exposure. Because patients are often older and more sensitive to anesthetics and surgical procedures, hemiarthroplasty requires a quick yet successful surgery with the least amount of stress and physiological disruption. There have been several surgical methods for the hip documented [3].

2. Indication

There is little doubt, and the evidence is convincing, that arthroplasty surgery, instead of internal fixation, should be performed for the elderly suffering from displaced intracapsular hip fractures.

This decision is often influenced not only by whether one implant is superior to another, but as surgeons, we must also take into account patient's medical comorbidities, functional demands, premorbid ambulatory status, and, inevitably, financial considerations. The debate on the choice of implant is, however, never-ending.

2.1 Arthroplasty vs internal fixation

The surgical treatment of patients with a femoral neck fracture should be based on the patient's age, walking ability, comorbidities, and life expectancy. Internal fixation or different types of hip arthroplasties are the available treatment modalities.

The degree of fracture displacement, the patient's age, functional demands, and risk profile, such as level of cognitive function and degree of physical fitness, should all be considered when deciding whether to treat displaced femoral neck fractures in the elderly with internal hemiarthroplasty, total hip artroplasty, or internal fixation [4].

For elderly patients with few functional demands who have displaced intracapsular fractures, unipolar or bipolar hemiarthroplasty appears to be the optimum technique, according to the orthopedic surgeon. However, treatment for the generally healthy, active, and cognitively alert old patient is still debatable [4].

Internal fixation is uncontroversial in patients with undisplaced fractures (Garden I-II), with a reasonable incidence of fracture healing problems and a favorable outcome in terms of function and health-related quality of life. Internal fixation is also seen to be the best treatment option for young patients with displaced fractures (Garden III-IV) [5].

Internal fixation causes less operative stress, but sequelae such as fracture displacement, non-union, and avascular necrosis may necessitate revision. Most surgeons now treat this fracture with arthroplasty, while internal fixation is still preferred in some countries.

A meta-analysis 1 of over 100 reports of displaced fractures of the neck of the femur reported a mean rate of nonunion of 33%, avascular necrosis of 16%, and a reoperation rate of 20–36% after internal fixation compared with 6–18% after hemiarthroplasty.

Randomized controlled trials (RCTs) have shown that a primary THR provides superior results to internal fixation in relation to the need for secondary surgery, hip function, and health-related quality of life for the active alert patient fractures(Garden III-IV) [6].

A recent multicenter randomized controlled trial shows THR should be thought of as the therapy of choice for the older patient in excellent condition with a displaced intracapsular fracture of the femoral neck when compared to internal fixation, bipolar hemiarthroplasty, and THR [7].

2.2 Hemiarthroplasty versus total hip arthroplasty

Hemiarthroplasty (HA) and total hip arthroplasty (THA) are still the most often used procedures of hip replacement following fracture. In the long term, some HA patients will require THA conversion owing to activity-limiting thigh discomfort caused by acetabulum wear. Reduced dislocation rates, less difficult surgery, shorter operation times, less blood loss, and cheaper initial expenditures are reported benefits of HA over THA [8].

THA yields superior functional outcomes than HA in the treatment of femoral neck fractures [9] and is, therefore, increasingly performed, notably in physically active patients. Nevertheless, the outcomes of THA used to treat a fracture differ from those of THA for osteoarthritis; blood transfusion is more often required; both the operative time and the hospital stays are longer; and the risks are higher for perioperative complications, infection, re-admission, and mortality [10].

Instabilities are more prevalent during total hip arthroplasty than hemiarthroplasty. The surgeon's competence, surgical approach, component alignment, and implant selection are all factors that influence hip arthroplasty outcomes [11] A femur neck fracture is a risk factor for instability in and of itself. Dislocation is also substantially more prevalent following THA to treat a fracture than in osteoarthritis patients [12] As a result, choosing an implant for THA for fracture treatment requires extraordinary prudence. Dual-mobility cups have been found to lower dislocation risk, outperforming large-diameter heads and Constrained implants [13].

The most serious long-term issue with hemiarthroplasty is severe acetabular erosion. Acetabular erosion rates have been observed to range from 0–26% for bipolar designs and from 2.2–36% for unipolar designs. According to one study, acetabular erosion necessitated the revision of 38% of unipolar prosthetic hips. Contrarily, dislocation is the most frequent early complication of total hip arthroplasty, and it is more likely when a posterior approach is used, and the prosthetic head size is smaller. After a complete hip replacement for a displaced intracapsular femoral neck fracture, dislocation rates have ranged from 2–20% [14].

Baker's findings suggest that for the treatment of individuals who are cognitively capable, independent, and active, total hip arthroplasty is preferred to hemiarthroplasty. After a three-year average follow-up, complete hip arthroplasty was associated with superior functional results, fewer problems, and fewer revisions. Both groups had functional decline postoperatively when compared to preoperative levels; however, individuals in the total hip arthroplasty group saw less deterioration and maintained their walking distances [14].

Meta-Analysis and systemic review of randomized trials comparing all forms of THA and hemiarthroplasty done by burger shows that total hip arthroplasty for displaced femoral neck fractures in the fit elderly may lead to higher patient-based outcomes but has higher dislocation rates compared with hemiarthroplastysty in a selected group of patients suffering displaced femoral neck fractures. This review, including the most recent evidence, shows that total hip arthroplasty may be advantageous over hemiarthroplasty [8].

Hedbeck's randomized controlled trial shows that complete hip arthroplasty produces superior results in terms of hip function and health-related quality of life than bipolar hemiarthroplasty in older, lucid patients with a displaced femoral neck fracture. The findings of this study and earlier research indicate that total hip arthroplasty should be the preferred form of treatment for this fracture in an active older patient with a long-life expectancy [9].

3. Types of hemiarthroplasty

3.1 Based on prosthesis head component

3.1.1 Bipolar vs unipolar hemiartroplasty

Hemiarthroplasty can be unipolar (the head is attached to the stem) or bipolar (in which there is an additional polyethylene bearing between the stem and the endoprosthetic head component). Previous systems, like the Moore, were unipolar arthroplasties with no modularity between the head and stem. Modularity is available in modern hip fracture arthroplasty systems for both unipolar and bipolar arthroplasties. In a bipolar arthroplasty, the second articulation ought to broaden the range of motion and reduce wear on the natural acetabulum, in principle. The production of particle wear debris as a result of the polyethylene might potentially result in osteolysis [15].

It is debatable that prosthesis should be used in hemiarthroplasty. Bipolar prosthesis is preferred by certain authors over unipolar prostheses by others. The motion at the inner bearing of the bipolar prosthesis, in addition to the prosthesis-acetabulum interface, is its potential benefit. The quantity of acetabular erosion should be reduced as a result. According to radiological proof and clinically proven pain reduction, however, investigations have revealed that the bipolar prosthesis acts similarly to the unipolar prosthesis and that the inner bearing loses mobility with time. Additionally, the bipolar prosthesis' two- to five-fold higher price tag than that of the unipolar prosthesis raises the question of whether it has an impact on older patients' quality of life and functional outcomes following fractures with high death rates [16].

Less wear on the acetabular cartilage is a putative benefit of the bipolar design. This has led to the suggestion that it might be a better option for patients who are more active and have longer life expectancies. Although there is a chance that the stem will become looser, and synovitis will develop as a result of polyethylene wear on the inner surface of the bipolar head covered in polyethylene. Despite the fact that several RCTs have failed to produce conclusive results on differences in clinical outcomes between the unipolar and the bipolar designs, there are few studies that report on acetabular wear using a grading system [17].

The results of unipolar and bipolar hemiarthroplasty procedures following femoral neck fracture have also been shown to be indistinguishable in several recent prospective investigations. Parker et al. revealed no variations in mortality or complication rates between unipolar and bipolar hemiarthroplasty treatment in a recent evidence-based Cochrane study [16].

3.2 Based on prostesis assembly

3.2.1 Monoblock vs modular

Monoblock and modular prostheses are the two main types of prosthesis assembly that can be used in hip hemiarthroplasty. The diameter of the patient's femoral head affects the prosthesis size for a monoblock hemiarthroplasty. The most popular monoblock hemi-arthroplasty is the collared Thompson. These implants usually fail to correctly restore the patient's original hip geometry because of the pre-fabricated design of the prosthesis, which limits its ability to be modified intra-operatively to accommodate for variations in femoral neck offset or leg length [18].

The stem, neck, and head components of a modular hemiarthroplasty are all manufactured separately. The surgeon can modify component size while assembling these intra-operatively, allowing for a more accurate restoration of the patient's original hip.

3.3 Based on technique of femoral stem insertion

3.3.1 Cemented vs uncemented hemiarthroplasty

According to the method of implant fixation, hemiarthroplasty prosthesis can be divided into two different types: cemented and uncemented hemiarthroplasty. However, controversy still exists regarding whether cemented or uncemented implant fixation is preferable in this patient population [19].

During hip arthroplasty, fixation of the femoral stem can be accomplished with cement or via bony growth into a porous-coated implant [2].

Design-wise, hemiarthroplasty stems can be either cemented or uncemented, both of which have a track record of effectiveness. Comparable to the debate over cement- or cementless-prostheses in primary hip arthroplasty, the controversy over cemented or non-cemented hemiar-throplasty is similar. Although each has advantages and disadvantages of its own, it is not clear which is better. Uncemented stems, which operate using the press-ft approach, may offer advantages in terms of less invasive and shorter surgery time, but they also carry a risk of periprosthetic fractures and thigh discomfort from implant loosening because they perform poorly when it comes to osteointegration with osteoporotic bone [20]. Due to the quality of younger patient bone stock, cementless hip arthroplasties are generally considered to be more suitable for them [21].

There is insufficient evidence from randomized studies to declare one method of hemiarthroplasty to be better than the other in hip fracture surgery. According to some researchers, patients with cemented stems recover more quickly and with less discomfort than those who had non-cemented press fits [22] Primary cementless complete hip arthroplasties usually result in reports of mid-thigh discomfort.

Bone quality is crucial for non-cemented prostheses, in elderly people, it is typically subpar. Inability to create a congruent fit and interference with bone in-growth are two relative contraindications for non-cemented total hip prostheses, both of which prevent the formation of rigid initial stability [21].

The use of a cemented stem, on the other hand, results in better implant fixation because the cement improves the anchor-age, with fewer chances of loosening and thigh pain but higher risks of cardiovascular and respiratory problems because of cement-related toxicity and embolization of cement monomer, or "cement disease." [23]. Furthermore, in cemented situations, revision procedures become quite challenging [24].

Cement implantation has a well-established impact on the cardiopulmonary system, ranging from temporary hypotension and hypoxemia to abrupt mortality [25]. Uncertainty surrounds the pathogenic mechanism behind this. The majority of experts feel that it is a direct result of fat and marrow emboli [26]; other ideas include cement toxicity, reflex autonomic effects, prostaglandin-induced vasodilatation, and thromboplast in activating the clotting cascade, lowering platelet count and oxygen tension [27]. No of the underlying mechanism, the small cardiopulmonary alterations seem to be temporary and not clinically meaningful. The prevalence of unexpected intraoperative death appears to be less than (0.2%) [28].

In choosing between these techniques, there is limited evidence contrasting the functional outcomes, morbidity, and mortality with cemented or uncemented stems [29]. The cemented group has been shown to be associated with greater blood loss and operative time, the revision rate is lower, with significantly less thigh pain and better mobility [29]. In some investigation, the cemented prosthesis provided stable early fixation with good functional outcomes at 1-year follow-up [30].

There are no differences between using current cemented and uncemented hemiarthroplasty for the treatment of intracapsular hip fractures in terms of mortality risk. The frequency of intraoperative and periprosthetic fractures is much lower with modern cemented hemiarthroplasty, but anesthesia and surgical time are prolonged [31].

4. Surgical approach

Hemiarthroplasty requires different considerations than complete hip arthroplasty. In the latter, clear exposure of both the femur and the acetabulum is essential, necessitating a very lengthy exposure. Because patients are often older and more sensitive to anesthetics and surgical procedures, hemiarthroplasty requires a quick yet successful surgery with the least amount of stress and physiological disruption. There have been several surgical methods to the hip documented [3].

Surgical approaches to the hip for hip hemiarthroplasty can be divided into three main categories: lateral approaches (LA), posterior approaches (PA), and anterior approaches (AA) [18].

According to the few national registers that collect data on surgical approaches for hemiarthroplasty, the direct lateral approach(DLA) and posterior approach(PA) are commonly used internationally. Anterior and anterolateral approaches are also used, but less often. Internationally, it appears that the choice of approach is frequently based on surgeon preference, as a result of training and experience, rather than rigid adherence to guidelines or evidence guide [32].

Posterior approaches commonly include the Moore, the Southern, the true posterior and the posterolateral approaches [18]. The division of the piriformis, and the short external rotators while preserving the hip abductor muscles are the major characteristics of this method. The approach permits the acetabulum and femur to be clearly visualized and exposed for as long as needed. There are advantages such as a lower risk of femoral shaft fracture, a shorter recovery period, a functional abductor, and reduced blood loss. The posterior technique can be used with or without the posterior joint capsule being repaired, along with additional muscle- and tendon-sparing adjustments [32].

There are two types of anterior approaches used to access the anterior part of the hip joint: direct anterior and Smith Peterson approach l. Both of them used the internervous plane in superficial dissection b/n sartorious muscle inervated by the femoral nerve and tensor facsia lata inervated by the superior gluteal nerve and in deep dissection bln gluteas medius muscle inervated by the superior gluteal nerve and rectus femoris muscle which is inerveted by the femoral nerve [18].

The major advantage of the anterior approach is that it has a lower risk of dislocation than other approaches; this advantage makes the rehabilitation program easier for the patient. There is also a minimal chance of sciatic nerve damage. The most common obstacle most surgeons face during an anterior approach is a restricted surgical field, which can result in extensive dissection of soft tissue, particularly the gluteas medius, as well as trouble reaming the femoral medulary cavity, which can result in femur fracture [32].

Lateral approaches commonly involve (partial or complete) division or retraction of the hip abductor muscles (gluteus medius and minimus) to enable access to the hip capsule. These include the Hardinge (direct lateral), the trans gluteal, and the Watson-Jones (anterolateral) approach [18].

There is solid evidence that the method affects the frequency and character of the complications. In individuals with FNF, the most commonly employed techniques are posterolateral and lateral or anterolateral. Data show that, as compared to the lateral or trans-gluteal approaches, the posterior route is linked with a significantly greater incidence of dislocation following both HA and conventional THA. When it comes to bipolar HA, the posterior approach is associated with an 8-fold increase in the risk of dislocation when compared to the lateral approach [12].

The risk of dislocation following traditional THA is also influenced by the surgical approach: documented dislocation rates are 2% for the anterolateral approach, 12% for the posterior approach, and 14% for the posterior technique without re-attachment of the posterior capsule (p 0.001) [12].

The combination of a dual-mobility cup with the posterior approach remains a reliable option, with a dislocation rate similar to that seen when conventional THA is performed via the antero lateral approach [12].

5. Conclusions

Hip fractures are classified according to their location: intracapsular and extra-capsular, with intra-capsular fractures being the most common, accounting for over 60% of all hip fractures. The patient's age and fracture displacement are taken into account when determining the procedure for a specific case. Fracture displacement raises the probability of femoral head blood supply interruption and, as a result, is associated with higher rates of non-union, fracture fixation failure, delayed union, and AVN of the femoral head. In old age (> 65 years), there is a high risk of non-union and fixation failure that leads to a high reoperation rate, which is not recommended in geriatric patients. As a result, current hip fracture treatment recommendations state that "displaced intracapsular neck of femur fractures in old age patients should be treated with arthroplasty."

There are two types of hip replacement procedures for the treatment of displaced femoral neck fractures of the intracapsular type: THA and HA. Its indication depends on the patient's age and the physiological as well as the general cognitive status of the patient. Hemiarthroplasty is recommended for the frail, low-preoperative mobility patient, and total hip arthroplasty is recommended for physically active and demanding patients.

Bipolar hemiarthroplasty and unipolar hemiarthroplasty showed comparable intraoperative blood loss, operative time, acetabular wear development, risk of instability, reoperation rates, systemic complications, mortality, and functional results. Given the lack of clinical data to support the superiority of either HA type, economic concerns should take precedence; bipolar implants are 2–5 times more expensive than unipolar implants; hence, unipolar implants are the preferable option when conducting HA [18].

Acronyms and abbreviations

THA	Total Hip Arthroplasty
HA	Hemiarthroplasty
DLA	Direct Lateral Approach
PA	Posterior Approach
AA	Anterior Approach
FNF	Femoral Neck Fracture

Author details

Beakal Gezahegn
Haramaya University, Harar, Ethiopia

*Address all correspondence to: beakalbogale2009@yahoo.com

References

[1] Sreekanta A, Eardley WGP, Wood H, Glanville JM, Cook J, Griffin XL. Surgical interventions for treating intracapsular hip fractures in adults: A network meta-analysis. Cochrane Database of Systematic Reviews. 2019;**2019**:1-3. DOI: 10.1002/14651858.CD013404

[2] Okike K, Chan PH, Prentice HA, Paxton EW, Burri RA. Association between uncemented vs cemented hemiarthroplasty and revision surgery among patients with hip fracture. Retrospective Cohort Study. DOI: 10.1001/JAMA.2020.1067

[3] Parker MJ, Pervez H. Surgical approaches for inserting hemiarthroplasty of the hip. Cochrane Database of Systematic Reviews. 2002;**3**:CD001707

[4] Blomfeldt R, Törnkvist H, Eriksson K, Söderqvist A, Ponzer S, Tidermark J. The randomized controlled trial of comparing bipolar hemiarthroplasty with total hip replacement for displaced intracapsular femur neck fracture in elderly patient. 2007. DOI: 10.1302/0301-620X.89B2.18576

[5] Bhandari M, Devereaux PJ, Tornetta P 3rd. et al, Operative management of displaced femoral neck fractures in elderly patients: An international survey. Journal of Bone and Joint Surgery. 2005;**87**(A):2122-2130

[6] Tidermark J, Ponzer S, Svensson O, Soderqvist A, Tornkvist H. Internal fixation compared with total hip replacement for displaced femoral neck fractures in the elderly. A randomised, controlled trial. Journal of Bone and Joint Surgery. British Volume (London). 2003;**85**(3):380-388. DOI: 10.1302/0301-620x.85b3.13609

[7] Keating JF, Grant A, Masson M, Scott NW, Forbes JF. Randomized comparison of reduction and fixation, bipolar hemiarthroplasty, and total hip arthroplasty: Treatment of displacedintracapsular hip fractures in healthy older patients. Journal of Bone and Joint Surgery. 2006;**88**(A):249-260

[8] Burgers PT, Van Geene AR, Van den Bekerom MP, Van Lieshout EM, Blom B, Aleem IS, et al. Total hip arthroplasty versus hemiarthroplasty for displaced femoral neck fractures in the healthy elderly: A meta-analysis and systematic review of randomized trials. International Orthopaedics. 2012;**36**(8):1549-1560. DOI: 10.1007/s00264-012-1569-7

[9] Hedbeck CJ, Enocson A, Lapidus G, Blomfeldt R, Tornkvist H, Ponzer S, et al. Comparison of bipolar hemiarthroplasty with total hip arthroplasty for displaced femoral neck fractures: A concise four-year follow-up of a randomized trial. The Journal of Bone and Joint Surgery. American Volume. 2011;**93**(5):445-450. DOI: 10.1007/s00264-013-2117-9

[10] Schairer WW, Lane JM, Halsey DA, Iorio R, Padgett DE, McLawhorn AS. Total hiparthroplasty for femoral neck fracture is not a typical DRG 470: A propensity-matched cohort study. Clinical Orthopaedics and Related Research. 2017;**475**:353-360. DOI: 10.1007/s11999-016-4868-2

[11] Guyen O. Hemiarthroplasty or total hip arthroplasty in recent femoral neck fractures? Orthopaedics & Traumatology, Surgery & Research. 2019;**105**(1S):S95-S101. DOI: 10.1016/j.otsr.2018.04.034

[12] Enocson A, Hedbeck CJ, Tidermark J, Pettersson H, Ponzer S,

Lapidus LJ. Dislo-cation of total hip replacement in patients with fractures of the femoral neck. Acta Orthopaedica. 2009;**80**:184-189. DOI: 10.3109/17453670902930024

[13] Terrier A, Latypova A, Guillemin M, Parvex V, Guyen O. Dual mobility cupsprovide biomechanical advantages in situations at risk for dislocation: A finiteelement analysis. International Orthopaedics. 2017;**41**:551-556. DOI: 10.1007/s00264-016-3368

[14] Baker RP, Squires B, Gargan MF, Bannister GC. Total hip arthroplasty and hemi-arthroplasty in mobile, independent patients with a displaced intracapsularfracture of the femoral neck. A randomized, controlled trial. J Bone Joint SurgAm. 2006;**88**:2583-2589. DOI: 10.2106/Jbjs.e01373

[15] Bhattacharyya T, Koval KJ. Unipolar versus bipolar hemiarthroplasty for femoral neck fractures: Is there a difference? Journal of Orthopaedic Trauma. 2009;**23**(6):426-427. DOI: 10.1097/bot.0b013e3181adb057

[16] Ayhan E, Kesmezacar H, Karaman O, Sahin A, Kir N. Bipolar or unipolar hemiarthroplasty after femoral neck fracture in the geriatric population. Balkan Medical Journal. 2013;**30**(4):400-405. DOI: 10.5152/balkanmedj.2013.8571

[17] Enocson A, Hedbeck CJ, Tornkvist H, Tidermark J, Lapidus LJ. Unipolar versus bipolar Exeter hip hemiarthroplasty: A prospective cohort study on 830 consecutive hips in patients with femoral neck fractures. International Orthopaedics. 2012;**36**(4):711-717. DOI: 10.1007/s00264-011-1326-3

[18] Robertson GA, Wood AM. Hip hemi-arthroplasty for neck of femur fracture: What is the current evidence? World Journal of Orthopedics. 2018;**9**(11):235-244. DOI: 10.5312/wjo.v9.i11.235

[19] Ning GZ, Li YL, Wu Q, Feng SQ, Li Y, Wu QL. Cemented versus uncemented hemiarthroplasty for displaced femoral neck fractures: An updated meta-analysis. European Journal of Orthopaedic Surgery and Traumatology. 2014;**24**(1):7-14. DOI: 10.1007/s00590-012-115-4

[20] Ayhan E, Kesmezacar H, Karaman O, Sahin A, Kir N. Bipolar or unipolar hemiarthroplasty after femoral neck fracture in the geriatric population. Balkan Medical Journal. 2013;**30**(4):400-405. DOI: 10.5152/balkanmedj.2013.8571

[21] Vochteloo AJ, Niesten D, Riedijk R, Rijnberg WJ, Bolder SB, Koeter S, et al. Cemented versus non-cemented hemiarthroplasty of the hip as a treatment for a displaced femoral neck fracture: Design of a randomised controlled trial. BMC Musculoskeletal Disorders. 2009;**10**:56. DOI: 10.1186/1471-2474-10-56

[22] Parker MJ, Gurusamy KS. Arthroplasties (with and without bone cement) for proximal femoral fractures in adults. Cochrane Database of Systematic Reviews. 2006;**2006**:4-7. DOI: 10.1002/14651858.CD001706.pub3

[23] Clark DI, Ahmed AB, Baxendale BR, Moran CG. Cardiac output during hemiarthroplasty of the hip. The Journal of Bone and Joint Surgery. 2001;**83**(3):414-418. DOI: 10.1302/0301-620x.83b3.11477

[24] Taylor F, Wright M, Zhu M. Hemiarthroplasty of the hip with and without cement: A randomized clinical trial. The Journal of Bone and Joint Surgery. American Volume. 2012;**94**(7):577-583. DOI: 10.2106/JBJS.K.00006

[25] Dandy DJ. Fat embolism following prosthetic replacement of the femoral head. Injury. 1972;**3**(2):85-88. DOI: 10.1016/s0020-1383(71)80190-0

[26] Pitto RP, Blunk J, Kößler M. Transesophageal echocardiography and clinical features of fat embolism during cemented total hip arthroplasty. Archives of Orthopaedic and Trauma Surgery. 2000;**120**(1-2):53-58. DOI: 10.1007/pl00021216

[27] Engesaeter LB, Strand T, Raugstad TS, Husebo S, Langeland N. Effects of a distal venting hole in the femur during total hip replacement. Archives of Orthopaedic and Trauma Surgery. 1984;**103**:328-331

[28] Parvizi J, Holiday AD, Ereth MH, Lewallen DG. Sudden death during hip arthroplasty. Clinical Orthopaedics and Related Research. 1999;**369**:39-48. DOI: 10.1097/00003086-199912000-00005

[29] Khan RJ, MacDowell A, Crossman P, Keene G. Cemented or uncemented hemiarthroplasty for displaced intracapsular fractures of the hip—A systematic review. Injury. 2002;**33**(1):13-17. DOI: 10.1016/s0020-1383(01)00101-2

[30] DeAngelis JP, Ademi A, Staff I, Lewis CG. Cemented versus uncemented hemiarthroplasty for displaced femoral neck fractures. Journal of Orthopaedic Trauma. 2012;**26**(3):135-140. DOI: 10.1097/bot.0b013e318238b7a5

[31] NanthaKumar N, Kunutsor SK, Fernandez MA, Dominguez E, Parsons N, Costa ML, et al. Effectiveness and safety of cemented and uncemented hemiarthroplasty in treatment of intracapsular hip fractures. DOI: 10.1302/0301-620X.102B9. BJJ-2020-0282

[32] Fullam J, Theodosi PG, Charity J, Goodwin VA. A scoping review comparing two common surgical approaches to the hip for hemiarthroplasty. BMC Surgery. 2019;**19**(1):32. DOI: 10.1186/s12893-019-0493-9

Chapter 4

Instability in Total Hip Arthroplasty

Kunal Panwar, Brenden Cutter, Michael Holmboe, Ryan Card, William Pistel and Jesua I. Law

Abstract

Total hip arthroplasty (THA) is becoming one of the most frequently sought-after surgeries in orthopedics. As the techniques and implants continue to evolve, the stability of the prosthesis is always at the forefront of the surgeon's mind. Multiple factors contribute to implant stability and there are many intraoperative decisions that can be made by the surgeon to increase stability. Techniques including approaches, adjusting length, adjusting offset, as well as implant choices can dictate stability in THA. There are multiple options that exist including different liners and constraint. One non modifiable variable which surgeons often struggle with is the spinopelvic relationship which can also affect stability post operatively. These factors include lumbar arthritis, variable pelvic tilt, and others that can make a routine approach to a total hip unsuccessful and increase the risk of post-operative complications. Ultimately there are many things to consider when approaching THA in patients, especially in the setting of abnormal pathology.

Keywords: instability, total hip arthroplasty, subluxation, dual mobility, dislocation

1. Introduction

Hip arthroplasty remains one of the most successful surgeries offered today; however, with a prosthetic hip component, a unique possibility of dislocation arises [1]. The incidence of instability within revision hip arthroplasty is estimated from 17 to 25% with a mean cost of care at $77.851.24 [2, 3]. With rates rates of primary hip arthroplasty increasing, the projected financial burden on the healthcare system remains large [4–6]. Historically, implant designs featured smaller femoral head articulations, such as the 22 mm femoral heads of the Charnley hip, which were associated with instability rates as high as 4.8% [7, 8]. Since the landmark Morrey article in 1982, improved implant designs and surgical techniques have evolved lowering the dislocation rate from 3.2% to less than 2% [9, 10]. Although a large percentage of instability can be managed nonoperatively, instability remains the most common indications for revision arthroplasty within the United States [4, 11]. Numerous risk factors exist including patient demographic variables, approach, surgeon learning curve, spinopelvic relationship, and indication for surgery. These factors should be

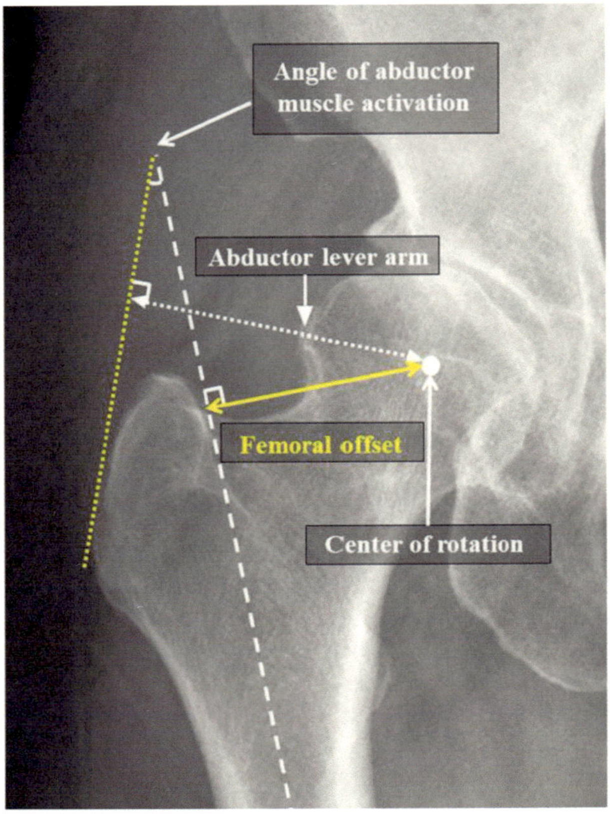

Figure 1.
Femoral offset and subsequent abductor moment arm [13].

taken into consideration when projecting a specific patients' potential risk of subsequent instability.

A stable THA relies on understanding the biomechanics of femoral head size and center of rotation (COR) [12]. Briefly, hip offset is defined as the linear distance from the femoral COR to the axis of the femoral shaft. A medial shift in the center of rotation decreases the moment arm of the abductors, thereby changing abductor tension and increasing potential risk of instability (**Figure 1**). Conversely, an increase in femoral offset adds to abductor tension and reduces potential instability [14]. Hip stability can also be achieved through modulation of femoral head size and consequently jump distance. The linear distance required for the femoral head to travel prior to dislocation is directly proportional to the femoral head size. By increasing the size of the femoral head a larger displacement is required prior to dislocation (**Figure 2**). Surgical manipulation of hip anatomy through biomechanics is central towards optimizing patient stability.

2. Risk factors

Several modifiable and nonmodifiable risk factors should be considered prior to undertaking hip arthroplasty. Modifiable risk factors include tobacco, alcohol use, and obesity [15, 16]. Modern hip arthroplasty utilizing press fit implants relies on

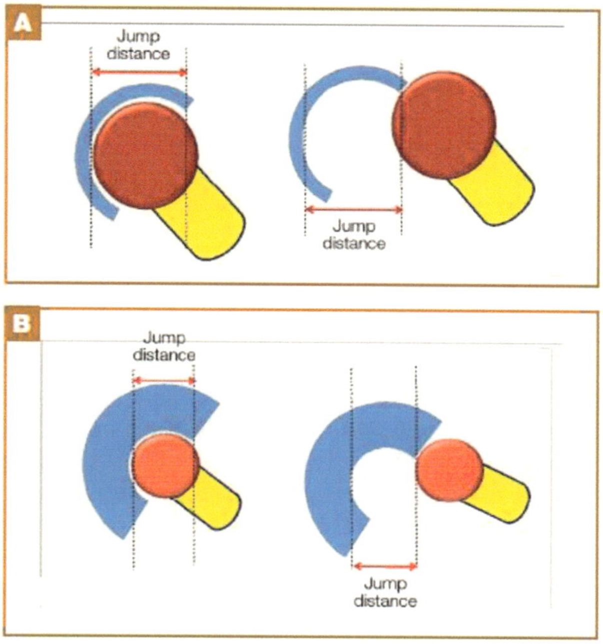

Figure 2.
*Large diameter femoral heads have larger jump distances than smaller diameter heads [14]. Of note, due to the fixed radius of the acetabular component, a larger femoral head will decrease the space available for polyethylene. This can be seen in **Figure 2A** versus **Figure 2B**.*

immediate stability at the bone/implant interface through a variety of tapers and coatings. Although the exact mechanism is not understood, this stability is weakened from tobacco use. Several researchers have demonstrated the adverse effects of delayed bone healing with tobacco use and this theory has been extended to include delayed bone-implant ingrowth [17, 18]. Elective arthroplasty offers a unique opportunity for patients to cease smoking, and some literature demonstrates continued abstinence [19]. A careful history with a targeted effort at reducing modifiable risk factors should be considered prior to hip arthroplasty.

Tobacco and alcohol use are correlated with wound complications and potential instability [16, 17]. Also, patients who abuse alcohol are less likely adhere to precautions and suffer more frequent falls, leading to interprosthetic instability. The immunosuppression from alcohol misuse has shown an increased risk of prosthetic joint infections thereby impairing bony ingrowth [17].

Currently, more than two-thirds of Americans are classified as obese (body mass index (BMI) $\geq$ 30 kg/m2) [20]. Groups with the highest BMI are increasing in size at the fastest rate, as evidenced by the greater than 50% annual increase in prevalence of patients with a BMI $\geq$ 40 kg/m^2 [21, 22]. Elevated BMI will increase the soft tissue envelope around the hip, thereby increasing the risk of implant malpositioning. This malpositioning along with soft tissue impingement are known risk factors for instability [23]. Patients with elevated BMI tend to be younger. Younger aged patients statistically place more stress on their implants and with the increased weight these patients may have elevated wear rates and higher risk of aseptic loosening [24].

Non modifiable risk factors include advanced age, cognitive impairment, and in some earlier studies, female sex [16]. Several comorbid conditions also predisposing patients to dislocation following THA include developmental dysplasia of the hip, neuromuscular disorders, and other connective tissue disorders. Abductor muscle deficiency, prior surgical revision, a history of instability, and prior spinal disease or surgery [25–28]. Previous instances of instability are also risk factors for future instability events.

3. Preoperative optimization of hip stability

Due to the numerous risk factors for instability, a thorough preoperative evaluation and identification of appropriate surgical approach should be performed. Several hip arthroplasty approaches exist with varied evidence on the risk of subsequent instability. Historically, the posterior approach was associated with highest rates of instability [29, 30]. This was reinforced with a subsequent large volume Kaiser series that demonstrated improved stability with the direct anterior approach over traditional posterior approaches [31]. However, recent literature has brought this into question, largely demonstrating that with capsular repair the posterior approach is no superior to alternate approaches [32–34]. Critics highlight the selection bias of these capsular repair/posterior approach papers stating they reflect academic practices and do not adequately reflect the community [35]. Further controversy exists when analyzing large joint registry databases. Both the Australian (122,345 primary THA) and Dutch (166,231 primary THA) Registries demonstrate a reduced risk of instability with the anterior approach [35, 36]. From a revision perspective, it appears that changing approach does not affect overall rate of instability [37]. Ultimately it is recommended that surgical approach be utilized at the discretion and comfort of the surgeon with the recognition that the anterior approach may have improved stability. If the posterior approach is preferred then careful capsular closure should be performed [38, 39].

Preoperative optimization of body mass index (BMI) continues to be an ongoing debate. Multiple studies demonstrate a slight preponderance for instability in cohorts with heavier BMI—with 5% increased risk for each BMI unit exceeding 35 kg/m^2 [40, 41]. Although the exact etiology of instability in heavier patients remains unknown, possibly resulting from combinations of deeper surgical field causing implant malposition versus muscular weakness; nonpharmacologic weight loss does seem to work at reducing BMI in some patients [42, 43]. From the perspective of instability, it remains unknown if weight loss causes a clinically significant risk reduction in postoperative instability; however, the generalized physical and mental health benefits certainly warrant an attempt at reducing BMI [44].

4. Intraoperative optimization of instability

4.1 Introductory statement

Surgeons should be aware of the impact their approach, implants, and implant positioning has on patient outcomes. When performing an arthroplasty for fracture, a hemiarthroplasty can be an option in a less active patient but this does not confer the longevity that a total hip offers. Studies note less morbidity, decreased operative time and decreased blood loss with a hemi versus total [45]. If the implant of choice is a hemiarthroplasty, a decision between a unipolar and a bipolar implant must be made. Proponents of a unipolar arthroplasty state that the hip stability primarily comes from the larger femoral head component and the dual articulation of the bipolar component provides negligible stability [46]. Yang et al. published a systematic review illustrating statistically significant decrease of cost and increased acetabular erosion with a unipolar arthroplasty [47].

Treatment of displaced femoral neck fractures in the elderly population continues to be a subject of controversy in recent literature. The New England Journal of Medicine recently published a study which included 1498 patients, ages 50 or older, across 80 centers, in 10 countries where patients were randomly assigned to either hemi or total hip arthroplasty group following a displaced femoral neck fracture. Despite only having a 2 year follow up, this cohort exhibited no significant difference in secondary procedures performed [48]. Some have critiqued this study questioning if a 2 year follow up was sufficient time to detect a difference. Another study noted no difference of revision rates at 5 years but improved quality of life favoring the THA cohort and reduced surgical time favoring the hemi arthroplasty cohort [49].

4.2 Femoral component: version + proper tensioning

Studies have shown large inconsistencies of the proximal femur from patient to patient. A patient's proximal femur may undergo morphological changes throughout their lifetime due to osteoporosis and age [50, 51]. Manufactures have designed the femoral component with variability to accommodate the irregularity of the native proximal femur [52, 53]. Hip dysplasia, while relatively common, can add up to 60 degrees variability in proximal femoral morphology and contract stress [54, 55].

Femoral anteversion is the angle between an axially projected line along the femoral neck and posterior condyles (**Figure 3**) [56]. This anteversion is essentially the extent the implants are "pointed "ventrally and has wide variation [57]. This angle can be measured preoperatively via CT scan or with a variety of different x-rays [58, 59]. Combined implant anteversion was popularized to improve hip stability and decrease intraprosthetic impingement while providing a functional range of motion for the patient [60]. Some surgeons have become proponents of "femur first" preparation since noncemented implants are constrained by the proximal femoral anatomy [61]. Once the femoral anteversion is measured, appropriate anteversion can then be "dialed into "the acetabular component as this is easier to change.

Femoral length is a measurement from the acetabular teardrop to the proximal femur [62]. This change is often easily noticed by patients and can often cause discomfort after a total hip replacement [63, 64]. Femoral length can be changed independently by changing the position of the implant within the femoral intermedullary

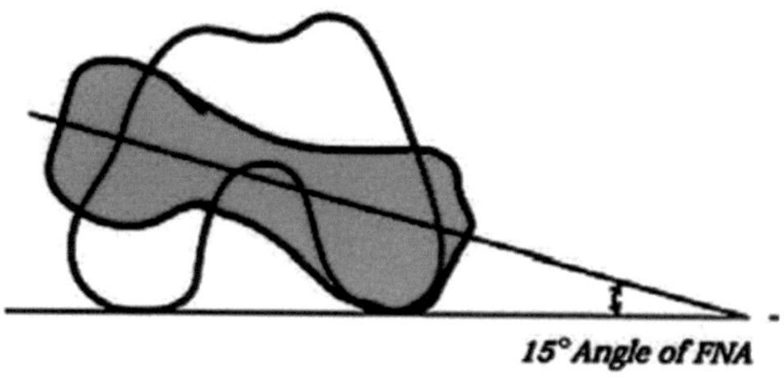

Figure 3.
Measurement of femoral Anteversion (FNA—Femoral neck angle) [56].

canal or changed in conjunction with offset when the surgeon changes the femoral neck component.

Femoral offset is a measurement of the distance from the femoral intermedullary canal to the center of rotation [12]. An increase in this measurement will allow the femur to sit further away from midline, thereby increasing the abductor lever arm [65]. Both femoral length and femoral offset will increase tension on the gluteal musculature and provide stability. The surgeon must take caution and balance hip stability with an increase in offset as excessive femoral offset will cause pain to the gluteal musculature, increase implant micromotion and overload the femoral component [66–68]. Femoral implants have different ways to increase offset. Some implants change offset based on a "medial shift" of the stem/neck takeoff while other implants change the neck shaft angle. The average neck/shaft angle in the Caucasian population is 130 degrees and by changing offset in different ways, the surgeon may restore "normal patient anatomy" and properly tension the soft tissues [52, 53]. It is important that the surgeon becomes familiar with how changes in the neck/shaft angle will change femoral neck length (**Figures 4** and **5**). In certain situations where a large femoral neck is needed a skirt may be required. This skirt is needed to properly engage the morse taper while moving the center of rotation away from the stem base. The "skirt" on the neck becomes necessary at differing + neck options based on manufacture designs and will vary based on skirt length and thickness. These femoral neck skirts decrease the head to neck ratio thereby possibly adding to hip impingement and instability [70].

Figure 5a shows 2 hip templates of the same implant with a change in neck shaft angle. Notice how the "offset" (125 degree) neck shaft angle will cause neck changes to primarily affect offset and little length is changed.

Figure 5b shows the "offset stem" in relation to the cup center of rotation. Notice the angle of the shaft is 125 degrees and changes in neck length primarily change offset with little change to length.

Figure 5c demonstrates a "standard offset" (131 degree) neck length. Notice how neck length changes will affect both length and offset more evenly.

4.3 Head size and instability

The value of larger femoral heads in THA has been increasingly recognized over the last 60 years. Since the 1960s, femoral head size increased from the original 22 mm to an average size of 32 mm by the mid 2000s [71]. Although some registry data reports the most common head diameter to be 32 mm, the use of 36 mm heads has been increasing. The AJRR recently reported a 36 mm head as the most commonly implanted size in the United States [72, 73]. Increasing femoral head size improves stability in THA through two main mechanisms. First, a larger diameter head is more deeply seated into the acetabular cup, requiring an increase in linear translation (also known as "jump distance") in order for a dislocation to occur [74]. Second, an increase in the femoral head diameter, while maintaining a constant neck diameter, increases the head to neck ratio allowing for a wider impingement-free arc of motion [75].

The stabilizing effect of large femoral heads is well documented in the literature. A randomized controlled trial of 644 patients found that 36 mm heads resulted in a significantly decreased rate of dislocation when compared to 28 mm heads (1.3% versus 5.4%, $p = 0.012$) at 1 year follow-up [76]. Several recent registry studies

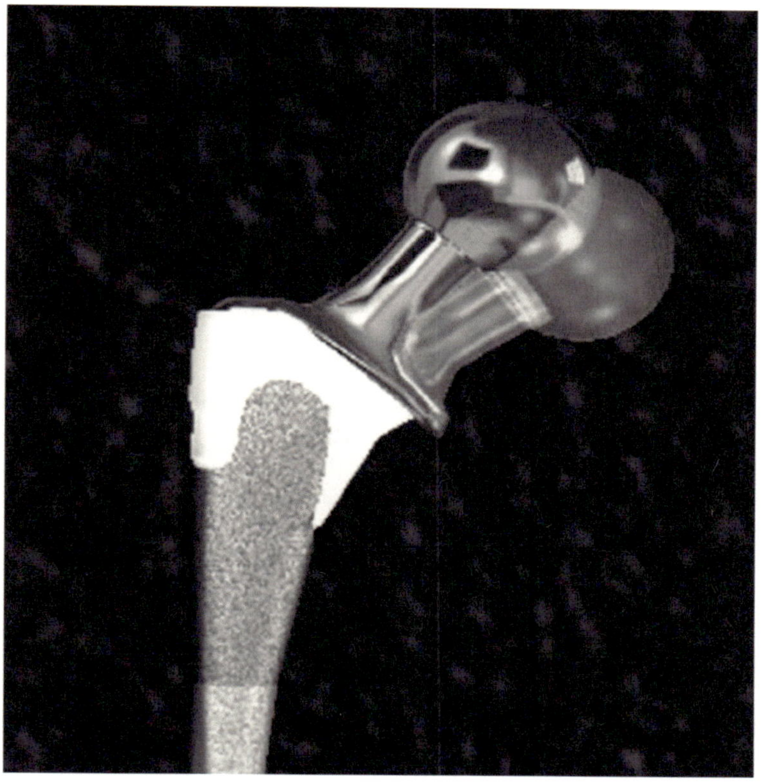

Figure 4.
A decrease in the femoral neck shaft angle will decrease the femoral height while increasing offset. This construct will increase the magnitude of the abductor lever arm [69].

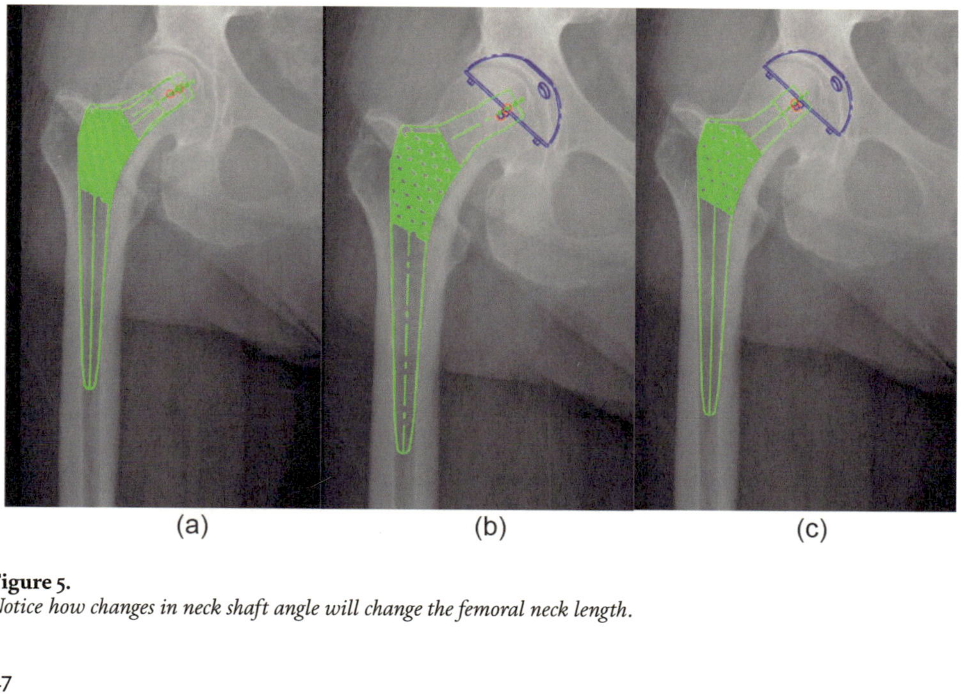

Figure 5.
Notice how changes in neck shaft angle will change the femoral neck length.

have further emphasized the advantage of large femoral heads [36, 72, 77]. A study published from the Dutch Arthroplasty Registry reported significantly decreased dislocation risk with 32 mm heads when compared to those using 22–28 mm [36]. These authors noted further improved stability with a 36 mm head compared to 32 mm when evaluating operations performed through the posterolateral approach. Another recent investigation using the Danish Hip Arthroplasty Register also favored 36 mm heads compared to 32 mm, demonstrating a reduced dislocation risk within 2 years of primary THA [77].

Although these studies emphasize the stabilizing advantage of a large femoral head, the surgeon must weigh this advantage against the concern for increased wear characteristics and late failure [78, 79]. Several studies have determined 36 mm and larger heads to exhibit increased frictional torque and volumetric wear versus heads of 32 mm and smaller [80, 81]. The surgeon must also be aware that with a fixed acetabular component the space available for polyethylene decreases as the femoral head size increases. This will lead to a thinner polyethylene liner implanted if a 36 mm head is used (**Figure 2A** and **B**). A recently published study from the Australian Regstristy found that 36 mm heads had a statistically higher risk of late revision when examining metal on cross-linked polyethylene constructs versus ceramic head components [79]. Although more long-term data is needed, this study suggests that when using femoral heads of 36 mm or more, the surgeon may consider ceramic femoral heads for the best combination of stability and longevity.

Several strategies can be employed to achieve the stabilizing advantage of a large femoral head in total hip arthroplasty. Although some authors advise reaming up to achieve an acetabular component of sufficient size to accommodate a 36 mm head, there are concerns that this can change the center of rotation and biomechanics of the hip [82]. Odri et al. found that patients experienced significantly more postoperative pain, especially anterior iliiopsoas impingement, when the implanted cup was 6 mm or more larger than the native femoral head [83]. Authors have therefore advised implanting a cup that is no larger than 4 mm above the measured diameter of the femoral head [82]. In patients whose anatomy cannot accomodate a large acetabular shell, surgeons can employ several strategies to achieve an increased head size. This includes the use of thin polyethylene liners, metal on metal bearings, and dual-mobility implants. Despite concerns for increased liner wear and fracture, a recent report evaluating the use of large femoral heads with thin polyethylene liners at average 8.5 year follow up, noted a 100% survival rate when using liner failure as an endpoint [84]. Metal on metal bearings, which allow a head size closer to that of the native femoral head. These implants have displayed low rates of dislocation but their utilization has waned due to concerns of adverse reactions to metal debris (ARMD) [85, 86]. Dual mobility constructs allow for large femoral head diameter in addition to an increased arc of motion, and will be discussed more thoroughly later in this chapter.

4.4 Acetabular component

Postoperative hip stability depends on accurate placement of the acetabular component [87]. Factors that contribute to malpositioning may include intraoperative patient-positioning, abnormal pelvic anatomy and body habitus [88]. Surgeons continue to aim for an acetabular position of 40 degrees +/− 10 degrees of abduction and 15 degrees +/− 10 degrees of anteversion [89]. One technique includes positioning the patient in the center of the room with the sides of the operating table paralleling the walls of the OR. This allows the surgeon to base the version and inclination from the walls and the floor of the operating room [90]. To perform this technique, the patient must be positioned in a stable lateral decubitus position with the pelvis directly perpendicular to the floor. However, variations in pelvic position make balancing and stabilizing the patient in this position difficult. Additionally, inconsistencies in the size and shape of the operating room may alter the surgeon's perception of patient orientation [90]. Therefore an alignment rod attached to the insertion handle of the cup has proven to be more accurate in comparison to free hand cup placement [91]. This rod allows the surgeon to more appropriately align the guide to visualize anteversion and inclination based on the floor and longitudinal axis of the patient. However, both techniques are sensitive to patient positioning and orientation of the pelvis.

Moreover, use of native pelvic anatomy increases accuracy in comparison to referencing external factors. One landmark often referenced to establish native pelvic anteversion is the transverse acetabular ligament (TAL) [92]. This landmark is independent of pelvic positioning and pelvic tilt. When using the TAL as a reference for anteversion and depth, Archbold et al. noted a 0.6% dislocation rate in 1000 consecutive patients [92, 93]. Other intrinsic pelvic landmarks such as the superior acetabulum, acetabular sulcus of the ilium and pubis have been reviewed but not widely adopted due to the large variability from osteophyte production [94]. Many are now starting to look towards intraoperative imaging and computer guidance to try to reduce surgeon error.

4.4.1 Acetabular Offset

Acetabular offset, defined as the distance between the COR of the femoral head and the center of the pelvis, can be an important contributor to the stability and overall forces on a total hip arthroplasty. Charnley's traditional techniques recommended medialization of the acetabular component in order to reduce the joint reactive force (JRF) on the hip [95]. However, this reduction in acetabular offset can result in increased impingement, reduced ROM, loss of soft tissue tension, and an increased risk of dislocation [96–99].

An astute surgeon should attempt to re-establish the patient's anatomic global offset (GO), the sum of femoral offset and acetabular offset. A decrease in GO after THA has been shown to result in loss of soft tissue tension and abductor function [100]. When medialization of the acetabulum is necessary, particularly in the setting of significant hip dysplasia, a stem with greater femoral offset is often required to restore the global offset and optimize stability of the hip joint [99]. Excessive medialization of the acetabular cup can increase the risk of impingement, a known risk factor for dislocation. In a computer model simulation, Kurtz et al. determined a decrease in acetabular offset to be the greatest risk factor for increased bony impingement [101]. Even restoration of global offset via increased femoral offset failed to fully restore range of motion before impingement. The study listed a deepened acetabular component leading to premature impingement of the femoral neck on either bone or soft tissue of the pelvis. With these ideas in mind, anatomic positioning of the cup with preservation of acetabular offset is advised.

4.5 Robotics/fluoroscopy and navigation cup position

With increased emphasis on proper positioning of components, there is growing interest in technology that allows more accurate and reproducible placement of total hip arthroplasty components. Free-hand cup positioning can be inaccurate and inconsistent, with one study finding that only 50% of the components were accurately placed in both anteversion and abduction target zones [23]. Techniques to improve component positioning can be separated into three categories: fluoroscopic guidance, computer navigation, and robotic-assisted total hip arthroplasty.

One advantage of the anterior approach is the ease of use of fluoroscopy during the operation. Rathod et al. found the use of fluoroscopy during an anterior approach significantly increased accuracy in cup placement compared to a non-guided posterior approach [102]. In addition, fluoroscopic guidance using the anterior approach has been shown to be more accurate than the use of fluoroscopy in the posterior approach due to the supine position allowing for a more accurate representation of a standing AP pelvis compared to the lateral position [103]. A recent study found the fluoroscopic assisted anterior approach to be as accurate at placing the cup into a target safe zone as a robotic-guided operation [104].

Computer navigation, used with or without the assistance of imaging, commonly relies on intra-operative anatomic landmarks and surgeon guided input reference points to aid in component positioning [99]. Several studies have reported computer navigation to result in more accurate acetabular component placement when compared to freehand methods [105, 106]. Robotic guidance combines computer navigation with the input of a robotic-assisted arm. Most contemporary designs are semi-active, where the robotic apparatus assists in certain actions while still requiring operation of the system by the surgeon [23, 104]. Similar to other technology guided techniques, robotic-assisted THA has shown increased accuracy of cup positioning versus manual techniques [107]. In addition to cup placement, these surgical technology enhancements can assist with achieving more accurate leg lengths, global offset, and combined anteversion measurements [108, 109].

Despite improved accuracy of component placement, the clinical advantages of technology assisted total hip arthroplasty continues to be debated. In a randomized controlled trial comparing 62 computer navigated THAs to 63 manual THAs, Lass et al. found no difference in dislocation rates at a minimum of 2 year follow up [110]. In their cohort of 2247 patients, Shaw et al. found robotic assisted THA to result in significantly lower rates of dislocation (0.6%) versus manual THA (2.5%, $p < 0.05$) [111]. Another recent study compared THAs performed through the posterior approach using robotic assisted, computer navigated, and manual techniques [112]. The authors found robotic-assisted posterior THA to have a statistically significant decrease in reoperation due to dislocation compared to the manual THA cohort ($OR = 0.3, p < 0.05$). Interestingly, this difference was not seen when comparing the computer navigated cohort to the manual group. The authors have proposed that the influence of robotic THA goes beyond improved cup positioning and warrants further study. These surgically assisted technology enhancements continues to increase in popularity, and continued high-level studies are needed to elucidate whether it provides sufficient advantages to outweigh the higher initial costs.

4.6 Acetabular liners: Added stability when needed

After satisfactorily implanting the acetabular component, the surgeon needs to make the decision on the type of liner used. Many manufacturers provide different acetabular liner options to allow the surgeon to recreate native anatomy and maximize hip stability. It is important that the surgeon become familiar with the liner options available when preparing for a case. Most implant manufactures allow for neutral, lipped, lateralized, oblique, constrained and dual mobility liners.

A neutral liner should be used when the surgeon is satisfied with the acetabular position, the hip stability, and in instances where the patient has no increased risk of dislocation. This liner allows the patient to have the greatest range of motion since the implant will sit flush with the acetabular component but does not give the surgeon any added stability [113]. Some surgeons prefer to use a "lipped or high walled liner" to allow for increased stability due to a larger jump distance in a discrete quadrant (**Figure 6**). With this liner option the surgeon can position the "elevated lip" to the area concern. This liner may increase intraoperative stability and allow the patient an additional 8 degrees of internal rotation if placed in the posterior quadrant [114]. From a posterior approach, the elevated liner should be placed in the "4 o'clock" position with a left hip and an "8 o'clock" position in the right hip [115]. It is important to note that this increased jump distance will also cause impingement in the area of increased elevation and may lead to dislocations.

In acetabular protrusio cases, native or iatrogenic from over reaming, or in cases where the patient has increased native offset, the surgeon may choose to use a lateralized liner. The lateralized liner has increased polyethelene in the medial portion of the implant and circumferential coverage. It is important to note that the lateralized liner will increase offset and length based on the acetabular implant position. In cases where the acetabular component is horizontal then the lateralized liner will increase overall hip length and in contrast in a vertical acetabular component orientation the lateralized liner will primarily increase offset. The lateralized liner should be considered when the abductor soft tissues are lax and the surgeon has already used a high offset implant [116]. It is important to note that a lateralized acetabular liner will increase the body weight moment arm and has been shown to increase joint reactive forces and thereby increase polyethelene wear rates [117].

In cases where the surgeon wishes to maintain a mildly malpositioned acetabular component an oblique liner may be used. When available, this option can become important in both primary and revision situations. The oblique acetabular insert has 180 degrees of coverage and reorients the range of motion in the direction of the obliquity [10]. Some surgeons have found this liner option to be quite useful in hip dysplasia since these patients may have highly irregular bone stock. This liner option allows the surgeon to place the acetabular component in a position that maximizes bony contact while reorienting the range of motion to a more functional "safe zone" [118].

Constrained liners are designed to physically lock the femoral head into the acetabular liner with the use of a metal ring [119]. These liners allow the surgeon the greatest amount of hip stability with the most amount of stress at the bone/implant

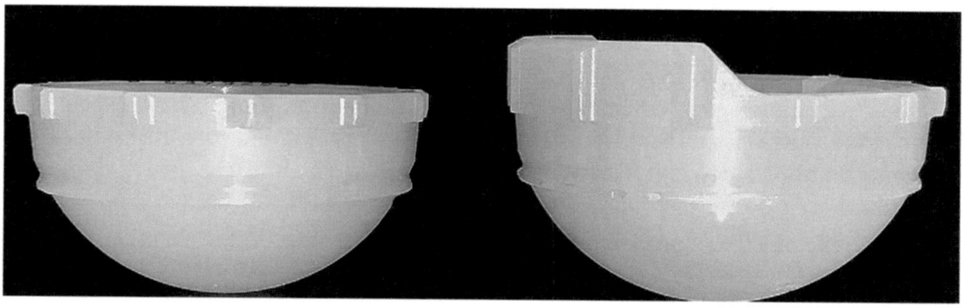

Figure 6.
Left is a neutral liner. Right is a high walled liner.

interface. Surgeons should be aware that these liners are not indicated in situations with implant malposition or hip impingement. The primary indication for these constraint liners is neuromuscular disorders, abductor deficiency or intraoperative multidirectional instability without hip impingement or implant malposition [113]. This increased constraint is commonly used in more difficult hips and has been shown to have higher revision rates from several mechanisms of failure [120]. Locking ring failure from polyethelene wear or repetitive impingement and aseptic loosening causing cup migration or pull out are known failure mechanisms [88, 121, 122].

4.7 Dual mobility

Dual Mobility (DM) articulations were first designed by Bousquet in 1974. This design capitalizes on the principle of low friction arthroplasty, which favors a small femoral head, and the improved stability given with increasing the femoral head size [123]. The DM articulation achieves both increased stability and decreases wear by featuring two articulating surfaces within a fixed acetabular shell. These shells articulate with a large polyethylene ball; within the polyethylene ball sits another small (generally 22–28 mm) metallic femoral head. The benefits of DM include reduced rates of instability while maintaining longevity [124].

Modern DM articulations offer modular highly polished liners that are compatible within prior titanium acetabular shell designs. Prior generations—sometimes referred to as anatomic DM—featured monoblock cobalt chrome acetabular components. A unique challenge of these anatomic components was implantation due to difficulty with verification of component seating. The primary benefit of a monoblock component is a theoretical decrease in metal ions due to the disappearance of differing metal interfaces; however, short term series have not found significant differences to date [125–127].

Perhaps the most pertinent application for a dual mobility liner is in the setting of femoral neck fracture. Femoral neck fractures present within a patient cohort of generalized muscular insufficiency, recurrent falls, spasticity from immobility, neurologic disorder, and cognitive decline. Dislocation rates for total hip arthroplasty within femoral neck fractures have been published as high as 9% but can be lowered to 1.2% with the use of a dual mobility construct [124, 128–131]. New literature has interestingly shown lower instability rates in DM total hips constructs over traditional hemiarthroplasty cohorts [129, 132]. It is therefore recommended to utilize DM constructs in total hips for femoral neck fracture [132, 133].

Fixed Spinopelvic alignment and its implications on hip stability has become an increasingly studied topic. In normal anatomy, the pelvis dynamically tilts posteriorly to increase acetabular coverage during a seated position to allow femoral clearance. In contrast while the patient is in the standing position the pelvis assumes a more neutral orientation [134, 135]. This native motion protects against femoral dislocation with hip flexion; however, patients with rigid spinopelvic alignment have repeatedly demonstrated to be at an increased risk of instability [136]. Dual mobility articulations have demonstrated significant improvement in hip stability within patients with fixed spinopelvic pathology [137].

Increasing data suggests that modern DM implants have longevity and appropriate wear characteristics; despite having two articulating surfaces which increases the risk of volumetric wear [138]. Limited retrieval studies demonstrate a wear rate similar to traditional cementless liners at 15 years [139]. Furthermore, systematic review suggests overall survivorship of 98% at mean followup of 8.5 years (2 to 16 years).

The most common cause of revision was aseptic loosening at 1.3% followed by intraprosthetic dislocation at 1.1% [124]. Overall, DM total hip arthroplasties are a viable option with a proven track record of longevity and an ideal clinical application for patients at increased risk of instability.

5. Soft tissue procedures

To optimize hip stability, attention should be drawn to the soft tissue integrity and tensioning around the hip. Approaches that utilize the lateral decubitus position require meticulous capsular repair. Critics have stated capsular repairs will ultimately fail or lead to an unnecessary increase in surgical time; however, this repair has demonstrated less blood loss, decreased dislocations, and better functional outcome scores [140, 141]. In contrast, supine approaches have not shown this increased benefit [142]. Schwartz et al. published a randomized controlled trial regarding capsular repair vs. capsulectomy utilizing the direct anterior approach noting no difference in outcomes [143]. The increased stability from the direct anterior muscle sparing approach maybe from the preservation of the short external rotators or from the fluoroscopic guidance of intraoperative implant positioning. Ultimately, the data is unclear whether capsular retention and repair is necessary for post-operative hip stability using the direct anterior approach.

Even when the femoral and acetabular components are appropriately oriented, restoration of length and offset are needed to recreate the mechanical advantage of the abductors [144]. Abductor tensioning is affected by the sizing and positioning of both the femoral and acetabular components. Poor abductor repair, failure of trochanter osteotomies, and destruction of the greater trochanter from fracture or osteolysis will adversely affect this tensioning [145]. In severe cases of abductor deficiency, soft tissue transfers may be needed to increase strength and stability of the hip joint. A transfer of the anterior ½ of the gluteus maximus to the greater trochanter has been described to increase lateral stability and to assist with Trendelenburg gait [146]. It is also possible to perform transfers such as transferring the anterior half of the gluteus maximus to the greater trochanter to increase lateral stability and to assist with issues of Trendelenburg gait [147].

Although rarely required for a primary hip arthroplasty, a greater trochanteric osteotomy is indicated to remove well fixed implants for hip revisions. Robust fixation of this osteotomy is crucial to avoid trochanteric nonunion which can result in pain, hip weakness, and hip instability [148]. In cases of abductor weakness or trochanteric nonunion, an advancement may be considered. Dennis and Lynch describe a greater trochanter advancement surgery specifically in patients who have postoperative hip weakness and instability [146].

6. Postoperative hip instability

6.1 Hip precautions and does anterior hip need precautions

Hip precautions have often been utilized to help aid in prevention of dislocation in the acute postoperative period. This is often done in patients who undergo a posterior approach where the short external rotators and the posterior capsule is compromised. Many physicians use these precautions. A recent prospective randomized trial from

Journal of Arthroplasty 2022 examined 346 consecutive patients all via posterior approach to the hip with a mean follow up of 2.3 years. This study demonstrated that if intraoperative hip stability was obtained at 90 degrees of flexion 45 degrees internal rotation and 0 degrees of abduction, postoperative hip precautions are no longer necessary. This study, however powerful, excluded patients with previous lumbar fusion, scoliosis or abductor insufficiency [149]. Mounts 2022 study is in accordance with another recently published a systematic review that included 6900 patients. This study demonstrated no statistically significant decrease in dislocations with the use of posterior hip precautions [150].

Since anteriorly based approachs are often regarded as a more stable approach post operatively, surgeons have questioned the need for precautions post operatively. Talbot et al. studied 499 cases of primary total hip arthroplasty done through an anterolateral approach and documented the dislocation rate when restrictions were not imposed. There were 3 early dislocations (within 6 weeks of surgery) all of which were close reduced, and every patient subsequently achieved a stable hip without further intervention [151]. Restrepo et al., also demonstrated a 0.16% dislocation rate which is significantly lower than the 2% overall that was found to occur within the 1st year by Maratt et al. in anterior and posterior approaches [34, 152]. The evidence for hip precautions after an anterior-based hip approach seems to be in favor of not requiring restrictions.

6.2 Recognition of postop instability from infection, poly wear, ALTR

To conclude, the surgeon must correctly identify the etiology of the instability to direct treatment. Early postoperative instability is likely due to component malpositioning or acute infection [116]. In cases of late stage instability the surgeon should consider component subsidence, aseptic loosening, osteolysis, indolent infection or the development of an adverse local tissue reaction (ALTR). Acute infection may be challenging to diagnose if obvious wound complications are not present [153, 154]. Both acute and chronic infection can present with loosening of one or both the acetabular and femoral components which may require staged revision. Another important cause of instability is aseptic loosening from polyethylene debris leading to macrophage induced osteolysis. This can ultimately lead to movement or dislodging of the implants which should be closely evaluated and may require revision surgery. Osteolysis can destroy available bone stock requiring the surgeon to become facile with bone grafting, cages, or even custom triflange implants for the acetabulum [155]. In the case of femoral bone loss there may be a need for diaphyseal engaging implants, bone grafting or even proximal femoral replacement [156]. Another potential cause of instability is the development of an ALTR from metal on metal (MOM) bearing surfaces. Diagnosis of ALTR is made from clinical history, radiography and serum metal ion levels. If surgery is deemed necessary, additional information may be obtained from ultrasound and metal artifact reduction sequence magnetic resonance imaging (MARS-MRI) to evaluate soft tissue destruction and possible need for augments or constraint due to abductor deficiency. Ultimately if serum ion levels continue to rise or patient functionality declines the patient will require revision surgery [157]. Although post-operative hip instability frequently requires revision surgery it is important to identify the root cause. This will allow the surgeon better surgical preparation, more readily available implants and the ability to manage infection with possible staged surgery or prolonged IV antibiotics.

Author details

Kunal Panwar*, Brenden Cutter, Michael Holmboe, Ryan Card, William Pistel and Jesua I. Law
Doctors Medical Center of Modesto, Modesto, CA, USA

*Address all correspondence to: kpanwar123@gmail.com

References

[1] Ferguson RJ, Palmer AJ, Taylor A, Porter ML, Malchau H, Glyn-Jones S. Hip replacement. The Lancet. 2018;**392**:1662-1671. DOI: 10.1016/S0140-6736(18)31777-X

[2] de Martino I, Triantafyllopoulos GK, Sculco PK, Sculco TP. Dual mobility cups in total hip arthroplasty. World Journal of Orthopedics. 2014;**5**:180-187. DOI: 10.5312/wjo.v5.i3.180

[3] Gwam CU, Mistry JB, Mohamed NS, Thomas M, Bigart KC, Mont MA, et al. Current epidemiology of revision total hip arthroplasty in the United States: National inpatient sample 2009 to 2013. The Journal of Arthroplasty. 2017;**32**:2088-2092. DOI: 10.1016/j.arth.2017.02.046

[4] Kelmer G, Stone AH, Turcotte J, King PJ. Reasons for revision: Primary total hip arthroplasty mechanisms of failure. The Journal of the American Academy of Orthopaedic Surgeons. 2021;**29**:78-87. DOI: 10.5435/JAAOS-D-19-00860

[5] Dobzyniak M, Fehring TK, Odum S. Early failure in total hip arthroplasty. Clinical Orthopaedics and Related Research. 2006;**447**:76-78. DOI: 10.1097/01.blo.0000203484.90711.52

[6] Schwartz AM, Farley KX, Guild GN, Bradbury TL. Projections and epidemiology of revision hip and knee arthroplasty in the United States to 2030. The Journal of Arthroplasty. 2020;**35**:S79-S85. DOI: 10.1016/j.arth.2020.02.030

[7] Older J. Charnley low-friction arthroplasty: A worldwide retrospective review at 15 to 20 years. The Journal of Arthroplasty. 2002;**17**:675-680. DOI: 10.1054/arth.2002.31973

[8] Berry DJ, von Knoch M, Schleck CD, Harmsen WS. The cumulative long-term risk of dislocation after primary Charnley total hip arthroplasty. The Journal of Bone and Joint Surgery. American Volume. 2004;**86**:9-14. DOI: 10.2106/00004623-200401000-00003

[9] Goel A, Lau EC, Ong KL, Berry DJ, Malkani AL. Dislocation rates following primary total hip arthroplasty have plateaued in the Medicare population. The Journal of Arthroplasty. 2015;**30**:743-746. DOI: 10.1016/j.arth.2014.11.012

[10] Woo RY, Morrey BF. Dislocations after total hip arthroplasty. The Journal of Bone and Joint Surgery. American Volume. 1982;**64**:1295-1306

[11] Bozic KJ, Kurtz SM, Lau E, Ong K, Vail TP, Berry DJ. The epidemiology of revision total hip arthroplasty in the United States. The Journal of Bone and Joint Surgery. American Volume. 2009;**91**:128-133. DOI: 10.2106/JBJS.H.00155

[12] Dastane M, Dorr LD, Tarwala R, Wan Z. Hip offset in total hip arthroplasty: Quantitative measurement with navigation. Clinical Orthopaedics and Related Research. 2011;**469**:429-436. DOI: 10.1007/s11999-010-1554-7

[13] Han Q, Xu X, Zhang A, Chen B, Qin Y, Wang J. Comparison of femoral offset measurement accuracy between three-dimensional-CT and X-ray in developmental dysplasia of the hip patients and normal. People. 2020. DOI: 10.21203/rs.3.rs-22041/v1

[14] Banerjee S, Pivec R, Issa K, Kapadia BH, Khanuja HS, Mont MA. Large-diameter femoral heads in total hip

arthroplasty: An evidence-based review. American Journal of Orthopedics (Belle Mead, N.J.). 2014;**43**:506-512

[15] Flick TR, Ross BJ, Sherman WF. Instability after total hip arthroplasty and the role of advanced and robotic technology. Orthopedic Clinics of North America. 2021;**52**:191-200. DOI: 10.1016/j.ocl.2021.03.001

[16] Kunutsor SK, Barrett MC, Beswick AD, Judge A, Blom AW, Wylde V, et al. Risk factors for dislocation after primary total hip replacement: A systematic review and meta-analysis of 125 studies involving approximately five million hip replacements. The Lancet Rheumatology. 2019;**1**:e111-e121. DOI: 10.1016/S2665-9913(19)30045-1

[17] Fini M, Giavaresi G, Salamanna F, Veronesi F, Martini L, de Mattei M, et al. Harmful lifestyles on orthopedic implantation surgery: A descriptive review on alcohol and tobacco use. Journal of Bone and Mineral Metabolism. 2011;**29**:633-644. DOI: 10.1007/s00774-011-0309-1

[18] Chen Y, Guo Q, Pan X, Qin L, Zhang P. Smoking and impaired bone healing: Will activation of cholinergic anti-inflammatory pathway be the bridge? International Orthopaedics. 2011;**35**:1267-1270. DOI: 10.1007/s00264-011-1243-5

[19] Akhavan S, Nguyen LC, Chan V, Saleh J, Bozic KJ. Impact of smoking cessation counseling prior to total joint arthroplasty. Orthopedics. 2017;**40**(2):e323-e328. DOI: 10.3928/01477447-20161219-02

[20] Haynes J, Nam D, Barrack RL. Obesity in total hip arthroplasty. The Bone & Joint Journal. 2017;**99-B**:31-36. DOI: 10.1302/0301-620X.99B1.BJJ-2016-0346.R1

[21] Smith KB, Smith MS. Obesity statistics. Primary Care: Clinics in Office Practice. 2016;**43**:121-135. DOI: 10.1016/j.pop.2015.10.001

[22] Mokdad AH, Ford ES, Bowman BA, Dietz WH, Vinicor F, Bales VS, et al. Prevalence of obesity, diabetes, and obesity-related health risk factors, 2001. JAMA. 2003;**289**:76. DOI: 10.1001/jama.289.1.76

[23] Callanan MC, Jarrett B, Bragdon CR, Zurakowski D, Rubash HE, Freiberg AA, et al. The John Charnley award: Risk factors for cup malpositioning: Quality improvement through a joint registry at a tertiary hospital. Clinical Orthopaedics and Related Research. 2011;**469**:319-329. DOI: 10.1007/s11999-010-1487-1

[24] Matziolis G, Brodt S. Total hip arthroplasty in young and obese patients. Zeitschrift für Orthopädie und Unfallchirurgie. 2020;**158**:184-187. DOI: 10.1055/a-0989-2765

[25] Yoshimoto K, Nakashima Y, Aota S, Kaneuji A, Fukui K, Hirakawa K, et al. Re-dislocation after revision total hip arthroplasty for recurrent dislocation: A multicentre study. International Orthopaedics. 2017;**41**:253-258. DOI: 10.1007/s00264-016-3127-1

[26] Jo S, Jimenez Almonte JH, Sierra RJ. The cumulative risk of re-dislocation after revision THA performed for instability increases close to 35% at 15years. The Journal of Arthroplasty. 2015;**30**:1177-1182. DOI: 10.1016/j.arth.2015.02.001

[27] Fessy MH, Putman S, Viste A, Isida R, Ramdane N, Ferreira A, et al. What are the risk factors for dislocation in primary total hip arthroplasty? A multicenter case-control study of 128 unstable and 438 stable hips. Orthopaedics & Traumatology, Surgery

& Research. 2017;**103**:663-668. DOI: 10.1016/j.otsr.2017.05.014

[28] Wetters NG, Murray TG, Moric M, Sporer SM, Paprosky WG, della Valle CJ. Risk factors for dislocation after revision total hip arthroplasty. Clinical Orthopaedics and Related Research. 2013;**471**:410-416. DOI: 10.1007/s11999-012-2561-7

[29] Masonis JL, Bourne RB. Surgical approach, abductor function, and total hip arthroplasty dislocation. Clinical Orthopaedics and Related Research. 2002;**405**:46-53. DOI: 10.1097/00003086-200212000-00006

[30] Angerame MR, Fehring TK, Masonis JL, Mason JB, Odum SM, Springer BD. Early failure of primary total hip arthroplasty: Is surgical approach a risk factor? The Journal of Arthroplasty. 2018;**33**:1780-1785. DOI: 10.1016/j.arth.2018.01.014

[31] Sheth D, Cafri G, Inacio MCS, Paxton EW, Namba RS. Anterior and anterolateral approaches for THA are associated with lower dislocation risk without higher revision risk. Clinical Orthopaedics & Related Research. 2015;**473**:3401-3408. DOI: 10.1007/s11999-015-4230-0

[32] Higgins BT, Barlow DR, Heagerty NE, Lin TJ. Anterior vs. posterior approach for total hip arthroplasty, a systematic review and meta-analysis. The Journal of Arthroplasty. 2015;**30**:419-434. DOI: 10.1016/j.arth.2014.10.020

[33] Huerfano E, Bautista M, Huerfano M, Nossa JM. Use of surgical approach is not associated with instability after primary total hip arthroplasty: A meta-analysis comparing direct anterior and posterolateral approaches. Journal of the American Academy of Orthopaedic Surgeons. 2021;**29**:e1126-e1140. DOI: 10.5435/JAAOS-D-20-00861

[34] Maratt JD, Gagnier JJ, Butler PD, Hallstrom BR, Urquhart AG, Roberts KC. No difference in dislocation seen in anterior vs posterior approach total hip arthroplasty. The Journal of Arthroplasty. 2016;**31**:127-130. DOI: 10.1016/j.arth.2016.02.071

[35] Hoskins W, Bingham R, Lorimer M, Hatton A, de Steiger RN. Early rate of revision of total hip arthroplasty related to surgical approach. Journal of Bone and Joint Surgery. 2020;**102**:1874-1882. DOI: 10.2106/JBJS.19.01289

[36] Zijlstra WP, de Hartog B, van Steenbergen LN, Scheurs BW, Nelissen RGHH. Effect of femoral head size and surgical approach on risk of revision for dislocation after total hip arthroplasty. Acta Orthopaedica. 2017;**88**:395-401. DOI: 10.1080/17453674.2017.1317515

[37] Harmer JR, Wyles CC, Larson DR, Taunton MJ, Pagnano MW, Abdel MP. Changing surgical approach from primary to revision total hip arthroplasty is not associated with increased risk of dislocation or re-revisions. The Journal of Arthroplasty. 2022;**37**(7S):S622-S627. DOI: 10.1016/j.arth.2022.03.007

[38] McLawhorn AS, Potter HG, Cross MB, Boettner F, Lim W, Lee Y, et al. Posterior soft tissue repair after primary THA is durable at mid-term followup: A prospective MRI study. Clinical Orthopaedics and Related Research®. 2015;**473**:3183-3189. DOI: 10.1007/s11999-015-4380-0

[39] Kwon MS, Kuskowski M, Mulhall KJ, Macaulay W, Brown TE, Saleh KJ. Does surgical approach affect total hip arthroplasty dislocation rates? Clinical Orthopaedics & Related Research.

2006;**447**:34-38. DOI: 10.1097/01.blo.0000218746.84494.df

[40] Wagner ER, Kamath AF, Fruth KM, Harmsen WS, Berry DJ. Effect of body mass index on complications and reoperations after total hip arthroplasty. Journal of Bone and Joint Surgery. 2016;**98**:169-179. DOI: 10.2106/JBJS.O.00430

[41] Azodi OS, Adami J, Lindström D, Eriksson KO, Wladis A, Bellocco R. High body mass index is associated with increased risk of implant dislocation following primary total hip replacement: 2,106 patients followed for up to 8 years. Acta Orthopaedica. 2008;**79**:141-147. DOI: 10.1080/17453670710014897

[42] Seward MW, Briggs LG, Bain PA, Chen AF. Preoperative nonsurgical weight loss interventions before total hip and knee arthroplasty: A systematic review. The Journal of Arthroplasty. 2021;**36**:3796-3806.e8. DOI: 10.1016/j.arth.2021.06.021

[43] Lui M, Jones CA, Westby MD. Effect of non-surgical, non-pharmacological weight loss interventions in patients who are obese prior to hip and knee arthroplasty surgery: A rapid review. Systematic Reviews. 2015;**4**:121. DOI: 10.1186/s13643-015-0107-2

[44] Payne ME, Porter Starr KN, Orenduff M, Mulder HS, McDonald SR, Spira AP, et al. Quality of life and mental health in older adults with obesity and frailty: Associations with a weight loss intervention. The Journal of Nutrition, Health & Aging. 2018;**22**:1259-1265. DOI: 10.1007/s12603-018-1127-0

[45] Lewis DP, Wæver D, Thorninger R, Donnelly WJ. Hemiarthroplasty vs total hip arthroplasty for the management of displaced neck of femur fractures: A systematic review and meta-analysis. The Journal of Arthroplasty. 2019;**34**:1837-1843.e2. DOI: 10.1016/j.arth.2019.03.070

[46] Ng DZW, Lee KBL. Unipolar versus bipolar hemiarthroplasty for displaced femoral neck fractures in the elderly: Is there a difference? Annals of the Academy of Medicine, Singapore. 2015;**44**:197-201

[47] Yang B, Lin X, Yin XM, Wen XZ. Bipolar versus unipolar hemiarthroplasty for displaced femoral neck fractures in the elder patient: A systematic review and meta-analysis of randomized trials. European Journal of Orthopaedic Surgery & Traumatology. 2015;**25**:425-433. DOI: 10.1007/s00590-014-1565-2

[48] Health Investigators. Total hip arthroplasty or hemiarthroplasty for hip fracture. New England Journal of Medicine. 2019;**381**:2199-2208. DOI: 10.1056/NEJMoa1906190

[49] Ekhtiari S, Gormley J, Axelrod DE, Devji T, Bhandari M, Guyatt GH. Total hip arthroplasty versus hemiarthroplasty for displaced femoral neck fracture. Journal of Bone and Joint Surgery. 2020;**102**:1638-1645. DOI: 10.2106/JBJS.20.00226

[50] Tanoğlu O. Determination of the gender-related differences on native femoral anatomy using three-dimensional computerized tomography models in Caucasian population. Cureus. 2021;**13**(7):e16235. DOI: 10.7759/cureus.16235 [Published 2021 Jul 7]

[51] Bozkurt M, Gursoy S, Shohat N, Simsek ME, Akkaya M, Parvizi J. Definition of a novel proximal femur classification in the sagittal plane according to the femur morphometric analysis. The Journal of Arthroplasty. 2019;**34**:1502-1508. DOI: 10.1016/j.arth.2019.03.005

[52] Boese CK, Jostmeier J, Oppermann J, Dargel J, Chang D-H, Eysel P, et al. The

neck shaft angle: CT reference values of 800 adult hips. Skeletal Radiology. 2016;**45**:455-463. DOI: 10.1007/s00256-015-2314-2

[53] van Houcke J, Yau WP, Yan CH, Huysse W, Dechamps H, Lau WH, et al. Prevalence of radiographic parameters predisposing to Femoroacetabular impingement in young asymptomatic Chinese and white subjects. The Journal of Bone and Joint Surgery. 2015;**97**:310-317. DOI: 10.2106/JBJS.M.01538

[54] Perry KI, Berry DJ. Femoral considerations for total hip replacement in hip dysplasia. Orthopedic Clinics of North America. 2012;**43**:377-386. DOI: 10.1016/j.ocl.2012.05.010

[55] Daniel M, Iglič A, Kralj-Iglič V. Hip contact stress during Normal and staircase walking: The influence of acetabular anteversion angle and lateral coverage of the acetabulum. Journal of Applied Biomechanics. 2008;**24**:88-93. DOI: 10.1123/jab.24.1.88

[56] Scorcelletti M, Reeves ND, Rittweger J, Ireland A. Femoral anteversion: Significance and measurement. Journal of Anatomy. 2020;**237**:811-826. DOI: 10.1111/joa.13249

[57] Sendtner E, Tibor S, Winkler R, Wörner M, Grifka J, Renkawitz T. Stem torsion in total hip replacement. Acta Orthopaedica. 2010;**81**:579-582. DOI: 10.3109/17453674.2010.524596

[58] Lee YK, Kim TY, Ha YC, Kang BJ, Koo KH. Radiological measurement of femoral stem version using a modified Budin method. The Bone & Joint Journal. 2013;**95-B**:877-880. DOI: 10.1302/0301-620X.95B7.31195

[59] Woerner ML, Weber M, Craiovan BS, Springorum HR, Grifka J, Renkawitz TF. Radiographic assessment of femoral stem torsion in total hip arthroplasty-a comparison of a caput-Collum-Diaphyseal angle-based technique with the Budin view. The Journal of Arthroplasty. 2016;**31**:1117-1122. DOI: 10.1016/j.arth.2015.11.013

[60] Blumenfeld TJ. Pearls: Clinical application of Ranawat's sign. Clinical Orthopaedics & Related Research. 2017;**475**:1789-1790. DOI: 10.1007/s11999-017-5376-8

[61] Dorr LD, Malik A, Dastane M, Wan Z. Combined anteversion technique for total hip arthroplasty. Clinical Orthopaedics & Related Research. 2009;**467**:119-127. DOI: 10.1007/s11999-008-0598-4

[62] Konyves A, Bannister GC. The importance of leg length discrepancy after total hip arthroplasty. The Journal of Bone and Joint Surgery British. 2005;**87-B**:155-157. DOI: 10.1302/0301-620X.87B2.14878

[63] Renkawitz T, Weber T, Dullien S, Woerner M, Dendorfer S, Grifka J, et al. Leg length and offset differences above 5 mm after total hip arthroplasty are associated with altered gait kinematics. Gait & Posture. 2016;**49**:196-201. DOI: 10.1016/j.gaitpost.2016.07.011

[64] Röder C, Vogel R, Burri L, Dietrich D, Staub LP. Total hip arthroplasty: Leg length inequality impairs functional outcomes and patient satisfaction. BMC Musculoskeletal Disorders. 2012;**13**:95. DOI: 10.1186/1471-2474-13-95

[65] Bjørdal F, Bjørgul K. The role of femoral offset and abductor lever arm in total hip arthroplasty. Journal of Orthopaedics and Traumatology. 2015;**16**:325-330. DOI: 10.1007/s10195-015-0358-7

[66] Blackley HR, Howell GE, Rorabeck CH. Planning and management of the difficult primary hip replacement: preoperative planning and technical considerations. Instructional Course Lectures. 2000;**49**:3-11

[67] O'Connor DO, Davey JR, Zalenski E, Burke DW, Harris WH. Femoral component offset: Its effect on micromotion in stance and stair climbing loading. Transactions 35th annual meeting of the Orthopaedic research. Society. 1989;**409**

[68] Davey JR, O'Connor DO, Burke DW, Harris WH. Femoral component offset. Its effect on strain in bone-cement. The Journal of Arthroplasty. 1993;**8**:23-26

[69] Charles MN, Bourne RB, Davey JR, Greenwald AS, Morrey BF, Rorabeck CH. Soft-tissue balancing of the hip: The role of femoral offset restoration. Instructional Course Lectures. 2005;**54**:131-141

[70] Yamaguchi M, Akisue T, Bauer TW, Hashimoto Y. The spatial location of impingement in total hip arthroplasty. The Journal of Arthroplasty. 2000;**15**:305-313. DOI: 10.1016/S0883-5403(00)90601-6

[71] Tsikandylakis G, Mohaddes M, Cnudde P, Eskelinen A, Kärrholm J, Rolfson O. Head size in primary total hip arthroplasty. EFORT Open Reviews. 2018;**3**:225-231. DOI: 10.1302/2058-5241.3.170061

[72] Jameson SS, Lees D, James P, Serrano-Pedraza I, Partington PF, Muller SD, et al. Lower rates of dislocation with increased femoral head size after primary total hip replacement. The Journal of Bone and Joint Surgery British. 2011;**93-B**:876-880. DOI: 10.1302/0301-620X.93B7.26657

[73] Heckmann N, Ihn H, Stefl M, Etkin CD, Springer BD, Berry DJ, et al. Early results from the American joint replacement registry: A comparison with other National Registries. The Journal of Arthroplasty. 2019;**34**:S125-S134.e1. DOI: 10.1016/j.arth.2018.12.027

[74] Sariali E, Lazennec JY, Khiami F, Catonné Y. Mathematical evaluation of jumping distance in total hip arthroplasty. Acta Orthopaedica. 2009;**80**:277-282. DOI: 10.3109/17453670902988378

[75] Blakeney WG, Epinette J-A, Vendittoli P-A. Reproducing the proximal femoral anatomy: Large-diameter head THA. In: Personalized Hip and Knee Joint Replacement. Cham: Springer International Publishing; 2020. pp. 65-73. DOI: 10.1007/978-3-030-24243-5_7

[76] Howie DW, Holubowycz OT, Middleton R. Large femoral heads decrease the incidence of dislocation after total hip arthroplasty. Journal of Bone and Joint Surgery. 2012;**94**:1095-1102. DOI: 10.2106/JBJS.K.00570

[77] Hermansen LL, Viberg B, Hansen L, Overgaard S. "True" cumulative incidence of and risk factors for hip dislocation within 2 years after primary total hip arthroplasty due to osteoarthritis. Journal of Bone and Joint Surgery. 2021;**103**:295-302. DOI: 10.2106/JBJS.19.01352

[78] Cooper HJ, della Valle CJ. Large diameter femoral heads. The Bone & Joint Journal. 2014;**96-B**:23-26. DOI: 10.1302/0301-620X.96B11.34342

[79] Shah SM, Walter WL, Tai SM, Lorimer MF, de Steiger RN. Late dislocations after total hip arthroplasty: Is the bearing a factor? The Journal of Arthroplasty. 2017;**32**:2852-2856. DOI: 10.1016/j.arth.2017.04.037

[80] Meneghini RM, Lovro LR, Wallace JM, Ziemba-Davis M. Large

metal heads and vitamin E polyethylene increase frictional torque in total hip arthroplasty. The Journal of Arthroplasty. 2016;**31**:710-714. DOI: 10.1016/j.arth.2015.09.020

[81] Lachiewicz PF, Soileau ES, Martell JM. Wear and osteolysis of highly crosslinked polyethylene at 10 to 14 years: The effect of femoral head size. Clinical Orthopaedics & Related Research. 2016;**474**:365-371. DOI: 10.1007/s11999-015-4319-5

[82] Beverland DE, O'Neill CKJ, Rutherford M, Molloy D, Hill JC. Placement of the acetabular component. The Bone & Joint Journal. 2016;**98-B**:37-43. DOI: 10.1302/0301-620X.98B1.36343

[83] Odri GA, Padiolleau GB, Gouin FT. Oversized cups as a Major risk factor of postoperative pain after total hip arthroplasty. The Journal of Arthroplasty. 2014;**29**:753-756. DOI: 10.1016/j.arth.2013.07.001

[84] Hagman DS, Smith AF, Presley TL, et al. Primary THA using thin polyethylene liners and large femoral heads: A minimum 5-year follow-up. The Journal of Arthroplasty. 2022;**37**(7S):S588-S591. DOI: 10.1016/j.arth.2022.02.117

[85] Semaan DJ, Rutledge-Jukes H, Berend KR, Lombardi AV Jr, Adams JB, Crawford DA. Survivorship of a metal-on-metal total hip implant with modular titanium adapter. The Journal of Arthroplasty. 2022;**37**(7S):S560-S565. DOI: 10.1016/j.arth.2022.01.053

[86] Palazzuolo M, Antoniadis A, Delaune L, Tornare I, Wegrzyn J. Comparison of the long-term cause of failure and survivorship of four hundred and twenty seven metal-on-metal hip arthroplasties: Resurfacing versus large head total hip arthroplasty. International Orthopaedics. 2021;**45**:3075-3081. DOI: 10.1007/s00264-021-05044-y

[87] Sanchez-Sotelo J, Berry DJ. Instability Amer Major Joint Replacement Epidemiology of Instability Af'ter Total Hip Replacement. n.d

[88] Khan RJK, Fick D, Alakeson R, Haebich S, de Cruz M, Nivbrant B, et al. A constrained acetabular component for recurrent dislocation. The Journal of Bone and Joint Surgery British. 2006;**88-B**:870-876. DOI: 10.1302/0301-620X.88B7.17644

[89] Abdel MP, von Roth P, Jennings MT, Hanssen AD, Pagnano MW. What safe zone? The vast majority of dislocated THAs are within the Lewinnek safe zone for acetabular component position. Clinical Orthopaedics & Related Research. 2016;**474**:386-391. DOI: 10.1007/s11999-015-4432-5

[90] Zhu J, Wan Z, Dorr LD. Quantification of pelvic tilt in total hip arthroplasty. Clinical Orthopaedics and Related Research. 2010;**468**:571-575. DOI: 10.1007/s11999-009-1064-7

[91] Bruce-Brand R, Magill P, O'Neill C, Karayiannis P, Hill J, Beverland D. Mechanical and anatomical alignment guide techniques are superior to freehand in achieving target orientation of an acetabular component. Arthroplasty Today. 2021;**11**:222-228. DOI: 10.1016/j.artd.2021.08.016

[92] Archbold HAP, Mockford B, Molloy D, Mcconway J, Ogonda L, Beverland D. The transverse acetabular ligament: An aid to orientation of the acetabular component during primary total hip replacement. In: A Preliminary Study of 1000 Cases Investigating Post-Operative Stability. 2006. p. 88. DOI: 10.1302/0301-620X.88B7

[93] Beverland DE, O'neill CKJ, Rutherford M, Molloy D, Hill JC, O'neill CKJ, et al. HIP arthroplasty: Avoiding

and managing problems. In: Placement of the acetabular component. 2016. p. 98. DOI: 10.1302/0301-620X.98B1

[94] Sotereanos NG, Miller MC, Smith B, Hube R, Sewecke JJ, Wohlrab D. Using intraoperative pelvic landmarks for acetabular component placement in total hip arthroplasty. Journal of Arthroplasty. 2006;**21**:832-840. DOI: 10.1016/j.arth.2005.12.001

[95] Charnley J. Low Friction Arthroplasty of the Hip. Berlin, Heidelberg: Springer Berlin Heidelberg; 1979. DOI: 10.1007/978-3-642-67013-8

[96] Brown TD, Callaghan JJ. (ii) impingement in total hip replacement: Mechanisms and consequences. Current Orthopaedics. 2008;**22**:376-391. DOI: 10.1016/j.cuor.2008.10.009

[97] Bonnin MP, Archbold PHA, Basiglini L, Fessy MH, Beverland DE. Do we medialise the hip Centre of Rotation in total hip arthroplasty? Influence of acetabular offset and surgical technique. Hip International. 2012;**22**:371-378. DOI: 10.5301/HIP.2012.9350

[98] Malik A, Maheshwari A, Dorr LD. Impingement with total hip replacement. The Journal of Bone & Joint Surgery. 2007;**89**:1832-1842. DOI: 10.2106/JBJS.F.01313

[99] Bhaskar D, Rajpura A, Board T. Current concepts in acetabular positioning in total hip arthroplasty. Indian Journal of Orthopaedics. 2017;**51**:386-396. DOI: 10.4103/ortho.IJOrtho_144_17

[100] Mahmood SS, Mukka SS, Crnalic S, Wretenberg P, Sayed-Noor AS. Association between changes in global femoral offset after total hip arthroplasty and function, quality of life, and abductor muscle strength. Acta Orthopaedica. 2016;**87**:36-41. DOI: 10.3109/17453674.2015.1091955

[101] Kurtz WB, Ecker TM, Reichmann WM, Murphy SB. Factors affecting bony impingement in hip arthroplasty. The Journal of Arthroplasty. 2010;**25**:624-634.e2. DOI: 10.1016/j.arth.2009.03.024

[102] Rathod PA, Bhalla S, Deshmukh AJ, Rodriguez JA. Does fluoroscopy with anterior hip Arthoplasty decrease acetabular cup variability compared with a nonguided posterior approach? Clinical Orthopaedics & Related Research. 2014;**472**:1877-1885. DOI: 10.1007/s11999-014-3512-2

[103] Ji W, Stewart N. Fluoroscopy assessment during anterior minimally invasive hip replacement is more accurate than with the posterior approach. International Orthopaedics. 2016;**40**:21-27. DOI: 10.1007/s00264-015-2803-x

[104] Stewart NJ, Stewart JL, Brisbin A. A comparison of component positioning between fluoroscopy-assisted and robotic-assisted total hip arthroplasty. The Journal of Arthroplasty. 2022. DOI: 10.1016/j.arth.2022.03.056

[105] Parratte S, Argenson J-NA. Validation and usefulness of a computer-assisted cup-positioning system in total hip arthroplasty. The Journal of Bone & Joint Surgery. 2007;**89**:494-499. DOI: 10.2106/JBJS.F.00529

[106] Kalteis T, Handel M, Bäthis H, Perlick L, Tingart M, Grifka J. Imageless navigation for insertion of the acetabular component in total hip arthroplasty. The Journal of Bone and Joint Surgery British. 2006;**88-B**:163-167. DOI: 10.1302/0301-620X.88B2.17163

[107] Ng N, Gaston P, Simpson PM, Macpherson GJ, Patton JT, Clement ND.

Robotic arm-assisted versus manual total hip arthroplasty. The Bone & Joint Journal. 2021;**103-B**:1009-1020. DOI: 10.1302/0301-620X.103B6.BJJ-2020-1856.R1

[108] Domb BG, Redmond JM, Louis SS, Alden KJ, Daley RJ, LaReau JM, et al. Accuracy of component positioning in 1980 total hip arthroplasties: A comparative analysis by surgical technique and mode of guidance. The Journal of Arthroplasty. 2015;**30**:2208-2218. DOI: 10.1016/j.arth.2015.06.059

[109] Chen X, Xiong J, Wang P, Zhu S, Qi W, Peng H, et al. Robotic-assisted compared with conventional total hip arthroplasty: Systematic review and meta-analysis. Postgraduate Medical Journal. 2018;**94**:335.1-335.33341. DOI: 10.1136/postgradmedj-2017-135352

[110] Lass R, Olischar B, Kubista B, Waldhoer T, Giurea A, Windhager R. Total hip arthroplasty using imageless computer-assisted navigation—2-year follow-up of a prospective randomized study. Journal of Clinical Medicine. 2020;**9**:1620. DOI: 10.3390/jcm9061620

[111] Shaw JH, Rahman TM, Wesemann LD, Z Jiang C, G Lindsay-Rivera K, Davis JJ. Comparison of postoperative instability and acetabular cup positioning in robotic-assisted versus traditional total hip arthroplasty. The Journal of Arthroplasty. 2022;S0883-5403(22)00113-9. DOI: 10.1016/j.arth.2022.02.002 [published online ahead of print, 2022 Feb 8]

[112] Bendich I, Vigdorchik JM, Sharma AK, Mayman DJ, Sculco PK, Anderson C, et al. Robotic assistance for posterior approach total hip arthroplasty is associated with lower risk of revision for dislocation when compared to manual techniques. The Journal of Arthroplasty. 2022;**37**:1124-1129. DOI: 10.1016/j.arth.2022.01.085

[113] Kunze KN, Premkumar A, Bovonratwet P, Sculco PK. Acetabular component and liner selection for the prevention of dislocation after primary total hip arthroplasty. JBJS Reviews. 2021;**9**(12):10. Published 2021 Dec 15. DOI: 10.2106/JBJS.RVW.21.00148

[114] Sultan PG, Tan V, Lai M, Garino JP. Independent contribution of elevated-rim acetabular liner and femoral head size to the stability of total hip implants. The Journal of Arthroplasty. 2002;**17**:289-292. DOI: 10.1054/arth.2002.30415

[115] Barrack RL. Dislocation after total hip arthroplasty: Implant design and orientation. Journal of the American Academy of Orthopaedic Surgeons. 2003;**11**:89-99. DOI: 10.5435/00124635-200303000-00003

[116] Werner BC. Instability after total hip arthroplasty. World Journal of Orthopedics. 2012;**3**:122. DOI: 10.5312/wjo.v3.i8.122

[117] Burke WV, Orishimo KF, McAuley JP, Engh CA. Midterm radiographic comparison of Cementless acetabular shells containing lateralized and nonlateralized liners. The Journal of Arthroplasty. 2006;**21**:1099-1104. DOI: 10.1016/j.arth.2006.01.029

[118] Zahos K, Mehendale S, Ward AJ, Smith EJ, Nichols M. The 15° face-changing acetabular component for treatment of osteoarthritis secondary to developmental dysplasia of the hip. The Journal of Bone and Joint Surgery British. 2012;**94-B**:163-166. DOI: 10.1302/0301-620X.94B2.27348

[119] van der Merwe JM. Comprehensive review of current constraining devices

in total hip arthroplasty. Journal of the American Academy of Orthopaedic Surgeons. 2018;**26**:479-488. DOI: 10.5435/JAAOS-D-16-00488

[120] Lewis PL, Graves SE, de Steiger RN, Cuthbert AR. Constrained acetabular components used in revision total hip arthroplasty: A registry analysis. The Journal of Arthroplasty. 2017;**32**:3102-3107. DOI: 10.1016/j.arth.2017.04.043

[121] Shah SN, Kaye RJ, Kelly NH, Su EP, Padgett DE, Wright TM. Retrieval analysis of failed constrained acetabular liners. The Journal of Arthroplasty. 2009;**24**:54-57. DOI: 10.1016/j.arth.2009.05.002

[122] Sathappan SS, Ginat D, Teicher M, Di Cesare PE. Failure of constrained acetabular liner without metal ring disruption. Orthopedics. 2008;**31**:275. DOI: 10.3928/01477447-20080301-34

[123] Farizon F, de Lavison R, Azoulai JJ, Bousquet G. Results with a cementless alumina-coated cup with dual mobility. A twelve-year follow-up study. International Orthopaedics. 1998;**22**:219-224. DOI: 10.1007/s002640050246

[124] Darrith B, Courtney PM, della Valle CJ. Outcomes of dual mobility components in total hip arthroplasty. The Bone & Joint Journal. 2018;**100-B**:11-19. DOI: 10.1302/0301-620X.100B1.BJJ-2017-0462.R1

[125] Sculco PK, Nocon AA, Selemon NA, Diane A, Demartino AM, Mayman DJ, et al. Dual mobility ADM versus MDM: Do differences in metal ions exist? Orthopaedic Proceedings. 2019;**101-B**:5. DOI: 10.1302/1358-992X.2019.12.005

[126] Greenberg A, Nocon A, de Martino I, Mayman DJ, Sculco TP, Sculco PK. Serum metal ions in contemporary Monoblock and modular dual mobility articulations. Arthroplasty Today. 2021;**12**:51-56. DOI: 10.1016/j.artd.2021.08.021

[127] Chalmers BP, Mangold DG, Hanssen AD, Pagnano MW, Trousdale RT, Abdel MP. Uniformly low serum cobalt levels after modular dual-mobility total hip arthroplasties with ceramic heads. The Bone & Joint Journal. 2019;**101-B**:57-61. DOI: 10.1302/0301-620X.101B6.BJJ-2018-1403.R1

[128] Cha Y-H, Yoo J-I, Kim J-T, Park C-H, Ahn Y-S, Choy W-S, et al. Dual mobility total hip arthroplasty in the treatment of femoral neck fractures. The Bone & Joint Journal. 2020;**102-B**:1457-1466. DOI: 10.1302/0301-620X.102B11.BJJ-2020-0610.R2

[129] Albanese KM, Deshmane P, Patil N, Larsen DA, Ordway NR. Dual-mobility articulations in femoral neck fractures: A systematic review of the literature and meta-analysis of the outcomes. Journal of the American Academy of Orthopaedic Surgeons. 2021;**29**:e618-e627. DOI: 10.5435/JAAOS-D-20-00407

[130] Burgers PTPW, van Geene AR, van den Bekerom MPJ, van Lieshout EMM, Blom B, Aleem IS, et al. total hip arthroplasty versus hemiarthroplasty for displaced femoral neck fractures in the healthy elderly: A meta-analysis and systematic review of randomized trials. International Orthopaedics. 2012;**36**:1549-1560. DOI: 10.1007/s00264-012-1569-7

[131] Cnudde PHJ, Nåtman J, Hailer NP, Rogmark C. Total, hemi, or dual-mobility arthroplasty for the treatment of femoral neck fractures in patients with neurological disease. The Bone & Joint Journal. 2022;**104-B**:134-141. DOI: 10.1302/0301-620X.104B1.BJJ-2021-0855.R1

[132] You D, Sepehri A, Kooner S, Krzyzaniak H, Johal H, Duffy P, et al.

Outcomes of total hip arthroplasty using dual mobility components in patients with a femoral neck fracture. The Bone & Joint Journal. 2020;**102-B**:811-821. DOI: 10.1302/0301-620X.102B7.BJJ-2019-1486.R1

[133] Ryu H-G, Roh YJ, Oh K-J, Hwang J-H, Kim Y, Cho H-W, et al. Dual mobility articulation total hip arthroplasty for displaced neck fracture in elderly with neuromuscular disorder. Injury. 2021;**52**:1480-1486. DOI: 10.1016/j.injury.2021.01.005

[134] Gorin M, Roger B, Lazennec J-Y, Charlot N, Arafati N, Bissery A, et al. Hip-spine relationship: A radio-anatomical study for optimization in acetabular cup positioning. Surgical and Radiologic Anatomy. 2004;**26**:136-144. DOI: 10.1007/s00276-003-0195-x

[135] Stefl M, Lundergan W, Heckmann N, McKnight B, Ike H, Murgai R, et al. Spinopelvic mobility and acetabular component position for total hip arthroplasty. The Bone & Joint Journal. 2017;**99-B**:37-45. DOI: 10.1302/0301-620X.99B1.BJJ-2016-0415.R1

[136] Heckmann N, McKnight B, Stefl M, Trasolini NA, Ike H, Dorr LD. Late dislocation following total hip arthroplasty. Journal of Bone and Joint Surgery. 2018;**100**:1845-1853. DOI: 10.2106/JBJS.18.00078

[137] Dagneaux L, Marouby S, Maillot C, Canovas F, Rivière C. Dual mobility device reduces the risk of prosthetic hip instability for patients with degenerated spine: A case-control study. Orthopaedics & Traumatology: Surgery & Research. 2019;**105**:461-466. DOI: 10.1016/j.otsr.2018.12.003

[138] Wegrzyn J, Antoniadis A, Sarshari E, Boubat M, Terrier A. Polyethylene wear of dual mobility cups: A comparative analysis based on patient-specific finite element modeling. International Orthopaedics. 2022;**46**:779-787. DOI: 10.1007/s00264-022-05305-4

[139] Boyer B, Neri T, Geringer J, di Iorio A, Philippot R, Farizon F. Long-term wear of dual mobility total hip replacement cups: Explant study. International Orthopaedics. 2018;**42**:41-47. DOI: 10.1007/s00264-017-3525-z

[140] Sun X, Zhu X, Zeng Y, et al. The effect of posterior capsule repair in total hip arthroplasty: a systematic review and meta-analysis. BMC Musculoskelet Disord. 2020;**21**(1):263. DOI: 10.1186/s12891-020-03244-y [Published 2020 Apr 21]

[141] Stähelin T, Drittenbass L, Hersche O, Miehlke W, Munzinger U. Failure of capsular enhanced short external rotator repair after total hip replacement. Clinical Orthopaedics. 2004;**420**:199-204. DOI: 10.1097/01.blo.0000119246.66584.4d

[142] Berry DJ, Bozic KJ. Current practice patterns in primary hip and knee arthroplasty among members of the american association of hip and knee surgeons. Journal of Arthroplasty. 2010;**25**:2-4. DOI: 10.1016/j.arth.2010.04.033

[143] Schwartz AM, Goel RK, Sweeney AP, Bradbury TL. Capsular management in direct anterior total hip arthroplasty: A randomized, single-blind, controlled trial. Journal of Arthroplasty. 2021;**36**:2836-2842. DOI: 10.1016/j.arth.2021.03.048

[144] Lim LA, Carmichael SW, Cabanela ME. Biomechanics of total hip arthroplasty. The Anatomical Record. 1999;**257**:110-116. DOI: 10.1002/(SICI)1097-0185(19990615)257:3<110::AID-AR8>3.0.CO;2-2

[145] Gomez PF, Morcuende JA. A historical and economic perspective on Sir John Charnley, Chas F. Thackray Limited, and the early arthoplasty industry. Iowa Orthopedic Journal. 2005;**25**:30-37

[146] Trochanteric Osteotomy and Advancement—A Technique for Abductor Related Hip Instability. n.d

[147] Whiteside LA. Surgical technique: Transfer of the anterior portion of the gluteus maximus muscle for abductor deficiency of the hip. Clinical Orthopaedics and Related Research, Vol. 470, Springer New York; 2012. p. 503-510. DOI: 10.1007/s11999-011-1975-y

[148] Hamad K, Konan S. Extended trochanteric osteotomy in revision hip arthroplasty: A case series study and systematic literature review. Arthroplasty (London, England). 2022;**4**:14. DOI: 10.1186/s42836-022-00115-w

[149] Mounts MR, Turner RA, Patel NB, et al. Patients achieving 90°/45°/0° intraoperative stability do not require hip precautions following posterior approach total hip arthroplasty: A prospective randomized study [published online ahead of print, 2022 Jan 31]. The Journal of Arthroplasty. 2022;S0883-5403(22)00045-6. DOI: 10.1016/j.arth.2022.01.028

[150] Crompton J, Osagie-Clouard L, Patel A. Do hip precautions after posterior-approach total hip arthroplasty affect dislocation rates? A systematic review of 7 studies with 6,900 patients. Acta Orthopaedica. 2020;**91**:687-692. DOI: 10.1080/17453674.2020.1795598

[151] Talbot NJ, Brown JHM, Treble NJ. Early dislocation after total hip arthroplasty. The Journal of Arthroplasty. 2002;**17**:1006-1008. DOI: 10.1054/arth.2002.34534

[152] Restrepo C, Javad Mortazavi SM, Brothers J, Parvizi J, Rothman RH. Hip dislocation: Are hip precautions necessary in anterior approaches? Clinical Orthopaedics & Related Research. 2011;**469**:417-422. DOI: 10.1007/s11999-010-1668-y

[153] Schmalzried TP. The infected hip: Telltale signs and treatment options. Journal of Arthroplasty. 2006;**21**:97-100. DOI: 10.1016/j.arth.2006.02.090

[154] Lee HD, Prashant K, Shon WY. Management of periprosthetic hip joint infection. Hip & Pelvis. 2015;**27**:63. DOI: 10.5371/hp.2015.27.2.63

[155] Siegel MA, Patetta MJ, Chen JY, Barragan Echenique DM, Gonzalez MH. The use of a triflange salvage system for catastrophic pelvic osteolysis after failed total hip arthroplasty. Journal of Orthopaedics. 2021;**25**:16-22. DOI: 10.1016/j.jor.2021.03.018

[156] Parvizi J, Sim FH. Proximal femoral replacements with megaprostheses. Clinical Orthopaedics and Related Research. 2004;**420**:169-175. DOI: 10.1097/00003086-200403000-00023

[157] Chalmers BP, Perry KI, Taunton MJ, Mabry TM, Abdel MP. Diagnosis of adverse local tissue reactions following metal-on-metal hip arthroplasty. Current Reviews in Musculoskeletal Medicine. 2016;**9**:67-74. DOI: 10.1007/s12178-016-9321-3

Chapter 5

Advanced, Imageless Navigation in Contemporary THA: Optimising Acetabular Component Placement

Andrew P. Kurmis

Abstract

Total hip arthroplasty (THA) stands as a reliable and effective way to manage end-stage hip disease secondary to a number of aetiologic conditions. While target 'safe zones' are widely quoted and endorsed, an increasingly robust body of evidence suggests that such idealised implantation goals have limited utility in patient-to-patient considerations and that even with a precise goal in mind, surgeons perform inconsistently in achieving these targets intra-operatively. Inter-patient variability, the concept of 'functional' safe zones and the largely under-appreciated impact of poor patient positioning (and progressive loss of position during the case) are all recognised and evidence-supported opponents of conventional '40/15' approaches. In an environment whereby accountable cost utility, maximised surgical consistency (i.e., outlier minimisation), improved attainment of target position, and awareness of the radiation exposure burden of many pre-operative templating regimes are all paramount, there appears to be an increasing role for the application of imageless 'mini' intra-operative navigation systems for primary (and revision) THA procedures. This chapter reviews the evolution of THA navigation and discusses contemporary applications, defines the challenges associated with unanticipated pelvic movement, and explores potential future directions in the use of this exciting technology.

Keywords: technology-assisted surgery, hip navigation, computer navigation, THA, total hip replacement

1. Introduction

Total hip replacement remains a tried-and-true method for managing hip pain and dysfunction resultant from end-stage degenerative disease and a number of other medical conditions [1–3]. It has a long-standing proven clinical track record with strong evidence to support consistent improvements in patient function and satisfaction—indeed primary total hip arthroplasty (THA) has been claimed as one of the most significant surgical advances of the 20th century [4].

In the late 1970s, Lewinnek and colleagues generated the landmark paper proposing the acetabular 'safe zone'—an idealised target orientation for component placement—suggested to be associated with decreased risk of prosthetic dislocation [5]. Nearly 45 years later, the paper stands as one of the most cited in the orthopaedic literature [6]. The '40/15 safe zone' of Lewinnek (inferring a target acetabular component insertion position of 40° of abduction and 15° of anteversion, each +/− 10°) (**Figure 1**) has largely become the 'ideal' cup orientation for hip replacement surgeons and forms the basis of most conventional implantation tools/aids. This fundamental premise of THA surgery has however been challenged extensively in the contemporary literature with many authors suggesting limited value for these targets on a patient-by-patient level—several larger, reputable, papers have shown large proportions of post-operative dislocations occurring well within the defined 'safe zone' [7, 8]. The suggestion that 'one size does *not* fit all' is gaining wider acceptance and a move towards 'functional' safe zones and/or 'patient-specific' acetabular component orientation is gaining momentum [9–12].

Acetabular prosthesis implantation angles have been shown to affect peri-articular muscle mechanical advantage, rates of dislocation, gait and gait efficiency, limb lengths, impingement, noise generation, loosening, postoperative range-of-movement, liner wear and overall revision rates [13–23]. Balanced biomechanical and anatomical reconstruction of the joint is therefore critical to achieve function, enduring longevity and prevention of avoidable complications following surgery [15, 16, 20]. Dislocation rates following primary THA are acknowledged to occur in 1–4% of cases, with 'instability' accounting for approximately 23% of all revisions and remains the most common reason for such surgery in the United States [24, 25]. Preoperative templating from a plain anterior-posterior radiograph is the primary method for initial evaluation and forms the cornerstone of pre-operative prosthesis position planning, however the value of such images are subject to degradation due to uncompensated patient pelvic malposition. Suboptimal acetabular component position can significantly negatively impact the results of a hip arthroplasty, including increased risk of instability, impingement, dislocation and cup failure [12, 14, 16, 19, 26–30]. Correct template positioning influences the accuracy of acetabular cup placement planning and hence the long-term success of the THA.

Traditional freehand THA techniques rely heavily upon surgeon judgement to manually place acetabular components accurately. Computer navigation to reduce acetabular malpositioning has been used for more than 20 years, demonstrating improved attainment of target cup placement and variable reports of improvement in clinical outcomes, including reducing rates of revision [31–33]. By comparison, the prestigious Australian Orthopaedic Association National Joint Replacement

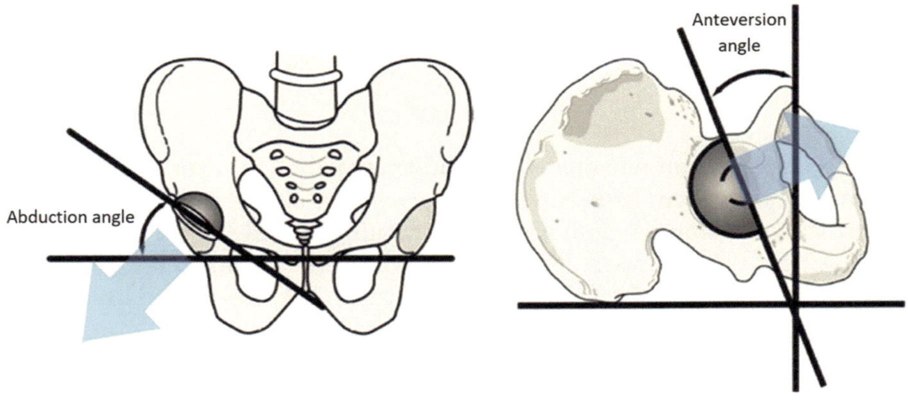

Figure 1.
Pelvic abduction angle (also known as 'inclination' or 'opening' angle) and anteversion angle determination.

Registry (AOANJRR) began collecting data on the use of computer-navigated total *knee* arthroplasty (TKA) in 2003 and has previously reported on the outcomes [31] which show clear outcome benefit in several patient demographics [34, 35]. The use of computer navigation has steadily increased in that setting for TKA, from 2.4% in 2003 to 33.2% in 2018. However, by comparison the AOANJRR shows that <2% of THAs recorded to date have utilised navigation-assistance [31, 36].

Historically two separate means of informing computer-assisted navigation systems have existed—those reliant upon pre-operative imaging and 'imageless' systems. Although plain X-ray-based renditions do exist [37], most 'image driven' systems rely on images generated from pre-operatively obtained computer tomography (CT) scans using proprietary image reconstruction and feature recognition. Common to 'imageless' systems is some method of anatomic feature recognition determined during the surgery itself which informs the surgical navigation plan. The use of CT-based navigation has been shown to be highly accurate, however it is burdened by the associated cost, the need for dedicated pre-operative imaging, and incumbent radiation exposure risk—all of which have been linked to low levels of clinical utilisation [38–41].

Imageless intra-operative navigation systems allow real-time, surgeon-controlled, determination of leg length and offset changes, and three-dimensional (3D) cup position [42]. The key features of these commercially-available systems are intended to overcome some of the recognised barriers to uptake associated with 'imaging-based' navigation, and are already in widespread use [3]. This chapter aims to review the rationale for, evolution of, and current evidence base supporting the use of such 'imageless' navigation tools and also provide understanding as to why pelvic positional variability makes such systems of high value, as well as exploring some of the exciting cutting-edge extensions of such technology into the foreseeable future.

2. Recognising the importance of optimised acetabular component orientation

Optimal insertional orientation of the acetabular component during THA is a critical determinant of many tangible outcomes, including construct stability [43]. At its extreme, malpositioning may lead to prosthetic dislocation. With the majority of THAs currently still being performed in a lateral decubitus patient position [43, 44], factors which introduce inconsistency or error in achieving the desired final cup position have been extensively explored. Sound previous research has confirmed the following: 1. there is great inconsistency and often poor reproducibility in the accuracy with which a true decubitus position is achieved during the 'set up' phase of a THA operation; 2. conventional positioning devices perform poorly in maintaining the initial set up position during the performance of a THA; 3. there is considerable patient loss-of-position during the operation itself (i.e. the position of the pelvis changes during surgery); 4. an erroneous pelvic position (from the start of the operation) and/or a loss of position during the procedure introduces a substantial potential for error in the ultimate insertional orientation of the cup; 5. suboptimal cup position has been strongly associated with a number of poor outcome measures, including wear, increased revision rate and dislocation.

A number of previous investigations have attempted to quantify the 'average' amount of unintended pelvic movement which occurs during the performance of a routine primary THA. These results are discussed in more detail later herein.

Interpretation of such information has however—in many instances—been clouded by inconsistent data collection methods or by unreliable measurement approaches.

3. Understanding the relationship between pelvic movement and resultant acetabular component position

While most surgeons agree that accurate implantation of the acetabular component of a THA is important for patient outcomes, the 'ideal' position is far from universally agreed upon [44, 45]. While the historic reference of Lewinnek's safe zone has formed the basis of most 'target' cup positions [46, 47], many contemporary authors suggest that there may be merit in a 'patient-specific' orientation goal and that 'one size' does not fit all [10, 11]. Indeed, many proponents advocate for individualised patient assessment—often in the form of pre-operative functional imaging [48–50]—to inform intra-operative decision making. Deviation from an 'anatomically neutral' starting position can have considerable negative impact on resultant cup insertion decision making. One key determinant 'pelvic tilt' (or 'roll') reflects the divergent angle between the anterior pelvic plane (APP) and a vertical line in the anatomical (standing) position [51] (**Figure 2**). The large recent study of 1517 THAs by Pierrepont and colleagues suggested that in nearly 20% of patients the extent of functional sagittal pelvic rotation (reflecting pelvic tilt) identified could potentially lead to construct instability using historical 'safe zone' targets [50]. This is a staggeringly high proportion.

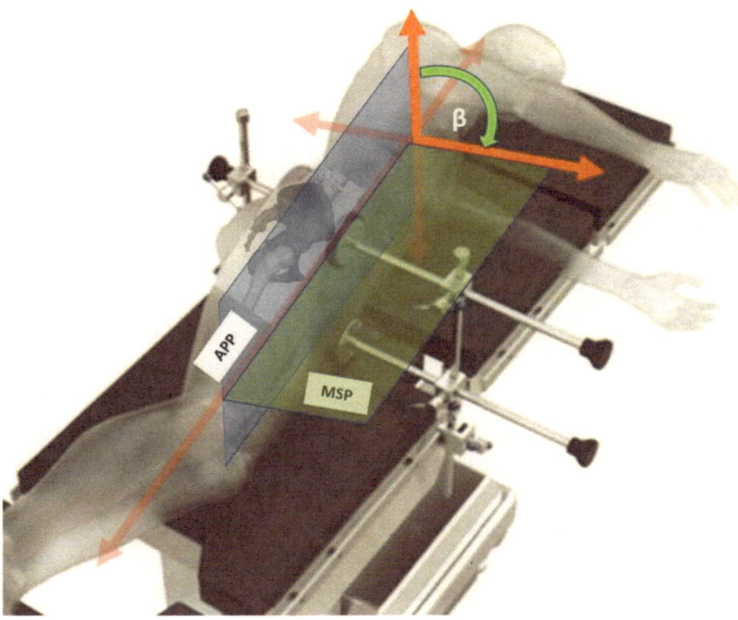

Figure 2.
Pelvic tilt. Measurement of the anterior tilt angle in a lateral decubitus position. Forward tilt is determined as the angle subtended by the difference in degrees from the true APP (i.e. the vertical starting position) to the measured APP as it approaches the MSP (i.e. as the pelvis rolls anteriorly) [43]. APP = anterior pelvic plane; MSP = mid-sagittal plane; β = anterior tilt angle.

The effects of changing pelvic position on pelvic tilt has been well studied [52–54]. When the pelvis tilts posteriorly during basic pre-operative functional screening, the respective anteversion and abduction angles of the final acetabular implant position increases, which may in turn lead to excessive wear due to neck impingement and edge loading, with an increased risk of dislocation [19]. Prediction of pelvic displacement before surgery has key importance for accurate placement of the acetabular implant despite historically being an under-valued consideration. Objectively, Babisch et al. demonstrated that acetabular cup positions are affected by pelvic tilt on CT models, with good accuracy and reproducibility [55]. Similarly, a previous study by Maratt et al. using a computer-generated 3D model also demonstrated the substantial effect of pelvic tilt on resultant acetabular angles [56]. In a practical sense, the functional angle of the acetabular implant is directly related to the pelvic tilt angle, with the anteversion angle of the acetabular implant changing by approximately 0.7° with every degree of change in pelvic inclination [43]. Therefore, only small linear magnitude changes can significantly affect endpoint cup version and contribute to construct instability.

In contrast, until recently there has been a lack of literature describing the isolated effects of radiographic pelvic rotation (PR) on preoperative acetabular planning angulation of acetabular prostheses. The recent work of Lourens et al. used high resolution 3D CT pelvis models generated from healthy controls and arthroplasty patients to quantify the effects of pelvic rotation on acetabular cup position in various static planes simulating radiographic errors in basic imaging used for component templating [2]. They concluded that pelvic rotation can also significantly impact on the perceived acetabular angles observed on an AP pelvic radiograph used for pre-operative planning, which can in turn result in poor prosthetic placement and subsequent poorer long-term clinical outcomes. Supportive of the reliability of conventional approaches, the presented data indicated that PR of less than 20° however was unlikely to have a clinical impact of preoperative measurements and therefore may serve as a guide for clinical application and operative planning.

4. Pre-operative assessment: setting a target position

Respecting that the optimal prosthetic position for an acetabular component is likely to be subtly (or not so subtly) different for each individual patient, establishing a clear target position for the acetabular component of a THA is of critical importance. Even once a 'target' is defined, attainment of this can be a challenging process. As discussed later herein, inaccurate patient set up, loss of pelvic position during the procedure (i.e. patient movement) and errors in intended implantation angles can all undermine the achieved outcome [2, 43]. Langston et al. [57] suggested that a change in pelvic tilt of 13° or more on pre-operative assessment may be deemed unfavourable as this will result in a change in the functional anteversion of the acetabulum of 10°. This has the potential to place even a well-orientated component outside of a +/−10° target safe zone [57]. In the same work, the authors suggested that unfavourable pelvic mobility was independently associated with limited lumbar flexion, a more posterior standing pelvic tilt and increasing age [57, 58]. Unsurprisingly, they strongly advocated for pre-operative functional X-ray imaging [57]. It is noteworthy that none of the three associated factors they determined are immediately amendable to peri-operative correction prior to elective THA and may also thus be considered immutable (albeit important perhaps to recognise and consider). In extreme such cases, there is already a trend for some surgeons to move towards large head and/or dual mobility bearings in an attempt to increase the functional safe range-of-movement [59] in instances whereby concerns regarding spinopelvic stiffness have been raised. Even with such informed pre-surgical patient data, what best to 'do' with this information is less clear. Simply centring the implanted cup to the middle of the functional movement range has inherent risk and may not necessarily result in the perfect construct orientation to accommodate the rigours of daily activity. Recognising that final construct stability is a composite of optimised component mechanics AND the concurrent effect of the static and dynamic elements of the surrounding soft tissue envelope is a far too often under-acknowledged reality.

The process of high precision data capture with pre-operative functional imaging is also not without its challenges. True lateral pelvic X-rays (required for accurate conventional angular measurement) can be technically challenging to obtain and—under present conditions—at best reflect a series of pre-determined static captures of the bony relationship between the lower lumbosacral spine, pelvis and proximal femur [43]. These are not dynamic measures and do not directly take into account the critical impact of the surrounding soft tissue envelopes. Using the more commonly employed proprietary functional x-ray series, the relationship of the key bony elements in the extremes of motion are not represented—likely the positions most vulnerable to permit prosthetic dislocation [43].

Undoubtedly, an awareness of spinopelvic movement parameters also allows informed consideration of customised/patient-specific cup implantation targets [50, 60–63]. Many centres now incorporate pre-operative spinopelvic movement assessment into routine work up pathways [64]. While it is clear that fundamental clinical assessment alone is insufficient to fully appreciate the linked movement characteristics of the human spine and pelvis on a patient-by-patient basis [64], how best to interpret often complex pre-operative imaging data and how to best apply this information to target cup planning [51] remains unclear and represents an opportunity for future investigation.

Recent work has suggested potential enhanced value with pre-operative simultaneous biplanar imaging [37, 64], as compared to conventional plain film X-rays. The proprietary EOS imaging system (Euronext: EOSI; Paris, France) is touted to reduce the radiation dose by two thirds as compared to equivalent plain X-ray imaging [64, 65]. Such technologies permit simultaneous capture of precisely orthogonal X-ray images in an upright, physiological load-bearing position and are claimed to be more accurate and less dependent on patient positioning [64]. Given that some have suggested limited practical utility of plain film X-rays in judging sagittal pelvic tilt [66] consideration of EOS (or other high precision imaging modalities) may hold merit. However, while the current science may suggest a role for EOS (or EOS-like imaging means) in replacing pre-operative radiographic assessment [64], the technology is not universally available and carries associated expense [43].

5. Intra-operative execution of the surgical plan

During the THA operation itself, three considerations become important with respect to the accuracy of definitive cup placement. Firstly, is the original position of the patient (as a surrogate for the true pelvis position). In the lateral (i.e. decubitus) set up, the surgeon/surgical team endeavour to ensure the patient's pelvic sagittal plane (PSP) is horizontally orientated. In most practical senses, this refers to this key alignment plane being parallel to the theatre floor [67, 68]. Classically, surgeons have relied on palpation of key bony landmarks (i.e. ASIS and pubic symphysis) [69–71] to determine if the vertically-orientated APP [72] is indeed perpendicular to the flat level surface of the operating table (**Figure 2**). Direct and accurate localisation of the contralateral ASIS for APP determination can be challenging in the lateral position [72], especially with increasing BMI. Unsurprisingly, there is considerable inaccuracy in this subjective process [73] which assumes both landmark symmetry and an ability of the surgeon to accurately appreciate the location of such landmarks. An array of commonly-used positioning aids are employed for achieving and maintaining the true lateral orientation for THA. These usually involve some combination of posterior sacral block [74] and an anterior symphyseal bolster or ASIS post [74]—the latter of which may involve single or paired extensions. More proprietary universal lateral positioners [75] or peg boards [76] are also used with reasonable quoted effect. Interestingly, in a 2019 UK nation-wide investigation however, Rutherford and colleagues explored surgeons' sentiment towards current positioning tools [77]. More than 35% of respondents were 'unhappy' with their current supports, while less than a third (31%) felt their current positioning supports were rigid and reliably stable [77]. The need for better positioning tools and supports is almost unanimously championed [74, 76].

Previous authors have proposed customised pelvic orientation devices for use during initial set up claiming simplicity of use and improved accuracy and reproducibility in achieving a pelvis horizontal in the sagittal plane [67]. To date, despite the potential value of such positioning aids, they have failed to attract mainstream uptake and use. Iwakiri and colleagues [78] reported a custom variation of an existing positioning device with the addition of an extra compression pad [78]. Described as 'simple, minimally invasive and cost effective' [78] the authors were able to show significant reductions in intra-operative sagittal pelvic tilt. Other studies have shown highly significant differences ($p < 0.001$) in the maintenance of pelvic position during surgery when comparing the type of mechanical support used [76].

Beyond blaming the tools, multiple studies have shown significant variation in the ability of surgeons/surgical teams to accurately position the pelvis for THA surgery [76]. The 2011 work of Nishikubo and colleagues used in-theatre fluoroscopy to check for pelvic positioning errors prior to commencement of surgery [79]. With a pelvis orientated with 0° of tilt versus the horizontal sagittal plane as the target standard, they reported a mean positioning error of nearly 6°—this before the operation had even begun [79]. The later study of Lambers et al. reported a more modest error of closer to 3° but a wider range of recorded starting errors as high as 13° [80]. In a sub-analysis the same authors suggest that malpositioning is indeed a common occurrence in everyday practice and is more likely with increasing patient body mass index (BMI) [80, 81]. Increased BMI is independently linked to increased rates of post-operative arthroplasty complications, compounded by errors in component placement resulting in suboptimal positioning [81].

The second critical element is the ability of the set up to *maintain* consistently the position of the patient during the operation itself. This too is a multi-factorial consideration. Pelvic movement affects perceived cup inclination and version and may lead to an unintended cup implantation error [82]. While the recommendations are not uniformly agreed, Otero and co-authors suggested that 'proper' (acceptable) positioning could perhaps be defined whereby there was <10° of subsequent pelvic positional change during the THA procedure itself [83]. The initial patient position is maintained by positioning devices presumed to be rigid and stable—in many instances however this is not the case. Especially with increasing BMI [84] and general patient size, the effectiveness with which these one-size-fits-all devices secure and maintain the position of the pelvis is poor. Further undermining this consideration, Milone and colleagues suggested that rigid positioning alone was an unreliable way of ensuring accurate final cup placement [75]. While almost all commonly employed such equipment is designed to provide stable support against unyielding bony landmarks (ASIS etc.), simply tightening them further to increase the rigidity of support is also not without risk. In their recent 2020 publication, Ueno and colleagues demonstrated a 2.64% rate of medically-important soft tissue ulceration secondary to pelvic positioner use for routine primary THAs [85].

The pelvis is exposed to many discrete deforming forces during a conventional THA which may result in iatrogenic pelvic tilt [3, 84]. The process of mechanical cup reaming and implant impaction are obvious examples [84], but 'strong' traction from exposure-permitting retractors are also a recognised culprit [84, 86]. While traction for safe exposure may be an unavoidable evil during primary THA, authors who have considered this important force mechanism recommend releasing or 'backing off' retractor tension during the critical stage of definitive cup impaction [85], which may permit some measure of tilt correction [84]. The 2019 work of Della Valle et al. however suggests that retractor removal is unlikely to facilitate complete correction of anterior roll which had been induced earlier during the case [82].

Thirdly, the surgeon must be able to accurately, consistently and reproducibly introduce the acetabular component with the correct intended 3D orientation and then impact it whilst precisely maintaining this. As a fundamental tenant of the assumption that surgeons can reliably perform this task Somerville et al. [86] explored the accuracy with which a cohort of experienced trauma and arthroplasty surgeons visually assessed cup anteversion and inclination insertion angles [86]. There was great variability amongst the group with results ranging from 'very poor' to 'very good' with only moderate inter-observer reproducibility [86]. There have been many proposed methods for improving the precision and/or reproducibility of cup insertion. Such measures have included: following anatomical landmarks [83], the use of intra-operative imaging [79], manual instrumentation jigs and alignment guides [67] or the use of computer-assisted navigation [87]. The most commonly cited anatomic landmark for cup insertion remains the transverse acetabular ligament (TAL) [44]. The value of this local feature has been questioned however, the earlier work of Epstein et al. suggesting the TAL was only appreciably present in 47% of osteoarthritic hips [88] and that, even when it was identified, its presence and recognition did not improve the attainment of target cup position [88]. They concluded that cup orientation using the TAL was no more accurate than an unassisted freehand insertion technique [88], with the subsequent work of Beverland et al. actively recommending against using the TAL to determine final cup inclination [44].

While the use of real-time imaging has been suggested as a potentially useful step to improve the accuracy of final cup position although this too is not without its inherent challenges. Difficulty in the physical process of introducing imaging equipment into sterile fields and capturing meaningful images (i.e. accurately perpendicular to the long axis of the pelvis), concerns regarding radiation exposure and fundamental problems with the interpretation of an image captured in a decubitus position (as compared to the 'routine' AP supine or standing states) are all noteworthy considerations. While some authors advocate the use of imaging routinely [89, 90] (most often fluoroscopy [80]) as an intra-operative aid—especially in the setting of a high BMI patient [80]—others have suggested limited utility through such means citing mismatch between apparent 'during surgery' and post-operative radiographic cup orientation [68]. Hayakawa et al. suggested mean errors of >5° in both cup inclination and anteversion perception using intra-operative radiographs versus the post-operative gold standard [91] concluding that in-theatre determinations may not reflect post-operative targets.

Using conventional instrumented cup implantation techniques there are many proprietary differences between implant systems which cloud comparability. In essence, the AP inclination angle (i.e. 'lateral opening' or 'abduction' angle) is visually-appreciated as the angle between the cup insertion handle and the sagittal plane [67] (**Figure 3**). Critically, if at the time of cup insertion the PSP is not (or is no longer) parallel to the floor, an error of component placement will occur [67]. Body axis alignment (or appreciation thereof) directly influences cup version, as can changes in pelvic flexion and extension.

Whilst a relatively recent addition to the arthroplasty surgeon's armamentarium in many parts of the world, the use of intra-operative computer-assisted hip navigation provides another means for aiding cup insertion [75, 92]. In its two most basic forms, such systems use either pre-operative 'imaging informed' or 'imageless' [73, 93] approaches. As with accepted total knee arthroplasty (TKA) applications, both portable (i.e. 'mini-nav' [94, 95]) and 'full navigation' systems are available for use during hip surgery. Whilst large volume data are still pending, early applications of navigated THA suggest consistent improvements in achieving the desired insertion orientation [93, 94, 96] with significantly less ($p < 0.001$) deviations from target [92, 97]. Most commercially-available navigation systems reference the APP which

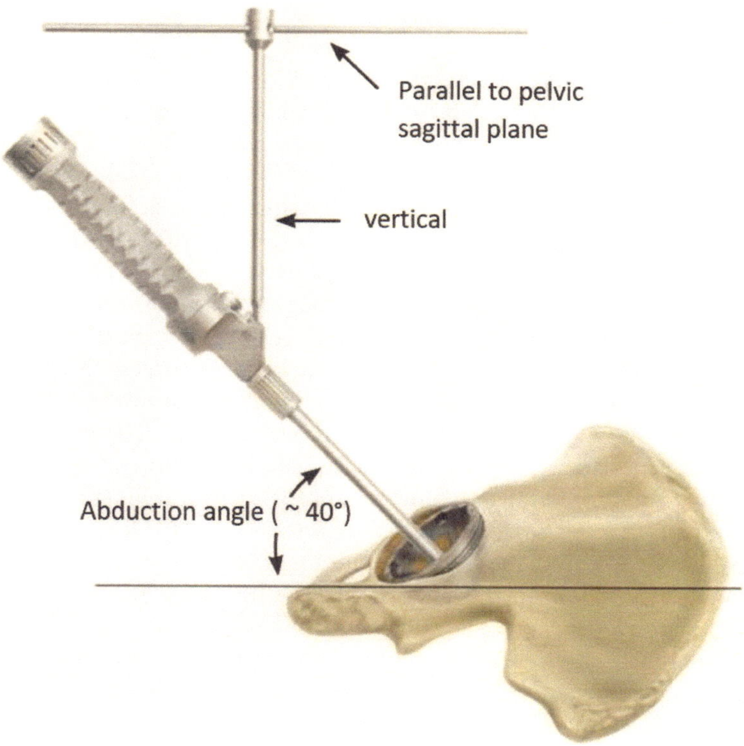

Figure 3.
Cup insertion angles using instrumented alignment towers.

provides the frame-of-reference orientation for later angular measurement [51, 73] although the paper by Vigdorchik and colleagues suggests that the perpendicular hip-shoulder-axis may actually be the more accurate and consistent registration plane [98]. The well-performed 2020 prospective randomised control trial by Tanino et al. compared the accuracy of a portable, accelerometer-based navigation system with that of conventional instrumented techniques [92]. While adding an average of 10 operative minutes to each case [92], the use of navigation was associated with significant improvements in attainment of target cup position [92]—a sentiment supporting the landmark earlier work of Jolles et al. in 2004 [99]. One of the key benefits of contemporary THA navigation [75, 92] likely lies in the ability of such systems to track pelvic movement during surgery and provide 'corrective' measurements [100]. In many cases, the system has the ability to recognise the occurrence and magnitude of pelvic positional changes, even when such movement is below the threshold of unaided surgeon perception. While many authors (and users) feel that intra-operative navigation stands as the best widely available tool for accurate cup implantation [73], such systems do have their own inherent shortcomings including a user learning-curve, system failures, loss of tracker position and poor reliability with increasing pelvic tilt [95, 101]. The integration of biplanar EOS-based imaging methods with existing navigation applications (NAVEOS; VA, USA) is an exciting novel pairing [69] which has been touted to further simplify cup placement with increased 3D accuracy in a lateral decubitus position [69] however, this technology needs further, rigorous, validation before wider adoption can be championed.

6. Discussion

Worldwide, the majority of primary THA is still performed in the lateral position [44] although it has been shown that this position is associated with the greatest degree of unintended intra-operative pelvic movement [74, 78, 92, 102]. Accurate acetabular cup orientation is critical in THA for good clinical results [103, 104] and most authors acknowledge that this can often be a difficult task [47]. Pelvic tilt alters apparent cup position [74] and may subsequently result in suboptimal placement [100]. While the operative approach itself whilst in the decubitus orientation is also an independent consideration for movement (more so with posterior versus antero-lateral approaches [76]), failure to recognise changes in pelvic position introduces the potential for erroneous cup placement [76], compounding surgeon insertion errors. Poor acetabular component placement has been linked to a number of post-operative adverse outcomes [49, 94] including accelerated bearing wear [23, 45, 70, 91, 105, 106] and dislocation risk [45, 70, 91, 92, 105, 107, 108] mechanical impingement [108], decreased functional range-of-movement [57, 70, 92, 105], component migration [91], poor joint function [106], and metal ion toxicity [106]. Regardless of the target orientation, the ability to reliably and predictably achieve the desired acetabular component position is crucial to successful THA [80, 83, 109].

As discussed previously herein, final cup position is substantially influenced by the 'on table' patient positioning [45, 77], including the initial set up [44, 76, 80]. Despite the best efforts of surgeons/theatre teams, it remains the case that a pelvis will often move unintendedly during the performance of a THA [46, 76]—in spite of seemingly well applied and tensioned positioning devices. Surgeons must remain cognisant to this reality [84]. While several novel devices have been proposed, to date, there exists no mainstream, low-risk accepted method for ensuring a 'true' lateral position at the start of each case [68]. Statistically, a pelvis is (far) more likely to roll anteriorly ($p < 0.001$) during a THA in the decubitus set up [46] and this forward tilt is likely progressive across the operation [82]. It has been demonstrated that the greatest source of error occurs when the PSP is no longer horizontal at time of cup insertion [110]. While it has been proposed that such sequential loss of starting position likely progresses until at least the point of definitive cup and liner insertion, few quantitative data support this at this stage—another inviting opportunity for future research. Pure anterior pelvic roll has been shown to influence cup anteversion to a greater extent than inclination [75]. It is accepted that major pelvic movement may have an effect on the final cup insertion position [85] through surgeon perceptual error. Given the common anterior roll mechanism seen, this consequently leads to an underestimation of cup anteversion [82], with the degree of error directly related to the magnitude of pelvic tilt [49, 78, 107].

How far does an average pelvis move during a routine, primary, THA? Several previous authors have attempted to quantify 'normal' ranges of unintended pelvic movement during THA [74, 76, 82, 85] and then to propose acceptable 'cut offs' to define clinically-important variation [75]. Anterior (or posterior) pelvic tilt alters the position of the cup in the sagittal plane [111] which has a direct impact on version perception. In case series' including 67–100 hips [74–76, 82, 85] previous works have reported median pelvic tilt values during surgery of >4° [46, 82], however mean values and maximum observed tilts ranged broadly between studies—often approaching 20° for the latter [82]. Such studies show 41–57% of cases rolling anteriorly >5° [74, 75, 80], with 21–38% by >10° [46, 75, 83]. Otero's paper reported 15.4% of cases with 10–20° of tilt and 2.8% with >20° [83]. In interpreting these errors, Grammatopoulos et al. suggested that a > 10° anteversion error had a 3.5 odds ratio of the final cup position falling outside of the target safe zone [46]. Using widely accepted mathematical conversion factors [111, 112], 1° of pelvic tilt results in a 0.7–0.8° change in final anteversion. Given the longstanding surgical goal of achieving target anteversion +/− 10° (see Lewinnek and others [113]), an unappreciated intra-operative pelvic tilt of just 13° would therefore be enough to see an otherwise perfectly centred cup fall outside of the 'safe' anteversion range.

Inconsistency in initial patient set up [76] (i.e. with non-perpendicular 'true' lateral decubitus positioning) linked with a subsequent change in the pelvic position during the operative process (i.e. movement) likely contributes a substantial burden of the variation seen in final cup position [76] despite otherwise technically sound surgical technique. Uniaxial pelvic tilt has been specifically associated with unintended errors in cup version [112]. A high correlation between direct pelvic tilt and version angle ($R^2 = 0.995$, $p < 0.001$) [112] has been confirmed and is intrinsically linked to the fact that the negative impact of pelvic tilt can be corrected with relative ease using simple (validated) mathematical algorithms with very high precision [112]. Until recently, the challenge however has remained the ability to *recognise* intra-operative pelvic tilt and to accurately quantify its magnitude. While the most common historical methods for determining implantation parameters for acetabular components have included mechanical alignment guides and reference against the TAL [77], both methods have been shown to be unreliable [103] and hinge on precise judgement 'as per the surgeons eye' [114]. Accurate determination of anteversion during conventional hip replacement surgery can be difficult [90], even in experienced hands. Technology-assisted surgical options—such as computer-navigation—however may provide a solution to the limitations of visual human assessment.

Using standard navigation, it is possible to determine pelvic inclination and tilt by calculating the angular difference between the anatomic frontal plane and true horizontal (i.e. floor) [87]. Modern navigation systems—especially those using accelerometer-based technologies—provide the valuable added benefit of measuring the relative change in the pelvic position independently from data captured from the fixed pelvic tracker(s). Measurement of pelvic tilt during THA allows corrective algorithms to re-calculate the cup insertion angles to correct for the error introduced by pelvic movement and have been shown to improve the accuracy of component placement as per the intended target [42, 111]. The large 2010 study by Zhu and colleagues explored the quantitative value of navigation during THA in a cohort approaching 500 hips [111]. While these authors reported a mean intra-operative tilt of just under 5°, the observed range was from 25° of posterior tilt through to 20° of anterior (i.e. a 45° unintended error range) [111]. Over 25% of patients rolled 6–9°, while over 16% moved more than 10°. It has not yet been definitively established what the perceptual tolerances of visual assessment of pelvic tilt may be by surgeons (or varying levels of experience) although it seems clear that deficiencies in this key skill likely have a negative influence on intended cup implantation position [57].

While much research, attention and interest has centred around pelvic tilt during surgery, the important role of pelvic adduction is rarely assessed or considered [82, 115]. Given that the acetabular cup is a 3D element, inserted with intended orientation goals in 3D, it is conceivable that unintended pelvic movement in any direction may have negative consequence on final cup position [86]. Mathematically, unappreciated pelvic adduction can increase radiographic inclination [114] which may have consequences for final bearing stability [115]. In a routine posterior approach to the hip (in a lateral decubitus position) the relatively wider pelvis as compared to the lower limbs tends to see the uppermost hemipelvis drift into adduction [114]. The previous work of O'Neill and colleagues (2018) assessed the pelvic movement in 270 consecutive primary THAs suggesting that none of their cases showed pelvic abduction with a mean adduction change of 4.4° [115]. This finding was similar to other authors who reported average adduction angles of 2.5–6.7° [82, 84]. It is generally felt that these smaller magnitude changes have a lesser impact on inclination than do comparable movements involving pelvic tilt.

Current research would support the notion that anterior pelvic roll occurs incrementally across the case from set up to definitive implant insertion. The descriptive work of Grammatopoulos et al. suggested a mean angular movement from set up to implant insertion of 9° (sd 6) [76]. Others have suggested similar changes [85]. The later work of Schloemann and colleagues suggested that more than just 5° of change may be 'clinically significant' [89] supporting the suggestion that such unaccounted for angular change may facilitate introduction of critical errors in target cup placement [75, 89]. Several authors have recommended that the highest (and most consistent) level of attainment of target cup position may perhaps be achieved using the combination of an assistive anatomical plane (pelvic) positioner and navigation [100, 103]. Iwakiri and colleagues suggested such an approach was reliably simple, consistent, economical and non-invasive [103].

Despite the focus of hip navigation on radiographic outcomes and intra-operative changes, the critical consideration of patient body habitus must be considered. Most authors agree that increasing patient BMI influences the likelihood of unintended pelvic positional change during surgery itself [84] and strongly correlates with subsequent errors in target cup orientation attainment [80, 85]. The extended size of bariatric tissue retractors for surgical exposure [84, 85] (and sometimes the force applied to them) and direct soft tissue impingement can worsen the magnitude of positional movement [116]. However, high BMI alone cannot be blamed for all of the issues noted with unintended pelvic positional change—the 2019 work of Schloemann et al. showed clinically-relevant anterior pelvic roll in a cohort with a mean BMI of just 20 [89]. Similarly, other authors have suggested no clear association between BMI and pelvic movement [75, 82, 117]. Regardless, obesity is just one factor so far linked to pelvic movement during THA surgery—with evidence to show that low volume surgeons and the surgical approach employed are also recognised cofactors [30, 118].

7. Looking to the future ...

The future for hip arthroplasty appears exciting, especially as appropriately-employed technologies facilitate further improvements in planning, precision and intra-operative execution. Historical two dimensional (2D) templating and planning has already been shown to be far less accurate than modern 3D equivalents [119–121]. The evolution to more universal 3D standards is likely to incrementally improve surgical planning [122–124] as such technologies become more mainstream. The cutting edge integration of artificial intelligence algorithms into the pre-operative decision making pathways may represent further advancement still [124]. Similarly, as real-time computer navigation is taken up more broadly many anticipate improved attainment of target cup placement [87] (in a similar fashion to accuracy improvements that were seen during the evolution of TKA navigation). Despite great enthusiasm in some spheres, navigated arthroplasty is not without its inherent problems and limitations. Tracker pin site placement and loosening [102] continue to undermine case-by-case precision with only small positional changes resulting in magnified degradation in accuracy. As with other bony-mounted navigation applications in other parts of the body, site fractures, wound and pin site issues post-operatively also plague use and present technique-specific challenges [101].

Some supporters of technology have suggested that formal ('full') hip navigation may be unnecessary, suggesting that less invasive and less time consuming alternatives are already available to improve operative precision. Using a simple off-the-self smartphone with basic accelerometer capability, Peters et al. in 2012 reported a series of 50 THAs suggesting their novel technique was simple, 'quick and accurate', reporting that 'all' cases were able to achieve less than 5% deviation from the intended pre-operative plan [47]. Similar work by O'Neill et al. using a simple digital inclinometer reported achieving target cup position within 2.5° in 88% of cases [110] and showed positive statistically-significant differences as compared to conventional instrumented approaches. Contrasting CT-based full navigation with 'imageless' accelerometer (mini) navigation however, the recent work by Testsunaga et al. suggested the latter lacked the accuracy of image-based techniques [102] but it was unclear whether the precision-versus-target cup position translated to meaningful clinical benefit. Equally, the potential improvement in accuracy must be weighed against the time, expense and radiation exposure associated with CT-based pre-op imaging. As point-of-care image registration approaches continue to improve with software and algorithm refinement, ease of use and reliable user accuracy will likely improve in parallel.

Regardless of the fundamental imaging method employed (i.e. plain X-ray, augmented X-ray, CT or MRI based), the concept of 'fusing' advanced or even 3D pre-operative templating with highly-precise intra-operative navigation means poses an exciting state-of-the-art possibility. Such novel approaches—already in clinical use in some domains—exploit the optimal elements of contemporary planning and surgical case execution. Some authors feel this may represent the best of both considerations [43].

Opponents of navigation frequently cite the 'is the extra angular precision actually worth it' argument. The now standard use of larger heads, and with increasingly-common selection of dual mobility bearings [59], has arguably improved the stability and mechanical characteristics in many instances perhaps negating the need for such high levels of cup orientation accuracy. Indeed, in their 2013 paper Eilander and colleagues suggested that hip navigation may be an 'unnecessary' technical burden, claiming that 82% of the hips included within their comprehensive study had cups within radiographic safe zones using conventional free hand techniques [105]. So far however, this has not been the sentiment shared by most. Finally, the progression to robot-assisted THA surgery [75]—arguably an evolutionary extension of computer-based navigation—may offer further clinical advantages with early science suggesting value, especially in complex cases [125]. This area too requires further research to ensure the evidence base underpinning wider uptake stays ahead of the enthusiastic hype.

8. Conclusions

This comprehensive review of the current literature highlights the following: 1. current techniques and equipment for patient set up in the lateral decubitus position are deficient and, if used poorly, have the potential to cause patient harm. As a result, sagittal plane movement during THAs (i.e. anterior pelvic roll) is currently an accepted shortcoming. Common patterns of sequential pelvic movement during surgery have not been well determined and represent an opportunity for future investigation; 2. the ability of surgeons/surgical teams to visually appreciate (often large) changes in pelvic position with any degree of quantitative precision—in a patient under exclusion draping—is universally unreliable. This is increasingly so in the setting of obesity/high BMI; 3. failure to appreciate such pelvic movement has a direct and tangible effect upon the ability to insert the definitive acetabular component accurately with the intended target position in mind; 4. such unintended component positioning errors likely have a subsequent negative effect on the mechanical parameters of the THA construct and previous evidence would suggest this may lead to increased risk of wear, instability and possibly dislocation (all key determinants of later revision surgery); 5. while the conventional/historical standard for cup insertion has been 'per the surgeon's eye' or using manual alignment jigs, both fail to reliably and accurately appreciate unintended patient movement during the operation itself. Evidence would suggest that—when used correctly—contemporary navigation systems can improve the precision of implant insertion versus target orientations by narrowing outlier ranges and by calculation of corrective parameters to compensate for computer-appreciated pelvic positional change; 6. while used widely in some international settings, intra-operative hip navigation (image informed or imageless) has not yet achieved widespread adoption and still requires rigorous scientific validation to confirm its utility in more general settings and to further refine optimised indications for use. The role of robot-assisted approaches in this context show promise but require more generalised validation.

Conflict of interest

The author declares no conflict of interest.

Author details

Andrew P. Kurmis[1,2]

1 Discipline of Medical Specialties, School of Medicine, University of Adelaide, Adelaide, SA, Australia

2 College of Medicine and Public Health, Flinders University, Bedford Park, SA, Australia

*Address all correspondence to: Andrew.Kurmis@sa.gov.au

References

[1] Kurmis AP. Thromboprophylaxis after total hip replacement. Journal of Orthopaedic Surgery (Hong Kong). 2010;**18**(1):92-97

[2] Lourens EC, Kurmis AP, Yin LW. Clinical impact of pelvic malrotation on radiograph-based preoperative planning for total hip arthroplasty: A proof-of-concept and prudent prediction of acceptable rotation. Indian Journal of Orthopaedics. 2022;**56**:1053-1060

[3] Lourens EC, Kurmis AP, Holder C, de Steiger RN. Early revision rates of total hip arthroplasty using Intellijoint HIP® computer navigation system: A Study from the Australian National Joint Replacement Registry of 1911 procedures. Journal of Arthroplasty. 2022 [In press]

[4] Learmonth ID, Young C, Rorabeck C. The operation of the century: Total hip replacement. The Lancet. 2007;**370**(9597):1508-1519

[5] Lewinnek GE, Lewis JL, Tarr R, Compere CL, Zimmerman JR. Dislocations after total hip-replacement arthroplasties. Journal of Bone and Joint Surgery. American Volume. 1978;**60**:217-220

[6] Lum ZC, Pereira GC, Giordani M, Meehan JP. Top 100 most cited articles in orthopaedic surgery: An update. Journal of Orthopaedics. 2020;**19**:132-137

[7] Esposito CI, Gladnick BP, Lee YY, Lyman S, Wright TM, Mayman DJ, et al. Cup position alone does not predict risk of dislocation after hip arthroplasty. The Journal of Arthroplasty. 2015;**30**:109-113

[8] Abdel MP, von Roth P, Jennings MT, Hanssen AD, Pagnano MW. What safe zone? The vast majority of dislocated THAs are within the Lewinnek safe zone for acetabular component position. Clinical Orthopaedics and Related Research. 2016;**474**(2):386-391

[9] Murphy WS, Yun HH, Hayden B, Kowal JH, Murphy SB. The safe zone range for cup anteversion is narrower than for inclination in THA. Clinical Orthopaedics and Related Research. 2018;**476**(2):325-335

[10] Tezuka T, Heckmann N, Bodner R, Dorr LD. Functional safe zone is superior to the Lewinnek safe zone for total hip arthroplasty: Why the Lewinnek safe zone is not always predictive of stability. The Journal of Arthroplasty. 2019;**34**:3-8

[11] Dorr LD, Callaghan JJ. Death of the Lewinnek "safe zone". The Journal of Arthroplasty. 2019;**34**(1):1-2

[12] Giachino M, Aprato A, Revetria TA, Vezzetti E, Massè A, Ulrich L, et al. Dynamic evaluation of THA components by prosthesis impingement software (PIS). Acta Bio-Medica. 2021;**92**(5):e2021295

[13] Kennedy JG, Rogers WB, Sullivan RJ, Griffen DG, Sheehan LJ. Effect of acetabular component orientation on recurrent dislocation, pelvic osteolysis, polyethylene wear, and component migration. The Journal of Arthroplasty. 1998;**13**(5):530-534

[14] Meftah M, Yadav A, Wong AC, Ranawat AS, Ranawat CS. A novel method for accurate and reproducible functional cup positioning in total hip arthroplasty. The Journal of Arthroplasty. 2013;**28**(7):1200-1205

[15] Ng VY, McShane MA. Understanding acetabular cup orientation: The importance of convention and defining

the safe zone. Hip International. 2011;**21**(6):646-652

[16] Merle C, Grammatopoulos G, Waldstein W, Pegg E, Pandit H, Aldinger PR, et al. Comparison of native anatomy with recommended safe component orientation in total hip arthroplasty for primary osteoarthritis. Journal of Bone and Joint Surgery. American Volume. 2013;**95**(22):e172

[17] McBride A, Flynn J, Miller G, Barnes M, Mackie S. Body mass index and acetabular component position in total hip arthroplasty. ANZ Journal of Surgery. 2013;**83**(3):171-174

[18] Grammatopoulos G, Thomas G, Pandit H, Beard D, Gill H, Murray D. The effect of orientation of the acetabular component on outcome following total hip arthroplasty with small diameter hard-on-soft bearings. Bone & Joint Journal. 2015;**97-B**(2):164-172

[19] Bhaskar D, Rajpura A, Board T. Current concepts in acetabular positioning in total hip arthroplasty. Indian Journal of Orthopaedics. 2017;**51**(4):386-396

[20] Scheerlinck T. Cup positioning in total hip arthroplasty. Acta Orthopaedica Belgica. 2014;**80**(3):336-347

[21] Jolles BM, Zangger P, Leyvraz PF. Factors predisposing to dislocation after primary total hip arthroplasty: A multivariate analysis. The Journal of Arthroplasty. 2002;**17**:282-288

[22] Miki H, Kyo T, Kuroda Y, Nakahara I. Sugano 367 N: Risk of edge-loading and prosthesis impingement due to posterior pelvic tilting after total hip arthroplasty. Clinical biomechanics. 2014;**29**:607-613

[23] Kilb BKJ, Kurmis AP, Parry M, Sherwood K, Keown P, Masri BA, et al. Frank Stinchfield award: Identification of the 'at risk' genotype for development of pseudotumours around metal-on-metal total hip arthroplasties. Clinical Orthopaedics and Related Research. 2018;**476**(2):230-241

[24] Upfill-Brown A, Hsiue PP, Sekimura T, Patel JN, Adamson M, Stavrakis AI. Instability is the most common indication for revision hip arthroplasty in the United States: National trends from 2012 to 2018. Arthroplasty Today. 2021;**11**:88-101

[25] Bozic K, Kurtz S, Lau E, Ong K, Vail T, Berry D. The epidemiology of revision total hip arthroplasty in the United States. Journal of Bone and Joint Surgery. American Volume. 2009;**91**(1):128-133

[26] Barrack RL, Krempec JA, Clohisy JC, McDonald DJ, Ricci WM, Ruh EL, et al. Accuracy of acetabular component position in hip arthroplasty. Journal of Bone and Joint Surgery. American Volume. 2013;**95**(19):1760-1768

[27] Domb BG, El Bitar YF, Sadik AY, Stake CE, Botser IB. Comparison of robotic-assisted and conventional acetabular cup placement in THA: A matched-pair controlled study. Clinical Orthopaedics and Related Research. 2014;**472**(1):329-336

[28] Korduba LA, Essner A, Pivec R, Lancin P, Mont MA, Wang A, et al. Effect of acetabular cup abduction angle on wear of ultrahigh-molecular-weight polyethylene in hip simulator testing. The American Journal of Orthopedics. 2014;**43**(10):466-471

[29] Barrack RL. Dislocation after total hip arthroplasty: Implant design and orientation. Journal of the American Academy of Orthopaedic Surgeons. 2003;**11**(2):89-99

[30] Callanan MC, Jarrett B, Bragdon CR, Zurakowski D, Rubash HE, Freiberg AA, et al. The John Charnley award: Risk factors for cup malpositioning: Quality improvement through a joint registry at a tertiary hospital. Clinical Orthopaedics and Related Research. 2011;**469**(2):319-329

[31] Agarwal S, Eckhard L, Walter W, Peng A, Hatton A, Donnelly B, et al. The use of computer navigation in total hip arthroplasty is associated with a reduced rate of revision for dislocation. Journal of Bone and Joint Surgery. American Volume. 2021;**103**(20):1900-1905

[32] Bohl D, Nolte M, Ong K, Lau E, Calkins T, Della VC. Computer-assisted navigation is associated with reductions in the rates of dislocation and acetabular component revision following primary total hip arthroplasty. Journal of Bone and Joint Surgery. American Volume. 2019;**101**(3):250-256

[33] Snijders T, van Gaalen S, de Gast A. Precision and accuracy of imageless navigation versus freehand implantation of total hip arthroplasty: A systematic review and meta-analysis. The International Journal of Medical Robotics and Computer Assisted Surgery. 2017;**13**(4):e1843

[34] Kurmis AP. Commentary & perspective: Understanding the role of computer-navigation in primary total knee arthroplasty. Journal of Bone and Joint Surgery. American Volume. 2019;**101**:e111(1-2)

[35] Kurmis AP. Commentary & perspective: Considering the value of imageless, accelerometer-based, intra-operative 'mini-' navigation systems in contemporary primary TKA. Journal of Bone and Joint Surgery. American Volume. 2020;**102**(22):e129

[36] de Steiger R, Liu Y-L, Graves SE. Computer navigation for total knee arthroplasty reduces revision rate for patients less than sixty-five years of age. Journal of Bone and Joint Surgery. American Volume. 2015;**97**(8):635-642

[37] Ghostine B, Sauret C, Assi A, Bakouny Z, Khalil N, Skalli W, et al. Influence of patient axial malpositioning on the trueness and precision of pelvic parameters obtained from 3D reconstructions based on biplanar radiographs. European Radiology. 2017;**27**(3):1295-1302

[38] Nobuhiko S, Takao M, Sakai T. Does CT-based navigation improve the long-term survival in ceramic-on-ceramic THA? Clinical Orthopaedics and Related Research. 2012;**470**(11):3054-3059

[39] Iwanna D, Nakamura N, Miki H. Accuracy of angle and position of the cup using computed tomography-based navigation systems in total hip arthroplasty. Computer Aided Surgery. 2013;**18**:187-194

[40] Yamada K, Endo H, Tetsunaga T. Accuracy of cup positioning with the computed tomography-based two-dimensional to three-dimensional matched navigation system: A prospective, randomized controlled study. The Journal of Arthroplasty. 2018;**33**:136-143

[41] Nakahara I, Kyo T, Kuroda Y. Effect of improved navigation performance on the accuracy of implant placement in total hip arthroplasty with a CT-based navigation system. Journal of Artificial Organs. 2018;**21**(3):340-347

[42] Paprosky WG, Muir JM. Intellijoint HIP: A 3D mini-optical navigation tool for improving intraoperative accuracy

during total HIP arthroplasty. Medical Devices: Evidence and Research. 2016;**9**:401-408

[43] Kurmis AP. Anterior pelvic roll during primary total hip arthroplasty in the lateral decubitus position: A systematic review. Journal of Orthopaedic Surgery. 2022 [In press]

[44] Beverland DE, O'Neill CKJ, Rutherford M, Molloy D, Hill JC. Placement of the acetabular component. Bone & Joint Journal. 2016;**98-B** (1 Suppl. A):37-43

[45] Daines BK, Dennis DA. The importance of acetabular component position in total hip arthroplasty. The Orthopedic Clinics of North America. 2012;**43**(5):e23-e34

[46] Grammatopoulos G, Gofton W, Cochran M, Dobransky J, Carli A, Abdelbary H, et al. Pelvic positioning in the supine position leads to more consistent orientation of the acetabular component after total hip arthroplasty. Bone & Joint Journal. 2018;**100-B**(10):1280-1288

[47] Peters FM, Greeff R, Goldstein N, Frey CT. Improving acetabular cup orientation in total hip arthroplasty by using smartphone technology. The Journal of Arthroplasty. 2012;**27**(7):1324-1330

[48] Attenello JD, Harpstrite JK. Implications of spinopelvic mobility on total hip arthroplasty: Review of current literature. Hawai'i Journal of Health & Social Welfare. 2019;**78**(11 Suppl 2):31-40

[49] Shon WY, Sharma V, Keon OJ, Moon JG, Suh DH. Can pelvic tilting be ignored in total hip arthroplasty? International Journal of Surgery Case Reports. 2014;**5**(9):633-636

[50] Pierrepont J, Hawdon G, Miles BP, O'Connor B, Baré J, Walter LR, et al. Variation in functional pelvic tilt in patients undergoing total hip arthroplasty. Bone & Joint Journal. 2017;**99-B**(2):184-191

[51] Blondel B, Parratte S, Tropiano P, Pauly V, Aubaniac JM, Argenson JN. Pelvic tilt measurement before and after total hip arthroplasty. Orthopaedics & Traumatology, Surgery & Research. 2009;**95**(8):568-572

[52] Mellano CR, Spitzer AI. How does pelvic rotation or tilt affect radiographic measurement of acetabular component inclination angle during THA? Journal of Orthopaedics. 2015;**12**(4):222-227

[53] Kyo T, Nakahara I, Miki H. Factors predicting change in pelvic posterior tilt after THA. Orthopedics. 2013;**36**(6):e753-e759

[54] Lembeck B, Mueller O, Reize P, Wuelker N. Pelvic tilt makes acetabular cup navigation inaccurate. Acta Orthopaedica. 2005;**76**(4):517-523

[55] Babisch JW, Layher F, Amiot LP. The rationale for tilt-adjusted acetabular cup navigation. Journal of Bone and Joint Surgery. American Volume. 2008;**90**(2):357-365

[56] Maratt JD, Esposito CI, McLawhorn AS, Jerabek SA, Padgett DE, Mayman DJ. Pelvic tilt in patients undergoing total hip arthroplasty: When does it matter? The Journal of Arthroplasty. 2015;**30**(3):387-391

[57] Langston J, Pierrepont J, Gu Y, Shimmin A. Risk factors for increased sagittal pelvic motion causing unfavourable orientation of the acetabular component in patients undergoing total hip arthroplasty. Bone & Joint Journal. 2018;**100-B**(7):845-852

[58] Heckmann N, McKnight B, Stefl M, Trasolini NA, Ike H, Dorr LD. Late dislocation following total hip arthroplasty: Spinopelvic imbalance as a causative factor. Journal of Bone and Joint Surgery. American Volume. 2018;**100**(21):1845-1853

[59] Kurmis AP. CORR insights: Is isolated mobile component exchange an option in the management of intraprosthetic dislocation of a dual mobility cup? Clinical Orthopaedics and Related Research. 2020;**478**:288-289

[60] Stefl M, Lundergan W, Heckmann N, McKnight B, Ike H, Murgai R, et al. Spinopelvic mobility and acetabular component position for total hip arthroplasty. Bone & Joint Journal. 2017;**99-B**(1 Supple A):37-45

[61] DelSole EM, Vigdorchik JM, Schwarzkopf R, Errico TJ, Buckland AJ. Total hip arthroplasty in the spinal deformity population: Does degree of sagittal deformity affect rates of safe zone placement, instability, or revision? The Journal of Arthroplasty. 2017;**32**:1910-1917

[62] Ike H, Dorr LD, Trasolini N, Stefl M, McKnight B, Heckmann N. Spine-pelvis-hip relationship in the functioning of a total hip replacement. Journal of Bone and Joint Surgery. American Volume. 2018;**100**:1606-1615

[63] Kleeman-Forsthuber LT, Elkins JM, Miner TM, Yang CC, Jennings JM, Dennis DA. Reliability of spinopelvic measurements that may influence the cup position in total hip arthroplasty. The Journal of Arthroplasty. 2020;**35**(12):3758-3764

[64] Lazennec JY, Rousseau MA, Rangel A, Gorin M, Belicourt C, Brusson A, et al. Pelvis and total hip arthroplasty acetabular component orientations in sitting and standing positions: Measurements reproductibility with EOS imaging system versus conventional radiographies. Orthopaedics & Traumatology, Surgery & Research. 2011;**97**(4):373-380

[65] Illés T, Somoskeöy S. The EOS™ imaging system and its uses in daily orthopaedic practice. International Orthopaedics. 2012;**36**(7):1325-1331

[66] Innmann MM, McGoldrick NP, Ratra A, Merle C, Grammatopoulos G. The accuracy in determining pelvic tilt from anteroposterior pelvic radiographs in patients awaiting hip arthroplasty. Journal of Orthopaedic Research. 2021;**40**(4):854-861

[67] McMahon SE, Magill P, Bopf DP, Beverland DE. A device to make the pelvic sagittal plane horizontal and reduce error in cup inclination during total hip arthroplasty: A validation study. Hip International. 2018;**28**(5):473-477

[68] Rutherford M, O'Connor JD, Gill HS, Hill J, Beverland D, Lennon AB, et al. Operative and radiographic acetabular component orientation in total hip replacement: Influence of pelvic orientation and surgical positioning technique. Medical Engineering & Physics. 2019;**64**:7-14

[69] Billaud A, Verdier N, de Bartolo R, Lavoinne N, Chauveaux D, Fabre T. Acetabular component navigation in lateral decubitus based on EOS imaging: A preliminary study of 13 cases. Orthopaedics & Traumatology, Surgery & Research. 2015;**101**(3):271-275

[70] Carcangiu A, D'Arrigo C, Topa D, Alonzo R, Speranza A, De Sanctis S, et al. Reliability of cup position in navigated THA in the lateral decubitus position

using the 'flip technique'. Hip International. 2011;**21**(6):700-705

[71] Rousseau M-A, Lazennec JY, Boyer P, Mora N, Gorin M, Catonné Y. Optimization of total hip arthroplasty implantation: Is the anterior pelvic plane concept valid? The Journal of Arthroplasty. 2009;**24**(1):22-26

[72] Dandachli W, Richards R, Sauret V, Cobb JP. The transverse pelvic plane: A new and practical reference frame for hip arthroplasty. Computer Aided Surgery. 2006;**11**(6):322-326

[73] Beckmann J, Lüring C, Tingart M, Anders S, Grifka J, Köck FX. Cup positioning in THA: Current status and pitfalls. A systematic evaluation of the literature. Archives of Orthopaedic and Trauma Surgery. 2009;**129**(7):863-872

[74] Kanazawa M, Nakashima Y, Ohishi M, Hamai S, Motomura G, Yamamoto T, et al. Pelvic tilt and movement during total hip arthroplasty in the lateral decubitus position. Modern Rheumatology. 2016;**26**(3):435-440

[75] Milone MT, Schwarzkopf R, Meere PA, Carroll KM, Jerabek SA, Vigdorchik J. Rigid patient positioning is unreliable in total hip arthroplasty. The Journal of Arthroplasty. 2017;**32**(6):1890-1893

[76] Grammatopoulos G, Pandit HG, da Assunção R, Taylor A, McLardy-Smith P, De Smet KA, et al. Pelvic position and movement during hip replacement. Bone & Joint Journal. 2014;**96-B**(7):876-883

[77] Rutherford M, O'Connor JD, Hill JC, Beverland DE, Lennon AB, Dunne NJ. Patient positioning and cup orientation during total hip arthroplasty: Assessment of current UK practice. Hip International. 2019;**29**(1):89-95

[78] Iwakiri K, Kobayashi A, Ohta Y, Takaoka K. Efficacy of the anatomical-pelvic-plane positioner in total hip arthroplasty in the lateral decubitus position. The Journal of Arthroplasty. 2017;**32**(5):1520-1524

[79] Nishikubo Y, Fujioka M, Ueshima K, Saito M, Kubo T. Preoperative fluoroscopic imaging reduces variability of acetabular component positioning. The Journal of Arthroplasty. 2011;**26**(7):1088-1094

[80] Lambers P, Jennings R, Bucknill AT. A novel fluoroscopic approach to assessing patient positioning in total hip arthroplasty: Accuracy and the influence of body mass index. Hip International. 2016;**26**(6):550-553

[81] Kurmis AP. CORR insights: Statistical methods dictate the estimated impact of body mass index on major and minor complications after total joint arthroplasty. Clinical Orthopaedics and Related Research. 2018;**476**:2430-2431

[82] Della Valle AG, Shanaghan K, Benson JR, Carroll K, Cross M, McLawhorn A, et al. Pelvic pitch and roll during total hip arthroplasty performed through a posterolateral approach. A potential source of error in free-hand cup positioning. International Orthopaedics. 2019;**43**(8):1823-1829

[83] Otero JE, Fehring KA, Martin JR, Odum SM, Fehring TK. Variability of pelvic orientation in the lateral decubitus position: Are external alignment guides trustworthy? The Journal of Arthroplasty. 2018;**33**(11):3496-3501

[84] Brodt S, Nowack D, Jacob B, Krakow L, Windisch C, Matziolis G. Patient obesity influences pelvic lift during cup insertion in total hip arthroplasty through a lateral transgluteal approach

in supine position. The Journal of Arthroplasty. 2017;**32**(9):2762-2767

[85] Ueno T, Kabata T, Kajino Y, Inoue D, Ohmori T, Yoshitani J, et al. Risk factors for pressure ulcers from the use of a pelvic positioner in hip surgery: A retrospective observational cohort study in 229 patients. Patient Safety in Surgery. 2020;**14**:10

[86] Somerville CM, Geddes JA, Tofighi M, Boddu K. Accuracy and reproducibility of visual estimation of the acetabular cup positioning in total hip arthroplasty on plain radiographs by orthopaedic surgeons. Journal of Perioperative Practice. August 16, 2021:17504589211026074. DOI: 10.1177/17504589211026074

[87] Chen E, Goertz W, Lill CA. Implant position calculation for acetabular cup placement considering pelvic lateral tilt and inclination. Computer Aided Surgery. 2006;**11**(6):309-316

[88] Epstein NJ, Woolson ST, Giori NJ. Acetabular component positioning using the transverse acetabular ligament: Can you find it and does it help? Clinical Orthopaedics and Related Research. 2011;**469**(2):412-416

[89] Schloemann DT, Edelstein AI, Barrack RL. Changes in acetabular orientation during total hip arthroplasty. Bone & Joint Journal. 2019;**101-B**(6_Supple_B):45-50

[90] Seo H, Naito M, Nakamura Y, Kinoshita K, Nomura T, Minokawa S, et al. New cross-table lateral radiography method for measuring acetabular component anteversion in total hip arthroplasty: A prospective study of 93 primary THA. Hip International. 2017;**27**(3):293-298

[91] Hayakawa K, Minoda Y, Aihara M, Sakawa A, Ohzono K, Tada K. Acetabular component orientation in intra- and postoperative positions in total hip arthroplasty. Archives of Orthopaedic and Trauma Surgery. 2009;**129**(9):1151-1156

[92] Tanino H, Nishida Y, Mitsutake R, Ito H. Portable accelerometer-based navigation system for cup placement of total hip arthroplasty: A prospective, randomized, controlled study. Journal of Arthroplasty. 2020;**35**(1):172-177

[93] Parvizi J, Benson J, Muir J. A new mini-navigation tool allows accurate component placement during anterior total hip arthroplasty. Medical Devices: Evidence and Research. 2018;**11**:95-104

[94] Tanino H, Nishida Y, Mitsutake R, Ito H. Accuracy of a portable accelerometer-based navigation system for cup placement and intraoperative leg length measurement in total hip arthroplasty: A cross-sectional study. BMC Musculoskeletal Disorders. 2021;**22**(1):299

[95] Asai H, Takegami Y, Seki T, Ishiguro N. Pelvic tilt reduces the accuracy of acetabular component placement when using a portable navigation system: An in vitro study. Arthroplasty Today. 2021;**7**:177-181

[96] Cross MB, Schwarzkopf R, Miller TT, Bogner EA, Muir JM, Vigdorchik JM. Improving registration accuracy during total hip arthroplasty: A cadaver study of a new, 3-D mini-optical navigation system. Hip International. 2018;**28**(1):33-39

[97] Mei XY, Etemad-Rezaie A, Safir OA, Gross AE, Kuzyk PR. Intraoperative measurement of acetabular component position using imageless navigation during revision total hip arthroplasty. Canadian Journal of Surgery. 2020;**64**(4):442-448

[98] Vigdorchik JM, Sculco PK, Inglis AE, Schwarzkopf R, Muir JM. Evaluating alternate registration planes for imageless, computer-assisted navigation during total hip arthroplasty. The Journal of Arthroplasty. 2021;**36**(10):3527-3533

[99] Jolles BM, Genoud P, Hoffmeyer P. Computer-assisted cup placement techniques in total hip arthroplasty improve accuracy of placement. Clinical Orthopaedics and Related Research. 2004;**426**:174-179

[100] Tsukamoto M, Kawasaki M, Suzuki H, Fujitani T, Sakai A. Proposal of accurate cup placement procedure during total hip arthroplasty based on pelvic tilt discrepancies in the lateral position. Scientific Reports. 2021;**11**(1):13870

[101] Kurmis AP. Retained pelvic pin site debris after navigated THA: Masquerading as an early-stage chondrosarcomatous lesion. Journal of Postgraduate Medicine. 2020;**66**(4):215-217

[102] Tetsunaga T, Yamada K, Tetsunaga T, Furumatsu T, Sanki T, Kawamura Y, et al. Comparison of the accuracy of CT- and accelerometer-based navigation systems for cup orientation in total hip arthroplasty. Hip International. 2021;**31**(5):603-608

[103] Iwakiri K, Kobayashi A, Ohta Y, Minoda Y, Takaoka K, Nakamura H. Efficacy of a pelvic lateral positioner with a mechanical cup navigator based on the anatomical pelvic plane in total hip arthroplasty. The Journal of Arthroplasty. 2017;**32**(12):3659-3664

[104] Sheridan GA, Hanlon M, Welch-Phillips A, Spratt K, Hagan R, O'Byrne JM, et al. Identification of protective and 'at risk' HLA genotypes for the development of pseudotumours around hip resurfacings—A case-control study. Journal of Arthroplasty. 2022 [In press]

[105] Eilander W, Harris SJ, Henkus HE, Cobb JP, Hogervorst T. Functional acetabular component position with supine total hip replacement. Bone & Joint Journal. 2013;**95-B**(10):1326-1331

[106] Tiberi JV, Pulos N, Kertzner M, Schmalzried TP. A more reliable method to assess acetabular component position. Clinical Orthopaedics and Related Research. 2012;**470**(2):471-476

[107] Yang G, Li Y, Zhang H. The influence of pelvic tilt on the anteversion angle of the acetabular prosthesis. Orthopaedic Surgery. 2019;**11**(5):762-769

[108] Foissey C, Batailler C, Fary C, Luceri F, Servien E, Lustig S. Transitioning the total hip arthroplasty technique from posterior approach in lateral position to direct anterior approach in supine position-risk factors for acetabular malpositioning and the learning curve. International Orthopaedics. 2020;**44**(9):1669-1676

[109] Goyal P, Lau A, Naudie DD, Teeter MG, Lanting BA, Howard JL. Effect of acetabular component positioning on functional outcomes in primary total hip arthroplasty. The Journal of Arthroplasty. 2017;**32**(3):843-848

[110] O'Neill CKJ, Hill JC, Patterson CC, Molloy DO, Gill HS, Beverland DE. Reducing variability in apparent operative inclination during total hip arthroplasty: Findings of a randomised controlled trial. Hip International. 2018;**28**(3):234-239

[111] Zhu J, Wan Z, Dorr LD. Quantification of pelvic tilt in total hip arthroplasty. Clinical Orthopaedics and Related Research. 2010;**468**(2):571-575

[112] Xu J, Su B, Zhang W, Sun H, Li D, Cai Z, et al. 3D simulation of radiographic projections to test and reduce the effect of pelvic tilt on the accuracy of cross-table lateral radiography. BMC Musculoskeletal Disorders. 2020;**21**(1):843

[113] Sharma AK, Cizmic Z, Dennis DA, Kreuzer SW, Miranda MA, Vigdorchik JM. Low dislocation rates with the use of patient specific "safe zones" in total hip arthroplasty. Journal of Orthopaedics. 2021;**27**:41-48

[114] Hill JC, Gibson DP, Pagoti R, Beverland DE. Photographic measurement of the inclination of the acetabular component in total hip replacement using the posterior approach. Journal of Bone and Joint Surgery. British Volume (London). 2010;**92**(9):1209-1214

[115] O'Neill CKJ, Magill P, Hill JC, Patterson CC, Molloy DO, Gill HS, et al. Correction of pelvic adduction during total hip arthroplasty reduces variability in radiographic inclination: Findings of a randomised controlled trial. Hip International. 2018;**28**(3):240-245

[116] Woerner M, Weber M, Sendtner E, Springorum R, Worlicek M, Craiovan B, et al. Soft tissue restricts impingement-free mobility in total hip arthroplasty. International Orthopaedics. 2017;**41**(2):277-282

[117] Kishimura Y, Minoda Y, Mizokawa S, Sugama R, Ohta Y, Nakamura H. Cup alignment in total hip arthroplasty using the muscle-sparing modified Watson-Jones approach-comparison between lateral and supine positions. International Orthopaedics. 2019;**43**(11):2477-2483

[118] Davda K, Smyth N, Cobb JP, Hart AJ. 2D measurements of cup orientation are less reliable than 3D measurements. Acta Orthopaedica. 2015;**86**(4):485-490

[119] Malik A, Jain N, Scharschmidt TJ, Li M, Glassman AH, Khan SN. Does surgeon volume affect outcomes following primary total hip arthroplasty? A systematic review. Journal of Arthroplasty. 2018;**33**:3329-3342

[120] Kurmis AP. Orthopaedic utilisation of three-dimensional image displays reconstructed from magnetic resonance imaging. The Radiographer. 2002;**49**(2):67-71

[121] Kurmis AP. The developing role of knee MRI in musculo-skeletal radiology: The progression to 3-D imaging. The Radiographer. 2001;**48**(1):21-28

[122] Kurmis AP, Slavotinek JP. Reconstructed three-dimensional MR images: Application to simulated tibial plateau depression fractures. Radiography. 2004;**10**(2):95-101

[123] Kurmis AP, Hearn TC, Grimmer K, Reynolds KJ. Dimensional measurement of structural features of the ovine knee using three-dimensional reconstructed imaging: Intra- and inter-observer repeatability. Radiography. 2004;**10**(4):269-276

[124] Kurmis AP, Ianunzio JR. Artificial intelligence in orthopaedic surgery: Evolution, current state and future directions. Art. 2022;**4**(1):9

[125] Zhou Y, Shao H, Huang Y, Deng W, Yang D, Bian T. Does robotic assisted technology improve the accuracy of acetabular component positioning in patients with DDH? Journal of Orthopaedic Surgery (Hong Kong). 2021;**29**(2):23094990211025325

Section 3

Knee Arthroplasty

Chapter 6

Total Knee Arthroplasty in Valgus Knee

Alessandro Rozim Zorzi, Wander Edney de Brito, Gustavo Constantino de Campos and João Batista de Miranda

Abstract

Total knee arthroplasty in valgus knee deformities continues to be a challenge. It comprises only 10% of patients who undergo total knee arthroplasty. The surgeon should be aware of the technical aspects that differentiate it from the varus deformity: surgical exposure, bone cuts, ligament balancing, gap balancing, joint line obliquity, patellar tracking, preserving fibular nerve function, and selection of the implant. The aim of this chapter is to provide step-by-step comprehensive knowledge about different surgical techniques for the correction of severe valgus deformity in total knee arthroplasty.

Keywords: knee, arthroplasty, deformity, valgus, prosthesis

1. Introduction

Valgus deformity of the knee occurs in the presence of a valgus alignment of the anatomical axes of the femur and tibia in the frontal plane greater than 10° [1]. Although osteoarthritis is the most common pathology related to this deformity in adults, other events and diseases, such as post-traumatic deformities, rickets, renal osteodystrophy, inflammatory pathologies such as rheumatoid arthritis, systemic lupus erythematous, psoriatic arthritis, or even hemophilic arthropathy are commonly associated [2].

Valgus deformity accounts for approximately 20% of the patients undergoing total knee arthroplasty (TKA) and can impose some challenges for the knee surgeon [1]. Proper coronal deformity correction is widely accepted as crucial for the success of a TKA [3]. It is recognized that the correction of a valgus deformity has technical particularities that need to be recognized by the knee surgeon when performing a TKA. It comprises surgical approach, bone cuts, and mostly ligament balance [1, 2, 4].

2. Preoperative evaluation

Patients diagnosed with end-stage primary or secondary osteoarthritis or other inflammatory arthritis, with refractory pain and loss of function that impair daily live activities, having failed conservative therapy, are elected to undergo TKA. It is important to emphasize that only a bad radiograph does not constitute an indication for arthroplasty.

A complete medical history, associated with a general medical examination, should be performed to rule out conditions and comorbidities that may contraindicate the procedure.

Every candidate should be clinically evaluated for weight-bearing alignment, flexion contracture, and ligamentous instability. Preoperative radiological assessment includes:

- weight-bearing anteroposterior view;
- stress radiographs in valgus and varus;
- lateral view;
- axial patellar view;
- limb axis deviation with long-standing views of the knee for overall coronal mechanical axis alignment;
- Nowadays, with the increase in the number of robotic surgeries and customized prostheses, especially in the knee, CT scans of the hip, knee, and ankle are also needed.

3. Classification

Many authors have proposed ways of classifying valgus deformities of the knee for the purpose of surgical correction with TKA. The idea is to stratify the patients in order to improve the surgical planning and the choice of the degree of constriction of the implants.

The Krakow classification [5] proposed in 1991 is one of the most famous classifications. It categorizes valgus knees based on the integrity of the medial soft tissues and on prior surgeries. Type 1 deformity has an intact medial collateral ligament (MCL). Type 2 has an insufficiency of the MCL with positive valgus stress test. Type 3 is a secondary valgus deformity created by an overcorrected high tibial osteotomy (HTO) in a previously varus-aligned limb.

The SOO classification, presented in 2003 (Societe d'Orthopedie de l'Ouest - Western France Orthopedics Society), recognizes four types of valgus knee, with increasing surgical difficulty. Type I can be completely reduced, without medial laxity. Type II is totally or partially irreducible, but without medial laxity. Lateral release is required, whereas Type III is reducible, but with medial distension laxity, and may require management of the medial laxity. Lastly, Type IV is irreducible, with medial distension laxity, combining the problems of types II and III [6].

Lombardi et al. in 2004 [7] proposed a slight modification of the Krakow classification, taking into account the degree of deformity, the status of the MCL, and the amount of release that must be performed. Variant I is characterized by mild deficiencies of the lateral femoral condyle and tibial plateau, with stable MCL and correction of the deformity with varus stress. In variant-II, the MCLs are intact, but they do not correct to neutral alignment with varus stress. Variant-III is distinguished by attenuation of the medial capsular ligament complex with opening of the medial joint line on valgus stress test.

Ranawat et al. in 2005 [1] added one more small modification, merging the previous classifications, adding the measure of the magnitude of the deformity to the Krakow classification. A type-I deformity has minimal valgus and medial soft-tissue stretching. A typical type-II fixed valgus deformity has a more substantial deformity (>10°) with medial soft-tissue stretching. A type-III deformity is a severe osseous deformity after a prior osteotomy with an incompetent medial soft-tissue sleeve.

Despite being widely used, the Krakow and the Ranawat classifications were designed with patients from developed countries, where most cases have minor deformities. In poorer countries, where the population has greater difficulty in accessing surgical treatment, there is a greater prevalence of severe cases and complex deformities. Therefore, new classifications have been proposed to better stratify severe cases.

In 2014, Mulaji et al. [8] proposed a classification into six types: type 1 reducible valgus, type 2 irreducible valgus, type 3 valgus associated with recurvatum, type 4 valgus associated with flexion contracture, type 5 valgus with MCL insufficiency, and type 6 extra-articular valgus.

Based on full-leg weight-bearing radiographs of 233 knees, the study of Mulaji et al. [9] identified four broad groups of valgus arthritic knees with nine phenotypes based on coronal plane variations in femoral and tibial morphology. Type 1 Neutral knees (12.5%) had almost normal values. Type 2 "Intra-articular valgus" (22.7%) showed lateral compartment bone loss. Type 3 "Extra-articular valgus" (35.2%) had extra-articular deformity: 3a showed valgus femoral bowing; 3b showed tibial valgus bowing; 3c showed tibial valgus bowing with lateral femoral condyle wear. Type 4 "Varus" type (29.6%) had features of varus knees: 4a had varus femoral bowing; distal femur in 4b was akin to varus knees with lateral tibial bone loss. 4c had varus tibial bowing and deficient lateral femoral condyle. 4d had varus tibial bowing and lateral tibial bone loss.

Yang et al. in 2021 [10] made deformity analysis on standing long-film radiographs and computed tomography (CT). Valgus deformities could be classified into five subtypes: the distal lateral femoral condyle (F1a), both distal and posterior lateral femoral condyle (F1b), the supracondylar region of the femur (F2), the tibial plateau (T1), or the metaphyseal segment of the tibia (T2). F2 and T1 (40.0% and 28.6%, respectively) were the most common two subtypes.

4. Surgical technique

4.1 Surgical approach

4.1.1 Anteromedial approach

As 90% of knee arthroplasties are associated with varus deformity, the anteromedial approach is more frequently practiced by surgeons. Therefore, even in valgus deformities, most surgeons opt for the anteromedial approach.

The advantage of this approach is that it allows a wide view of the joint cavity and does not require any additional training by the surgeon.

The disadvantage of this approach is that it does not directly address the lateral contracture structures. In cases of mild deformity, Ranawat grade 1, small surgical gestures such as releasing the iliotibial band (ITB) and pie crusting the lateral capsule may be sufficient. In developed countries in Europe and North America, this is perhaps the majority of cases. But in Latin American, African, and Asian countries, severe cases classified as Ranawat grade 2 or 3 are frequent. To correct these major deformities, the medial approach can cause problems not only with ligament balance, but mainly with patellar tracking.

To compare the clinical and radiological outcomes of anteromedial and anterolateral approaches for valgus TKA, a pilot randomized clinical trial evaluated the radiographic patellar tilt, the visual analog scale of pain, postoperative levels of hemoglobin, and clinical aspect of the operative wound. Mean lateral tilt of the patella was 3.1° (SD ± 5.3) in the lateral approach group and 18° (SD ± 10.2) in the medial approach group ($p = 0.02$). There were no differences regarding other outcomes [4].

In severe deformities, release of lateral patellar retinaclum is necessary in most cases in order to prevent patellar instability. Lateral release in combination with medial capsulotomy results in significant impairment of the extensor mechanism blood supply and could cause avascular necrosis of the patela [11].

4.1.2 Anterolateral approach

The anterolateral approach proposed by Keblish in 1991 allows for a better exposure of the lateral and posterolateral structures, which are contracted in valgus deformities and should be released for proper ligament balance; it also has the advantage of including the release of lateral patellar retinaculum, which is necessary in most cases with valgus deformity [12].

After proper preparation and placement of drapes and with the knee positioned at 90°, the technique begins with the skin incision, which must follow the direction of the deformity (so that at the end of the procedure and consequent correction of the deformity, the incision is straight). An incision between 15 and 20 centimeters is usually sufficient, starting over the superior pole of the patella, going to the anterior tibial tuberosity (ATT) (laterally). Skin and subcutaneous tissue should be detached together and to a sufficient extent just to access the lateral border of the patella, avoiding unnecessary tissue damage. The arthrotomy is performed starting at the center of the quadriceps tendon, going down the lateral border of the patella, to the lateral border of the ATT. It is essential to maintain Hoffa's fat connected by its pedicle to the lateral portion of the capsule, as this tissue will be necessary for its closure. Nikolopoulos et al. in 2015 provided a detailed description of the lateral approach technique, along with its advantages and disadvantages [6].

As in the classic medial arthrotomy, in which the deep medial collateral is released as part of the approach, we recommend, in the lateral approach, desperiostization of the lateral portion of the tibia, thus detaching the distal insertion of the iliotibial tract from the tubercle of Gerdy. This step already releases one of the three major soft tissue structures involved in valgus deformity (the other two being the lateral collateral ligament and the popliteal tendon). In cases of mild and reducible deformity, this already resolves the ligament balance. For this reason, we strongly believe that the indication of the lateral approach is advantageous even in milder cases, solving at the same time the ligament balance and patellar tracking.

Exposing the tibia is actually a little more difficult with this access. This is mainly due to the fact that the TAT is lateralized, which opens a smaller window of vision (the space between the TAT and the lateral collateral is much smaller than the space between the TAT and the medial collateral). For the same reason, patellar eversion is a more difficult maneuver to perform, which makes the exposure of the tibia more difficult. We recommend spending a little more time on this step for adequate exposure of the tibia and consequent correct understanding of the structures and their relationships.

Keblish's original description includes an anterior tibial tubercle osteotomy (ATT) for further exposure. We do not believe it to be necessary in the vast majority of cases. However, in certain situations such as in severe valgus knees or after a previous tibial osteotomy, patella's eversion may be compromised and the patellar ligament may be particularly prone to spontaneous avulsion by forceful retraction, especially if patella cannot be everted with the knee flexed at 90°. In these situations, the surgeon should not hesitate to perform an ATT. This is a safe and effective procedure. It also may simplify proper positioning of the tibial component in severe valgus knees, avoiding internal rotation of the tibial component. However, careful fixation of the tuberosity is mandatory [11].

4.2 Soft tissue balancing

The goal of ligament balance is to achieve symmetrical rectangular extension and flexion gaps. This can be achieved through several techniques, summarized in just two main philosophies: "Mesaured ressection" and "Gap balancing." Gap balancing relies on ligament releases prior to bone cuts. There are basically two gap balancing sequences. One relies on balancing the flex gap first, and the other technique initially balances the knee in extension. On the other hand, bony landmarks such as the transepicondylar axis and the posterior condylar axis are used to set femoral component rotation when using a measured resection technique. Bone cuts are initially made independent of soft tissue tension.

Regardless of the philosophy used, gap balancing, or measured resection or a combination of both, in general we can say that the ligament balance of valgus deformity depends on the release of tense lateral structures and the tensioning of attenuated medial structures. Unfortunately, many authors have described several sequences for the serial release of these structures, and there is still no consensus on the best technique.

4.2.1 Release of lateral structures

Ligaments can be released through pie-crusting, subperiosteal release, transverse section, or osteotomy. Unfortunately, there is no consensus among the authors on a sequence for carrying out the releases. The releases should be performed in full extension, by using spreaders to check the tension of the medial and lateral compartments. After each release, the surgeon should evaluate the alignment and the stability of the knee, in order to achieve a symmetrical rectangular extension and flexion gaps [6].

Krackow et al. [5] advocate the release of the ilio tibial band (ITB), followed by the lateral colateral ligament (LCL), next by the posterolateral corner structures (PLC) and the gastrocnemius muscle lateral head (LHG).

Buechel [13] presented a sequential three-step lateral release, which included elevation: (1) the ITB from Gerdy's tubercle; (2) the LCL and popliteous tendon (POP); and (3) the entire periosteum of the fibular head.

Ranawat et al. [1] described a stepwise technique in which the first structure to be released is the posterior cruciate ligament (PCL). When necessary, the ITB and the LCL are released with multiple stab incisions, the so-called "pie-crusting" technique. The POP is normally preserved.

Favorito et al. [14] proposed that LCL is the first structure to be released. The next sequential release follows the POP (an important structure for rotational and valgus stability in flexion), the PLC, the femoral insertion of the LHG, and finally, the ITB.

Whiteside [15] described a release sequence based on the tension of ligaments in flexion and extension: For tight knees both in flexion and extension, the LCL and POP tendon are released. For those knees, tightness remains in extension and only ITB is released. Posterior capsular release is performed only when necessary for persistent lateral tightness.

An alternative technique for lateral structure release was described by Brilhault et al. [16]. A sliding osteotomy of the lateral epicondyle contains LCL and POP insertions.

4.2.2 Tensioning of medial structures

As described by Krackow et al. [17], when the MCL is attenuated and there is a residual medial laxity, the authors suggest tightening of the medial structures. The advancement of the MCL from the epicondyle or a division and imbrication in order to tighten, it can be performed.

4.2.3 The fibular nerve dilemma

Fibular nerve palsy (FNP) is a feared complication after valgus TKA. The reported incidence of FNP after valgus TKA in the literature ranges between 0.3% and 9.5%. Injury of the Fibular nerve can be caused by indirect damage due to stretch or ischemia after correction, or by direct injury due to laceration during lateral soft tissue release. As FNP has serious consequences, some orthopedic surgeons advocate to prevent this complication by a concomitant fibular nerve release (FNR). Due to the limited number of studies investigating FNR, no consensus has yet been reached on the value and indication of the procedure. A systematic review demonstrated no significant differences in FNP rate between valgus TKA with and without FNR (2.4% vs 2.1%) [18]. Therefore, the authors of this chapter do not recommend the routine use of FNR.

4.3 Bone resection

Valgus deformity has particularities that need to be recognized so that bone cuts can be made properly. In most cases, the origin of the deformity is located in the distal femur, as opposed to the varus deformity. Lateral condyle hypoplasia is frequently present and needs to be recognized, as it directly interferes with several parameters of femoral bone cuts. A smaller number of cases may have lateral tibial plateau sinking, either due to fracture sequelae or in very advanced cases with deformity > 20° and MCL insufficiency.

Extra-articular deformities such as external torsion of the tibia and remodeling with valgus deviation of the femoral and tibial shafts may also coexist [19].

4.3.1 Tibial resection

We recommend that the first bone cut is the tibial one, parallel to the ground. The main reason is that we can use the tibia as a parameter for the posterior cut of the femur through the gap balancing technique, in which the cut is performed parallel to the tibial cut with the knee at 90° under symmetrical soft tissue tension. This is important because, due to hypoplasia of the lateral condyle, we cannot rely on the classic parameter of 3° of external rotation in relation to the posterior condyles, which will be discussed later.

A marked valgus deformity of the tibial diaphysis is frequently observed in valgus knee, which makes it impossible to use an intramedullary guide for the tibia in most cases. Therefore, we recommend the use of the extramedullary guide for all cases. In addition, tibial cutting guides are usually sided (left or right). In these cases, it will be necessary to use the guide on the opposite side. Another important detail of this step is the amount of bone to be cut. Traditionally, in varus knee prosthesis, 9–10 mm of bone can be removed using the healthy plateau as a parameter. However, the healthy tibial plateau in valgus knee is the medial plateau. It turns out that the medial plateau is 3 mm more distal than the lateral plateau. Therefore, we must discount this 3 mm when making the cut, otherwise we will inadvertenltly cut more tibia than ideal. Therefore, make the tibial cut 6 or 7 mm from the medial plateau.

4.3.2 Femural resection

Next, we will make the distal cut of the femur. Instead of the 7° of valgus traditionally used in varus knees, we used 5° in the distal cut of the femur, in order not to under-correct the deformity. The surgeon may also choose to use the exact difference

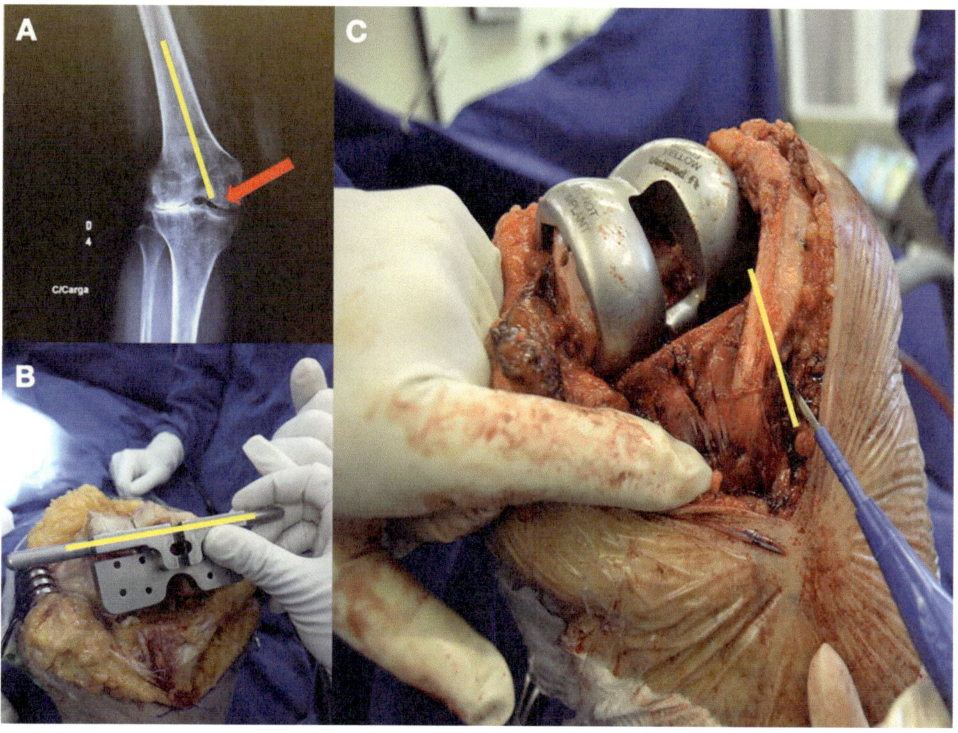

Figure 1.
Tips and tricks for appropriate bone resection in valgus TKA. (A) Weight-bearing knee radiography demonstrating lateral condyle hypoplasia and the adjusted entry point for IM guide at the medial condyle (red arrow), in the prolongation of the anatomical axis of the femur; (B) determination of the rotation of the femoral component by the Whiteside line (yellow), parallel to the transepicondylar axis. Do not use the support guide on the posterior condyles; (C) When determining the rotation of the tibial component, 1 centimeter medial to the TTA, the less experienced surgeon with the Keblish approach must be careful because the tibia is being viewed "in a mirror."

measured between the anatomical and mechanical axis of the femur in the preoperative panoramic X-ray. Caution should be taken with the entry point of the intramedular guide. Because of hypoplasia of the lateral femoral condyle, the entry point must be medialized, sometimes not above the intercondylar notch as usually done in varus cases, but in the medial femural condyle.

Regarding the adjustment of the femoral rotation, one more point of attention: The existence of hypoplasia of the lateral femoral condyle is very common. Therefore, the use of a guide based on the posterior condylar line will incur in excessive internal rotation of the femoral component. If the technique used is measured resection that considers the anatomical points, the correct way is to base it on the trans-epicondylar axis or on the Whiteside line. An alternative, as already described, is to use the gap balancing technique in this step.

Figure 1 brings some tips and tricks to keep in mind as they are common causes of errors.

4.4 Implant choice

Some surgeons consider it inappropriate or almost impossible to preserve the posterior cruciate ligament (PCL) in severe valgus deformities. The use of intramedullary nails and implants with revision concepts is also frequently indicated by some surgeons whenever they are faced with a severe valgus deformity [19]. But what is the logical reasoning that should guide the choice of implant? **Figure 2** shows the algorithm for implant choice in valgus TKAs.

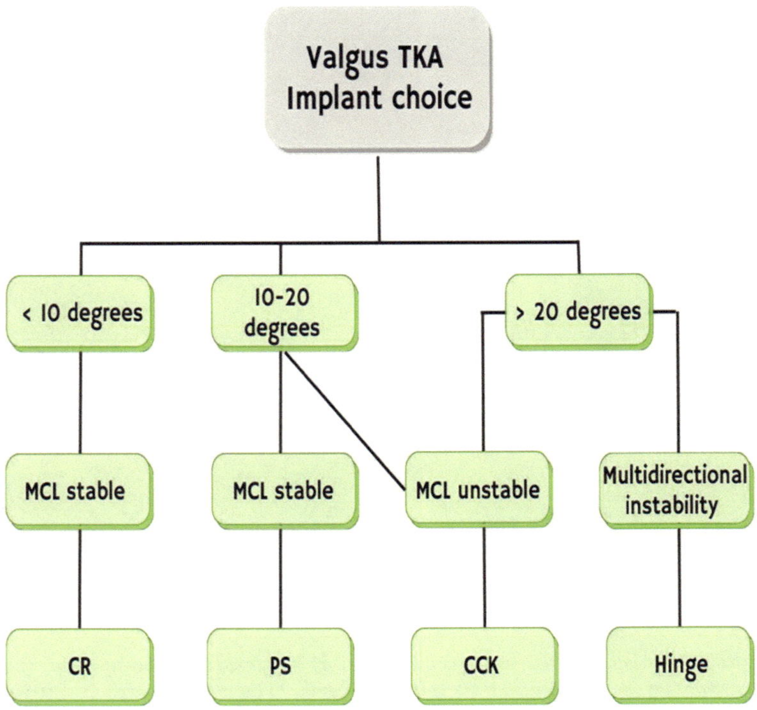

Figure 2.
Algorithm for implant choice in valgus TKAs.

The choice of implant must be based on the degree of joint instability and the presence of bone defects. Taking into account the Ranawat classification, for Grade I valgus knees (<10° deformity and intact MCL), Cruciate Retaining (CR) implants can be used, with proper bony resections and adequate soft tissue balancing for TKA long-term survival. The advantage of CR implants is the preservation of bone stock and improvement in knee proprioception [5, 6, 20–22].

For grade I or II valgus knees, mild-to-moderate coronal deformity is mild (<20°), and the MCL tension is inadequate, posterior stabilized (PS) implant can be used. In young patients, it is possible to preserve bone stock through the use of ultracongruent polyethylene insert, thus avoiding the resection of a box in the distal femur [7, 23–25].

In the presence of MCL insufficiency or >20° deformity (grade III), a greater constraint implant such as condylar constrained knee (CCK) or hinged implants should be used. CCK implants show good results at 10 years of follow-up, with a survival rate of around 97% [23, 26, 27]. Caution should be taken in younger patients, because it is necessary to remove a larger portion of distal femoral bone to accommodate the femoral box, which decreases the remaining bone stock available for revisions. In the case of elderly patients with severe ligamentous insufficiency and multiplanar instability or major bone defects, a hinged implant should be the choice [19].

5. New technologies

5.1 Computer-assisted navigation in valgus knee

Computer-assisted navigation (CAN) was developed to improve the position of the implants, achieving more accurate postoperative alignment through more precise and reproducible bony resection and ligament balancing [28].

Regarding the use of CAN in valgus TKAs, there are some published case series. Hadjicostas et al. [29] described the results of 15 knees with a mean valgus deformity of 21° (17–27°) and a mean follow-up of 28 months (24–60). All the knees were corrected to a mean of 0.5° of valgus (0–2 degrees).

Shao et al. [30] presented the results of six cases of CAN-assisted valgus TKA, in which ideal mechanical and prosthetic alignment was achieved with an image-free, computer-assisted navigation system. A primary, posterior-stabilized prosthesis was utilized in all cases. The average preoperative overall mechanical axis of the seven knees was 19.6° ± 4.6° of valgus, and the average postoperative mechanical axis was 0.4° ± 0.7°.

Between 2002 and 2009, Huang et al. [31] reported in a retrospective study, the results of 62 patients (70 knees) with Ranawat type-II valgus deformity who underwent primary TKA with or without CAN. At a mean follow-up of 6.2 years, both groups had significant postoperative improvements in clinical performance.

Unfortunately, there are still no good-quality randomized clinical trials that demonstrate evidence for the routine use of CAN in valgus TKAs. The decision remains based on the surgeon's common sense and experience.

5.2 Robotics and 3D printed implants in valgus knee

In recent years, the launch of new robotic platforms has caused great interest on the part of orthopedic surgeons. The use of robotic surgery in TKA improves the accuracy of knee alignment, implant positioning, and ligament balance, although it does not demonstrate superiority in clinical-functional outcome [32]. However, surgeons new to the robotics technique have been advised by more experienced ones to avoid valgus deformities at the beginning of the learning curve. The opinion of experts is that this is a challenge that requires more experience with the technique.

Marchant et al. [33] analyzed a series of cases with complex deformities undergoing knee arthroplasties and noted that robotic devices can help correct severe deformities, both in valgus with varus and in cases of flexion contracture. New studies should be carried out to analyze the clinical superiority of the use of robots in cases of valgus deformity. It was observed in another study that in seven knees with valgus deformity, all were corrected for alignment in neutral and without overcorrection [34].

Another recent technology is the manufacture of personalized implants. The use of 3D modeling techniques based on computed tomography in challenging cases of valgus deformity allows components to be placed in positioning according to the patient's anatomy in the coronal, sagittal, and transverse planes. This type of technology allows surgeons to make intraoperative adjustments and can place components outside of preoperative planning guidelines based on each patient's clinical need [35].

6. Rehabilitation

Rehabilitation of patients undergoing total valgus knee arthroplasty should follow common rehabilitation protocols. They should be focused on strength recovery, proprioception, and range of motion. Exercise therapy techniques, balance training, aquatic therapy, cryopneumatic therapy, and neuromuscular and transcutaneous electrical stimulation can be used [36].

The contact of the surgical and physical therapy team should be close. Consideration should be given to the surgical technique, implant design and constriction, release technique (osteotomy or soft tissue), and care in the possible neurological injury of the peroneal nerve.

7. Conclusion

Surgical treatment of the valgus arthritic knee presents a number of specific challenges. Multiple techniques have been described to treat this dysfunction with satisfactory clinical results. However, it is important for the surgeon to recognize the particularities and different techniques and practice a systematic approach to deformity correction.

Author details

Alessandro Rozim Zorzi[1,2]*, Wander Edney de Brito[1],
Gustavo Constantino de Campos[2] and João Batista de Miranda[2]

1 São Leopoldo Mandic Medical School, Campinas, SP, Brazil

2 Department of Orthopedics, Rheumatology and Traumatology, Campinas State University (UNICAMP), Campinas, SP, Brazil

*Address all correspondence to: arzorzi@hc.unicamp.br

References

[1] Ranawat AS, Ranawat CS, Elkus M, Rasquinha VJ, Rossi R, Babhulkar S. Total knee arthroplasty for severe valgus deformity. The Journal of Bone and Joint Surgery. 2005;**87**(Pt 2):271-284

[2] Zhou K, Zhou Z, Shi X, Shen B, Kang P, Yang J, et al. Effect of individual distal femoral valgus resection in total knee arthroplasty for patients with valgus knee: A retrospective cohort study. International Journal of Surgery. 2018;**52**:309-313

[3] Thienpont E, Schwab PE, Cornu O, Bellemans J, Victor J. Bone morphotypes of the varus and valgus knee. Archives of Orthopaedic and Trauma Surgery. 2017;**137**(3):393-400

[4] Tonelli Filho JR, Passarelli MC, Brito JA, Campos GC, Zorzi AR, Miranda JB. Keblish's lateral surgical approach enhances patellar tilt in valgus knee arthroplasty. Revista Brasileira de Ortopedia. 2016;**51**(6):680-686

[5] Krackow KA, Jones MM, Teeny SM, Hungerford DS. Primary total knee arthroplasty in patients with fixed valgus deformity. Clinical Orthopaedics and Related Research. 1991;**273**:9-18

[6] Nikolopoulos D, Michos I, Safos G, Safos P. Current surgical strategies for total arthroplasty in valgus knee. World Journal of Orthopedics. 2015;**6**(6):469-482. DOI: 10.5312/wjo.v6.i6.469

[7] Lombardi AV, Dodds KL, Berend KR, Mallory TH, Adams JB. An algorithmic approach to total knee arthroplasty in the valgus knee. The Journal of Bone & Joint Surgery. 2004;**86**(suppl. 2):62-71

[8] Mullaji AB, Shetty GM. Preoperative planning. In: Mullaji AB, Shetty GM, editors. Deformity Correction in Total Knee Arthroplasty. New York: Springer; 2014. pp. 5-7

[9] Mullaji A, Bhoskar R, Singh A, Haidermota M. Valgus arthritic knees can be classified into nine phenotypes. Knee Surgery, Sports Traumatology, Arthroscopy. Sep 2022;**30**(9):2895-2904. DOI: 10.1007/s00167-021-06796-1. Epub: 9 Nov 2021. PMID: 34750671

[10] Yang D, Zhou Y, Shao H, Deng W. Different deformity origins and morphological features in subtypes of valgus knees: A radiological classification system. Orthopedic Surgery. 2022;**14**(1):96-103. DOI: 10.1111/os.13178

[11] Apostolopoulos AP, Nikolopoulos DD, Polyzois I, Nakos A, Liarokapis S, Stefanakis G, et al. Total knee arthroplasty in severe valgus deformity: Interest of combining a lateral approach with a tibial tubercle osteotomy. Orthopaedics & Traumatology, Surgery & Research. 2010;**96**(7):777-784. DOI: 10.1016/j.otsr.2010.06.008

[12] Keblish PA. The lateral approach to the valgus knee. Surgical technique and analysis of 53 cases with over two-year follow-up evaluation. Clinical Orthopaedics and Related Research. 1991;**271**:52-62

[13] Buechel FF. A sequential three-step lateral release for correcting fixed valgus knee deformities during total knee arthroplasty. Clinical Orthopaedics and Related Research. 1990;**260**:170-175

[14] Favorito PJ, Mihalko WM, Krackow KA. Total knee arthroplasty in the valgus knee. The Journal of the American Academy of Orthopaedic Surgeons. 2002;**10**:16-24

[15] Whiteside LA. Selective ligament release in total knee arthroplasty of the knee in valgus. Clinical Orthopaedics and Related Research. 1999;**367**:130-140. DOI: 10.1097/00003086-199910000-00016

[16] Brilhault J, Lautman S, Favard L, Burdin P. Lateral femoral sliding osteotomy lateral release in total knee arthroplasty for a fixed valgus deformity. Journal of Bone and Joint Surgery. British Volume (London). 2002;**84**:1131-1137. DOI: 10.1302/0301-620X.84B8.12824

[17] Krackow KA, Holtgrewe JL. Experience with a new technique for managing severely overcorrected valgus high tibial osteotomy at total knee arthroplasty. Clinical Orthopaedics and Related Research. 1990;**258**:213-224. DOI: 10.1097/00003086-199009000-00027

[18] Puijk R, Rassir R, Kok LM, Sierevelt IN, Nolte PA. Common peroneal nerve palsy after TKA in valgus deformities; a systematic review. Journal of Experimental Orthopology. 2022;**9**(1):12. DOI: 10.1186/s40634-021-00443-x

[19] Alesi D, Meena A, Fratini S, Rinaldi VG, Cammisa E, Lullini G, et al. Total knee arthroplasty in valgus knee deformity: Is it still a challenge in 2021? Musculoskeletal Surgery. 2022;**106**(1):1-8. DOI: 10.1007/s12306-021-00695-x

[20] Rajgopal A, Dahiya V, Vasdev A, et al. Long-term results of total knee arthroplasty for valgus knees: Soft-tissue release technique and implant selection. Journal of Orthopaedic Surgery (Hong Kong). 2011;**19**:60-63. DOI: 10.1177/230949901101900114

[21] McAuley JP, Collier MB, Hamilton WG, et al. Posterior cruciate-retaining total knee arthroplasty for valgus osteoarthritis. Clinical Orthopaedics and Related Research. 2008;**466**:2644-2649. DOI: doi.org/10.1007/ s11999-008-0436-8

[22] Politi J, Scott R. Balancing severe valgus deformity in total knee arthroplasty using a lateral cruciform retinacular release. The Journal of Arthroplasty. 2004;**19**:553-557. DOI: doi.org/10.1016/j.arth.2003.12.083

[23] Elkus M, Ranawat CS, Rasquinha VJ, et al. Total knee arthroplasty for severe valgus deformity. Five to fourteen-year follow-up. Journal of Bone Joint Surgery. 2004;**86**:2671-2676. DOI: doi.org/10.2106/00004623-200412000-00013

[24] Easley ME, Insall JN, Scuderi GR, Bullek DD. Primary constrained condylar knee arthroplasty for the arthritic valgus knee. Clinical Orthopaedics and Related Research. Nov 2000;**380**:58-64. DOI: 10.1097/00003086-200011000-00008. PMID: 11064973

[25] Anderson JA, Baldini A, MacDonald JH, et al. Primary constrained condylar knee arthroplasty without stem extensions for the valgus knee. Clinical Orthopaedics and Related Research. 2006;**442**:199-203. DOI: doi.org/10.1097/01.blo.0000185675.99696.29

[26] Lachiewicz PF, Soileau ES. Ten-year survival and clinical results of constrained components in primary total knee arthro- plasty. The Journal of Arthroplasty. 2006;**21**:803-808. DOI: 10.1016/j. arth.2005.09.008

[27] Feng X-B, Yang C, Fu D-H, et al. Mid-term outcomes of primary constrained condylar knee arthroplasty for severe knee deformity. Journal of Huazhong University of Science

and Technology. Medical Sciences. 2016;**36**:231-236. DOI: 10.1007/s11596-016-1572-0

[28] Bae DK, Song SJ. Computer assisted navigation in knee arthroplasty. Clinics in Orthopedic Surgery. 2011;**3**(4):259-267. DOI: 10.4055/cios.2011.3.4.259

[29] Hadjicostas PT, Soucacos PN, Thielemann FW. Computer-assisted osteotomy of the lateral femoral condyle with non-constrained total knee replacement in severe valgus knees. Journal of Bone and Joint Surgery. British Volume (London). 2008;**90**(11):1441-1445. DOI: 10.1302/0301-620X.90B11.20092

[30] Shao JJ, Zhang XL, Wang Q, Chen YS, Shen H, Jiang Y. Total knee arthroplasty using computer assisted navigation in patients with severe valgus deformity of the knee. Chinese Medical Journal. 2010;**123**(19):2666-2670

[31] Huang TW, Lee CY, Lin SJ, Peng KT, Huang KC, Lee MS, et al. Comparison of computer-navigated and conventional total knee arthroplasty in patients with Ranawat type-II valgus deformity: Medium-term clinical and radiological results. BMC Musculoskeletal Disorders. 2014;**15**:390. DOI: 10.1186/1471-2474-15-390

[32] Batailler C, Shatrov J, Sappey-Marinier E, Servien E, Parratte S, Lustig S. Artificial intelligence in knee arthroplasty: Current concept of the available clinical applications. Art. 2022;**4**(1):17. DOI: 10.1186/s42836-022-00119-6

[33] Marchand RC, Khlopas A, Sodhi N, Condrey C, Piuzzi NS, Patel R, et al. Difficult cases in robotic arm-assisted total knee arthroplasty: A case series. Journal of Knee Surgery. 2018;**31**(4):371-372

[34] Marchand RC, Sodhi N, Khlopas A, Sultan AA, Higuera CA, Stearns KL, et al. Coronal correction for severe deformity using robotic-assisted total knee arthroplasty. The Journal of Knee Surgery. 2018;**31**(1):2-5. DOI: 10.1055/s-0037-1608840

[35] Marchand RC, Scholl L, Bhowmik-Stoker M, Taylor KB, Marchand KB, Chen Z, et al. Total knee arthroplasty in the valgus knee: Can new operative technologies affect surgical technique and outcomes? Surgical Technology International. 2021;**39**:389-393. DOI: 10.52198/21.STI.39.OS1462

[36] Mistry JB, Elmallah RD, Bhave A, Chughtai M, Cherian JJ, McGinn T, et al. Rehabilitative guidelines after total knee arthroplasty: A review. The Journal of Knee Surgery. 2016;**29**(3):201-217. DOI: 10.1055/s-0036-1579670

Chapter 7

Primary Total Arthroplasty in Stiff Knees

Rogério Teixeira de Carvalho

Abstract

Knee with less than a 50° arc of motion can be considered "stiff." The surgical exposure in total knee arthroplasty (TKA) is technically challenging in the stiff knees. Other problems like longer operative time, patellar maltracking, rupture or avulsion of patellar tendon, difficulty in flexion-extension gap balancing, bone avulsion, or fracture in the distal femur can occur during TKA. It is not uncommon, and the surgeon needs an extensile surgical approach as early quadriceps release or tibial tubercle osteotomy for adequate exposure. The TKA postoperative outcome is suboptimal with less arc of motion, superficial wound problems, deep infection, and higher late revision surgeries. The rehabilitation protocol should take into account improvements in the range of motion in comparison with the preoperative status, and the patient expectations must be realistic.

Keywords: total knee arthroplasty, stiffness, knee osteoarthritis

1. Introduction

The stiff knee (SKN) is considered as a clinical situation that the range of motion (ROM) is less than a 50° arc of movement [1, 2]. SKN causes a variable level of functional disability, painful discomfort during scarce knee mobility, limp in the gait cycle, and hamper with activities of daily living [3]. Normal walking requires 70°–80° of ROM, stairs require 80°–90° of ROM, and squatting requires at least 130° of ROM [4].

The main causes of SKN are previous surgery on the knee, advanced primary knee ostearthritis, secondary posttraumatic ostearthrosis, reflex sympathetic dystrophy (RSD), neuromuscular disorder, sequelae of previous infection, inflammatory diseases (rheumatoid and psoriatic arthritis), arthrofibrosis, and hemofilic arthropathy. Ankylosis is more common in patients who had their knee immobilized or who are wheelchair bound. The common clinical characteristics in patients with SKN are patela baja, quadriceps contracture, intra-articular adhesions, posterior capsule contracture, poor patellar gliding, and heterotopic ossification [5, 6]. Total knee arthroplasty (TKA) in SKN is a challenging procedure. One of the goals of TKA is to improve knee mobility, including ambulatory ability in the gait [7, 8]. Other goals of TKA in patients with SKN are to relieve pain, improve the alignment to correct the knee deformity, and provide knee stability.

The most relevant factor that predicts knee mobility after TKA is preoperative range of motion [9, 10]. Young age, female sex, and obese patients are more susceptible to achieve less mobility after TKA [11, 12]. In patients with SKNs, the predominant symptom is not mechanical pain. Functional disabilities like impairments in stair climbing, unable to sit on a chair, and inability to walk a long distance are common complaints. Psychological and cosmetic harms are associated with decline in the quality life. TKA is considered a valuable option to improve functional capacity and obtain a mobile knee.

2. Classification

The SKN can be presented clinically in loss of extension (LOE), loss of flexion (LOF), mixed or ankylosed. The major troubles in LOE are adhesions in suprapatellar pouch and in medial and lateral gutters, contracture of extensor mechanism, patellofemoral joint fusion, and loss of tibiofemoral joint space. The SKN in LOF, the extensor mechanism that is elongated with posterior capsule, posterior cruciate ligament (PCL), and collaterals ligaments are contractured. The posterior osteophytes causes a mechanical barrier to achieve complete ROM. Ankylosed knee can be associated with knee arthrodesis, infection, reconstruction after tumor ressection, after severe trauma with distal femur, and tibial plateau fractures. The classification proposed by Sharma [13] is based on the degree of loss of ROM in the knee joint, as shown in **Table 1**.

Type 1: Stiffness/fibrous ankylosis in flexion
• 1a: Stiffness/fibrous ankylosis in 30°–60°
• 1b: Stiffness/fibrous ankylosis in 60°–90°
Type 2: Stiffness/fibrous ankylosis in extension
• 2a: Stiffness/fibrous ankylosis in 0°–15°
• 2b: Stiffness/fibrous ankylosis in 15°–30°
Type 3: Bony ankylosis/arthrodesis
• 3a: Bony ankylosis in flexion >30°
• 3b: Bony ankylosis in extension (flexion <30°)

Table 1.
Classification for stiff/ankylosed knees proposed by Sharmal [13].

This classification provides a guidance for surgeons related to surgical approach, type of prosthetic implants, and helps to presume functional outcome after TKA.

3. Indications

- Advanced primary knee osteoarthritis (Kellgren-Lawrence 3 or 4);
- Posttraumatic knee osteoarthitis and/or previous knee surgery;
- After knee osteotomy (distal femur and/or proximal tibia);

- Arthrofibrosis (post-surgery and/or prolonged immobilization);
- Inflammatory osteoarthritis (rheumatoid arthritis and psoriasis);
- Hemophilic arthropathy;
- Ankylosis (after knee arthrodesis);
- Heterotopic ossification (HO);
- Reflex sympathetic dystrophy (RSD);
- Neurologic arthropathy;
- Postinfection arthropathy.

4. Contra indications

- Neuromuscular disease (s) with RSD;
- Paralysis after brain vascular stroke;
- Patient inability to follow the postoperative rehabilitation protocol;
- Active infection without clinical control.

5. Preoperative evaluation

A through clinical history must include questions about previous conservative treatment and surgeries, period of time that stiffness started, comorbidities, medications, and psychological profile. The physical examination must comprise the preoperative passive and active ROM (flexion and extension), patellar gliding, the amount of flexion contracture, scars, type and flexibility of the angular deformity, gait pattern, and extensor mechanism status (elongated or contractured). Osteoporosis is frequent in SKNs. Complete motor, sensory, and vascular assessment should be performed. Ankle/brachial index and Doppler ultrasound can be useful to estimate the function of blood circulation in the legs.

The imaging exams of the knee should include radiographic evaluation in anteroposterior (AP) and lateral at 30° of flexion (**Figures 1** and **2**). Special views with maximal and minimal flexion in the sagittal plane should be documented. Long-axis anteroposterior (AP) view can be useful to determine the mechanical and anatomical axis of the lower limbs. The sunrise patellar view at 45° of flexion can demonstrate a severe arthritic involvement, where the patella usually is fused with the anterior femur [2, 5]. A stress view in the coronal plane can be helpful to determine if the angular deformity is rigid or correctable. Presence of hardware is not uncommon in STK patients. Computed tomography (CT) scan may be used to assess bone stock and rule out infections [3].

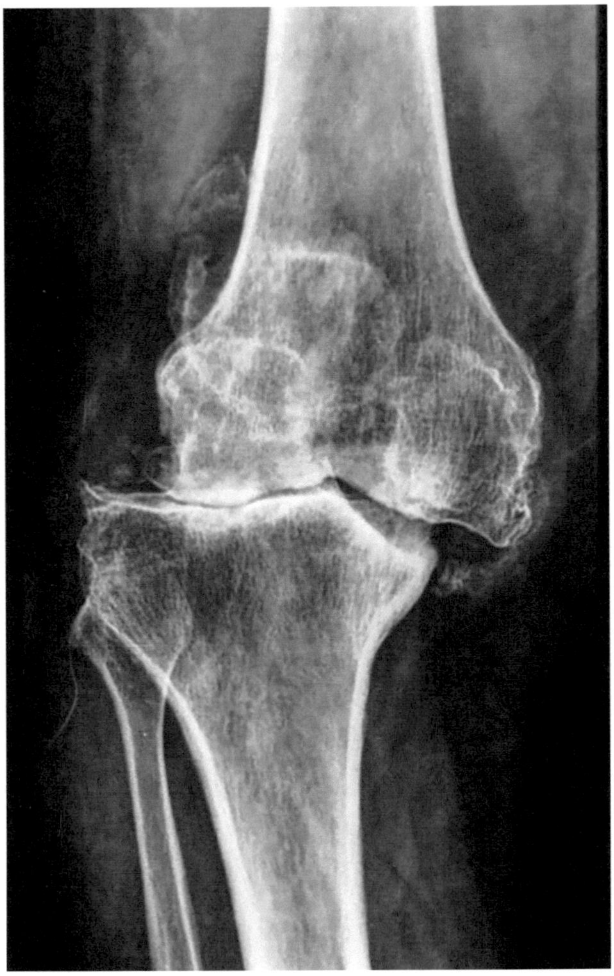

Figure 1.
Radiography in anteroposterior view with stiff knee.

The surgeon must select which type of knee prosthesis will be required. A broad assortment of modular systems are disposable according to each patient. More constrained implants can be considered in cases with bone loss, ligamentous insufficiency, or after extensive soft tissues releases. A custom prosthesis must be fabricated for a particular situation as a very small or large knees and ankylosed knees in rheumatoid patients. In a previous infected STK, a staged procedure can be recommended to decrease the risk of serious complications [14, 15].

6. Surgical technique

The type of anesthesia should emphasize the muscle relaxation and minimize blood loss. Usually, the epidural anesthesia associated with peripheral nerve block as adductor canal provide decrease of narcotic usage and postoperative pain. The tranexamic acid (20–60 mg/kg) can be administrated intravenous during the anesthetic induction in attempt to reduce the blood loss. The use of tourniquet is

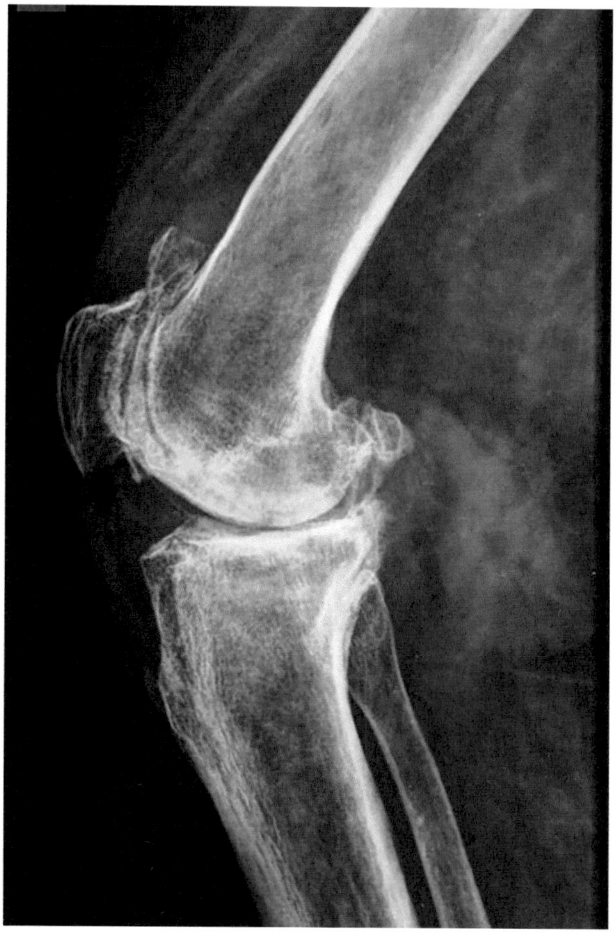

Figure 2.
Radiography in lateral view with 30° of flexion.

questionable and can be avoidable in STK patients [16, 17]. The use of sterile drape is recommended, and the leg should be free to move during the TKA. The range of motion (ROM) and ligamentous stability should be addressed prior the incision and documented.

A straight midline incision should be used, if there is not prior surgical scar. If an anterior longitudinal knee scar is found, the skin incision starts more proximally. Usually, the skin is adherent to the subcutaneous tissue and careful dissection may be required to mobilize the skin. This step assists the deep subfascial dissection and facilitates the dermis and epidermis closure. A medial parapatellar arthrotomy is performed with capsule opening and releases the adhesions in the suprapatellar pouch and plane between anterior distal femur underneath the quadriceps tendon. After this step, cleaning the medial and lateral gutters may be required to gain adequate exposure. All the fibrotic tissues should be removed. The patellar tendon is identified and protected during the TKA, and the space posterior to the tendon freed by sharp dissection with the scalpel or eletrocautery.

The next step is the patellar eversion. The difficulty to dislocate the patella laterally, in SKN, remains a problem. The lateral retinacular release can be performed, if the knee remains stiff with flexion less than 40° and the lateral patellofemoral ligament is cut to assist the patellar eversion. An extensive transquadricipital approach, the rectus snip, can be performed to improve and provide good exposure with low risk related to the extensor mechanism damage. The rectus tendon is transected in an oblique fashion, around 45°, in a superior and lateral direction [18]. Orienting the rectus snip distally allows for conversion to a V-Y quadricepsplasty that the surgeon incises the rectus tendon and vastus lateralis, but not the lateral retinaculum [19, 20]. This approach preserves the superior lateral geniculate artery, which provides the major blood supply to the patella, when a medial arthrotomy has been performed. However, this technique is not recommended in the presence of subluxated or dislocated patella laterally. In this scenario, an extensive lateral retinacular release can be performed and the patella is everted and knee is flexed gently. It is recommended to be cautious during this maneuver to avoid patellar tendon avulsion from the tibia tubercle, bone avulsion, and medial collateral ligament (MCL) tear in the progression for the knee flexion [21]. The placement of a metallic pin through the tibial tubercle can decrease the stress over the patellar tendon and hinder the avulsion. The combination of a quadriceps snip and lateral release provides an adequate exposure for most SKNs. The rectus tendon and vastus lateralis muscle are repaired, but the lateral retinacular incision is left open. This approach has the advantage of not requiring modification of postoperative rehabilitation [22].

In the varus deformity, the subperiosteal medial release is then continued, with a sharp scalpel, an electrocautery or an osteotome, as the knee is further flexed and the tibia externally rotated. Dissection should begin in extension on the bone surfaces in attempt to mobilize the soft tissues. Then, skeletonization of the tibia and femur has been performed to allow knee flexion for adequate exposure. For severe varus SKNs, a medial transepicondylar femoral osteotomy may be required. In the valgus deformity with SKNs, a decision must be made to choose an anterior longitudinal traditional incision or lateral approach described by Keblish [23].

The tibial tubercle osteotomy (TTO) can be performed to extend the incision distally for the most difficult SKNs. The osteotomy should encompass at least 8 centimeters (cm) distal to the top of the tibial tubercle. The bone cut is made with an oscillating saw from medial to lateral, and then the lateral cortex is transected with an osteotome. Muscle attachments to the lateral tibial crest with a periosteal soft tissues hinge are left preserved. Two or three wires are passed to encompass the tubercle during closure [24]. Furthermore, two or three screws can be used to stabilize the TTO, in patients with good bone quality. In osteoporotic bone, TTO is not recommended. Before wound closure, the knee was taken through a passive ROM to assure osteotomy fixation and patellofemoral tracking. Postoperatively, the patients wore a protective knee immobilizer while up and walking for the first 6 weeks.

For the ligament balancing, sequential soft tissue release can be performed to correct the angular deformity; if posterior cruciate ligament (PCL) appears to be functional and balanced, cruciate retaining (CR) prosthesis can be used, but this is an uncommon scenario. For a rigid or severe flexion, contracture may be necessary to cut more distal femur (2 mm) to achieve a straight knee in extension. It is not a feasible solution to cut more distal femur than 2 mm due to the high risk to raise the joint line. Then, the tibial and femoral bone cuts are recommended to place the laminar spreaders in extension and flexion in 90°. A curved osteotome is used to remove the posterior osteophytes and release the posterior capsule (**Figure 3**). This maneuver is essential to open the flexion gap [25] (**Figures 4** and 5).

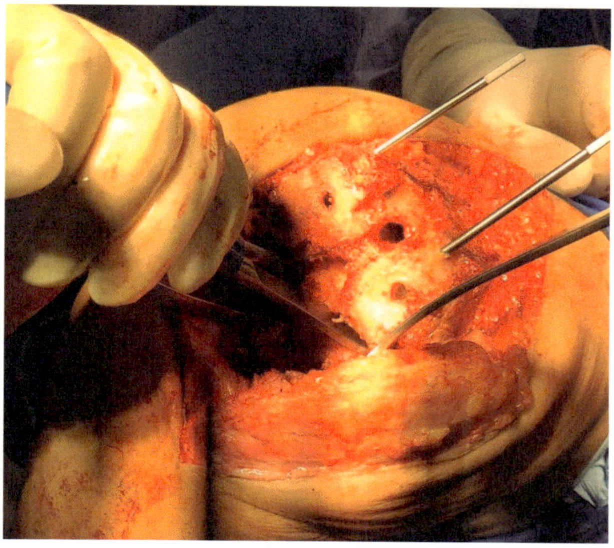

Figure 3.
Removal of posterior osteophytes in the femoral condyles.

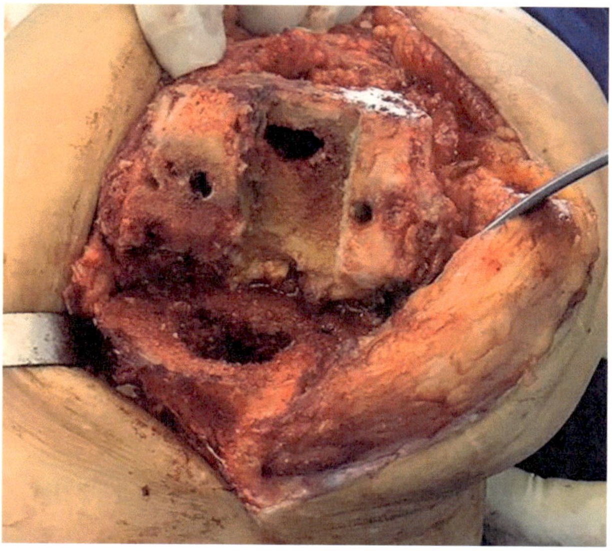

Figure 4.
Narrow flexion gap prior the posterior release.

Moreover, more constrained implants as posterior stabilized (PS) models with an elevated polyethylene post are considered as the implant of choice due to the PCL contracture in SKNs. If during insertion of trial components, the knee is unstable in both coronal and sagittal plane, and a more constrained modular component with augments and stems or hinged prosthesis can be chosen. It is recommended to place the femoral component more posterior to decrease the flexion gap, mainly in PS implants. The level of constriction will depend the extent of the ligamentous releases and the amount of bone loss encountered during the TKA. A tumor prosthesis or custom

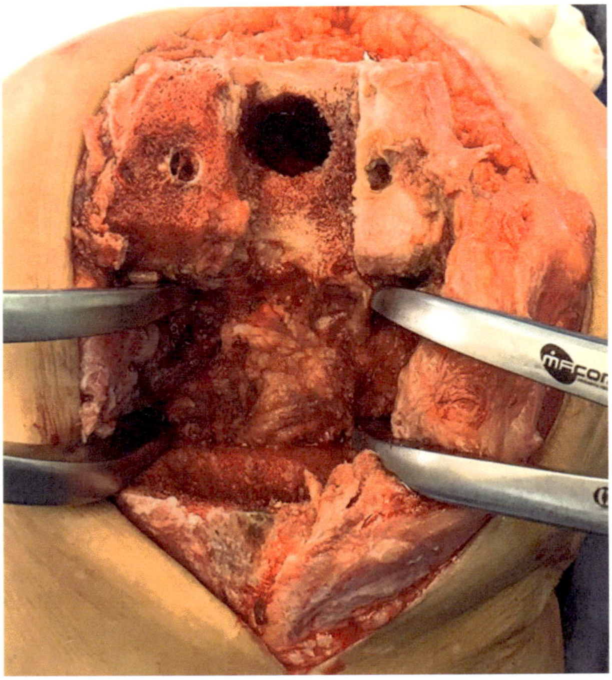

Figure 5.
Opening of the flexion gap with laminar spreaders.

implants may be needed in extremely SKNs, especially in extension. The prosthesis chosen should have options available for femoral and tibial implants in attempt to re-establish the anatomic joint line with available metallic augments (**Figures 6** and 7). Care should be taken to avoid overstuff in the patellofemoral articulation that can lead to a flexion contracture and anterior knee pain.

In ankylosed and after knee arthrodesis, the patellar and proximal tibial cut can be performed in the beginning to obtain more space and promote a better exposure during the TKA. A posterior capsule release with the electrocautery and the laminar spreaders positioned in extension can help after the bone cuts to achieve zero degrees. For a more severe contracture above 30°, the quadricepsplasty may be needed in attempt to elongate the extensor mechanism and to re-establish the joint line. In patients with MCL insufficiency and bone loss in the metaphysis, a hinge TKA can be considered.

The closure of the quadriceps tendon should be performed between 30° and 60° of knee flexion, depending on the preoperative gravity of the SKN. The type of quadriceps release or TTO performed should be taken into account to consider the angulation of knee flexion during the closure. The intraoperative ROM after this surgical step should be documented with a photograph to demonstrate for the patient and the physiotherapist [26].

7. Postoperative management

A light pressure dressing is applied, and cryotherapy can be used to reduce swelling and knee pain. The effectiveness of rehabilitation on functional outcomes

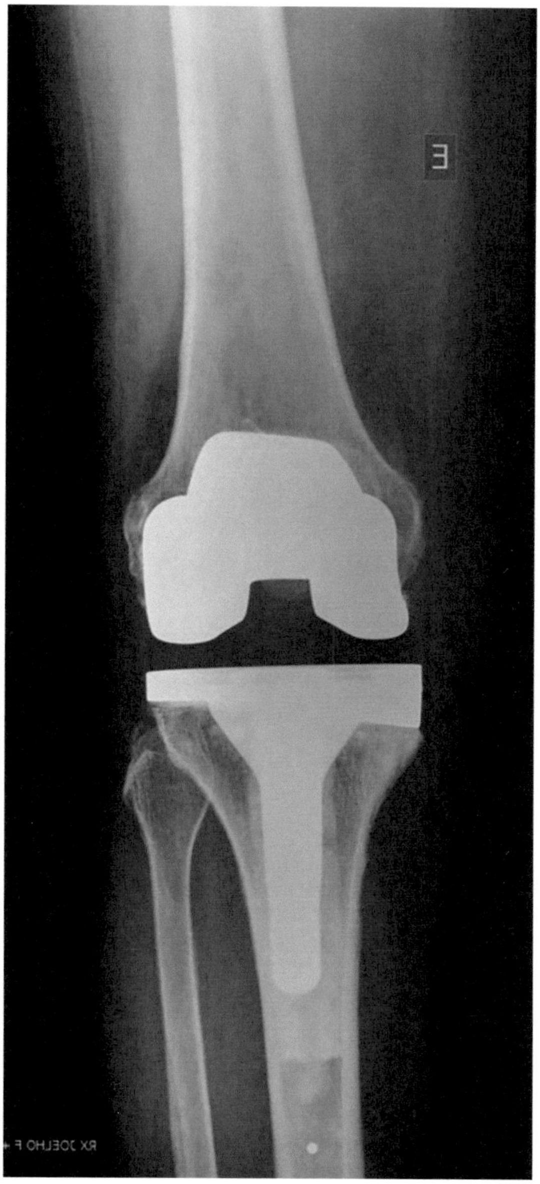

Figure 6.
Postoperative radiography in anteroposterior view after TKA in stiff knee.

depends on the appropriate timing, intensity, and progression of the ROM, accounting for the patient's ability and level of pain. The use of the removable knee orthosis is debatable. It can be used in static or dynamic manner in attempt to avoid loss of motion after TKA [27]. The patient is immediately placed in a continuous passive motion (CPM) machine from 0° to 30° of flexion in the recovery room. The flexion is increased 10° a day or as tolerated. The physical therapy can be prescribed in the early stage of the postoperative rehabilitation protocol intercalated with the CPM to optimize the gain of knee motion [28]. The pain control is crucial to achieve the progressive ROM. The use of spinal or epidural catheters with analgesic infusion can

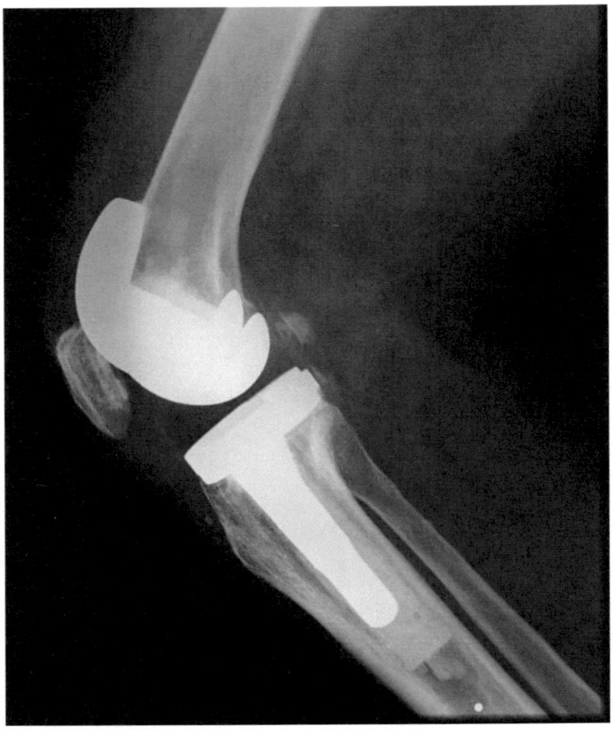

Figure 7.
Postoperative radiography in lateral view after TKA in stiff knee.

be helpful after TKA in SKNs. The early quadriceps activation is recommended with physical methods (sensory transcutaneous electrical stimulation), active isometric contraction, and early deambulation with walker or crutches. After TTO and V-Y quadricepsplasty, the rehabilitation protocol is delayed to preserve bone and soft tissue healing, mainly between 4 to 6 weeks. A long orthosis is recommended in the lower limb to keep the gait secure. The recovery of quadriceps function is essential to achieve a satisfactory outcome during the day life activities, improve ROM, and obtain a stable gait [29].

8. Clinical results and complications

The clinical results of TKA in SKNs are inferior in comparison with non-stiff knees with higher complication rates [21, 30]. The rate of complications ranges from 21–35% [31, 32]. The common complications are patellar tendon avulsion, partial or complete tear of MCL, bone fracture or avulsion (epicondyle (s), patella), stiffness after TKA, wound dehiscence, ligamentous imbalance between extension, and flexion gap. Gentle knee flexion and progressive subperiosteal soft tissue releases with the electrocautery can prevent intraoperative bone fracture. It is not uncommon a painful TKA in SKNs that can be a challenging situation to achieve a better functional outcome. Extension lag is associated with V-Y quadricepsplasty [32]. Aseptic loosening in the tibial component has been described in some SKNs [32, 33]. Osteoporotic bone can be considered as a risk factor for fractures around the knee.

The functional scores applied after TKA like Hospital for Special Surgery (HSS), Knee Society Score (KSS), Knee Society Functional Score (FS) have improved due to gain in postoperative ROM in comparison with preoperative status [11, 30–33]. The range of improvement in ROM after TKA in SKNs is around 50°–70°. The range of improvement in KSS after TKA is between 30 and 45 points [30–33]. In spite of the enhancement in motion, some residual flexion contracture is predictable in type 2 and 3 SKNs and can affect the pattern of the gait. A limp with overload in the lumbar spine can be expected in this scenario.

The TKA in SKNs is technically demanding with a time-consuming rehabilitation protocol. Patient expectation should be realistic according to the level of SKNs. The complication rate is greater than conventional TKA. A good preoperative evaluation is mandatory to avoid unexpected intra- and postoperative hassle.

Author details

Rogério Teixeira de Carvalho[1,2,3,4]

1 Hospital do Servidor Público Estadual (HSPE), Brazil

2 Hospital Israelita Albert Einstein(HIAE), Brazil

3 Federal University of São Paulo (Unifesp), Brazil

4 Orthopaedic Department of Unifesp, Brazil

*Address all correspondence to: rtcarv27@gmail.com

References

[1] Aglietti P, Windsor RE, Buzzi R, Insall JN. Arthroplasty for the stiff or ankylosed knee. The Journal of Arthroplasty. 1989;**4**(1):1-5

[2] Rajgopal A, Ahuja N, Dolai B. Total knee arthroplasty in stiff and ankylosed knees. The Journal of Arthroplasty. 2005;**20**(5):585-590

[3] Cuckler JM. The stiff knee: Evaluation and management. Orthopedics. 2002;**25**(9):969-970

[4] Laubenthal KN, Smidt GL, Kettelkamp DB. A quantitative analysis of knee motion during activities of daily living. Physics Therapaphy. 1972;**52**(1):34-43

[5] Kelly MA, Clarke HD. Stiffness and ankylosis in primary total knee arthroplasty. Clinical Orthopaedics and Related Research. 2003;**416**:68-73

[6] Montgomery WH 3rd, Insall JN, Haas SB, Becker MS, Windsor RE. Primary total knee arthroplasty in stiff and ankylosed knees. The American Journal of Knee Surgery. 1998;**11**(1):20-23

[7] Lange T, Schmitt J, Kopkow C, Rataj E, Günther KP, Lützner J. What do patients expect from total knee arthroplasty? A Delphi consensus study on patient treatment goals. The Journal of Arthroplasty. 2017;**32**(7):2093-2099

[8] Gibon E, Goodman MJ, Goodman SB. Patient satisfaction after total knee arthroplasty: A realistic or imaginary goal? Orthop Clinics. 2017;**48**(4):421-431

[9] Ritter MA, Harty LD, Davis KE, Meding JB, Berend ME. Predicting range of motion after total knee arthroplasty. The Journal of Bone and Joint Surgery. American. 2003;**85A**:1278-1285

[10] Lizaur A, Marco L, Cebrian R. Preoperative factors influencing the range of movement after total knee arthroplasty for severe osteoarthritis. Journal of Bone and Joint Surgery. British Volume (London). 1997;**79**(4):626-629

[11] Gatha NM, Clarke HD, Fuchs R, Scuderi GR, Insall JN. Factors affecting postoperative range of motion after total knee arthroplasty. The Journal of Knee Surgery. 2004;**17**(4):196-202

[12] Winemaker M, Rahman WA, Petruccelli D, de Beer J. Preoperative knee stiffness and total knee arthroplasty outcomes. The Journal of Arthroplasty. 2012;**27**(8):1437-1441

[13] Sharma M, Sharma S, Upadhyaya AR. Classification-based management of stiff/ankylosed knees. Indian Journal of Orthopology. 2021;**55**(5):1158-1174

[14] Bae DK, Yoon KH, Kim HS, Song SJ. Total knee arthroplasty in stiff knees after previous infection. Journal of Bone and Joint Surgery. 2005;**87**(3):333-336

[15] Hsu CH, Lin PC, Chen WS, Wang JW. Total knee arthroplasty in patients with stiff knees. The Journal of Arthroplasty. 2012;**27**(2):286-292

[16] Liu Y, Si H, Zeng Y, Li M, Xie H, Shen B. More pain and slower functional recovery when a tourniquet is used during total knee arthroplasty. Knee Surgery, Sports Traumatology, Arthroscopy. 2020;**28**(6):1842-1860

[17] Ahmed I, Chawla A, Underwood M, Price AJ, Metcalfe A, Hutchinson CE, et al. Time to reconsider the routine

use of tourniquets in total knee arthroplasty surgery: An abridged version of a Cochrane systematic review and meta-analysis. Bone Joint Journal. 2021;**103**(5):830-839

[18] Garvin KL, Scuderi G, Insall JN. Evolution of the quadriceps snip. Clinical Orthopaedics and Related Research. 1995;**321**:131-137

[19] Scott RD, Siliski JM. The use of a modified VY quadricepsplasty during total knee replacement to gain exposure and improve flexion in the ankylosed knee. Orthopedics. 1985;**8**(1):45-48

[20] Trousdale RT, Hanssen AD, Rand JA, Cahalan TD. VY quadricepsplasty in total knee arthroplasty. Clinical Orthopaedics and Related Research. 1993;**286**:48-55

[21] Debette C, Lustig S, Servien E, Lording T, Villa V, Demey G, et al. Total knee arthroplasty of the stiff knee: Three hundred and four cases. International Orthopaedics. 2014;**38**(2):285-289

[22] Barrack RL, Smith P, Munn B, Engh G, Rorabeck C. Comparison of surgical approaches in total knee arthroplasty. Clinical Orthopaedics and Related Research. 1998;**356**:16-21

[23] Keblish PA. The lateral approach to the valgus knee. Surgical technique and analysis of 53 cases with over two-year follow-up evaluation. Clinical Orthopaedics and Related Research. 1991;**271**:52-62

[24] Whiteside LA. Exposure in difficult total knee arthroplasty using tibial tubercle osteotomy. Clinical Orthopaedics and Related Research. 1995;**321**:32-35

[25] Fosco M, Filanti M, Amendola L, Savarino LM, Tigani D. Total knee arthroplasty in stiff knee compared with flexible knees. Musculoskeletal Surgery. 2011;**95**(1):7-12

[26] Pinsornsak P, Kanitnate S, Boontanapibul K. The effect of immediate post-operative knee range of motion photographs on post-operative range of motion after total knee arthroplasty. International Orthopaedics. 2021;**45**(1):101-107

[27] McElroy MJ, Johnson AJ, Zywiel MG, Mont MA. Devices for the prevention and treatment of knee stiffness after total knee arthroplasty. Expert Review of Medical Devices. 2011;**8**(1):57-65

[28] Richter M, Trzeciak T, Kaczmarek M. Effect of continuous passive motion on the early recovery outcomes after total knee arthroplasty. International Orthopaedics. 2022;**46**(3):549-553

[29] Ha CW, Park YB, Song YS, Kim JH, Park YG. Increased range of motion is important for functional outcome and satisfaction after total knee arthroplasty in Asian patients. The Journal of Arthroplasty. 2016;**31**(6):1199-1203

[30] McAuley JP, Harrer MF, Ammeen D, Engh GA. Outcome of knee arthroplasty in patients with poor preoperative range of motion. Clinical Orthopaedics and Related Research. 2002;**404**:203-207

[31] Bhan S, Malhotra R, Kiran EK. Comparison of total knee arthroplasty in stiff and ankylosed knees. Clinical Orthopaedics and Related Research. 2006;**451**:87-95

[32] Choi YJ, Seo DK, Lee KW, Ra HJ, Kang HW, Kim JK. Results of total knee arthroplasty for painless, stiff knees. Knee Surgery Related Research. 2020;**32**(1):1-7

[33] Naranja RJ, Lotke PA, Pagnano MW, Hanssen AD. Total knee arthroplasty in a previously ankylosed or arthrodesed knee. Clinical Orthopaedics and Related Research. 1996;**331**:234-237

Chapter 8

Complications after Total Knee Arthroplasty: Stiffness, Periprosthetic Joint Infection, and Periprosthetic Fracture

Atthakorn Jarusriwanna and Chaturong Pornrattanamaneewong

Abstract

Total knee arthroplasty (TKA) is one of the most successful surgical procedures with effective treatment in patients suffering from end-stage knee osteoarthritis. The goal of the operation is to improve pain, correct the deformity, and increase function. However, complications after surgery are the important factors related to dissatisfied TKA. Stiffness, periprosthetic joint infection (PJI), and periprosthetic fracture are among the most common complications following TKA and usually raise issues as concern points for both patients and the surgeons. Each complication needs precise assessment and specific care to prevent further serious issues. In this chapter, the authors will focus and describe all of these three frequent complications in details from their definition to management.

Keywords: total knee arthroplasty, complications, stiffness, periprosthetic joint infection, periprosthetic fracture

1. Introduction

There is approximately 20 percent of the patients with dissatisfaction following TKA whether pain or having postoperative problems [1, 2]. In the previous literatures, reporting of complications and adverse events after TKA was not standardized with several definitions being proposed. Healy et al. published a list of 22 TKA complications and their standardized definitions including these three common problems, which were endorsed by The Knee Society to improve quality measurement and consistent with ICD-9 codes [3]. Stiff TKA could produce pain and diminish functional ability, whereas PJI and periprosthetic fracture might cause severe morbidity. Early detection and appropriate management are the key success to resolve these problems which would enhance patient's outcome and improve satisfaction.

2. Stiffness

Normal knee range of motion (ROM) ranges from 0 to 140 degrees, while achievement of postoperative ROM from 0 to 110 degrees can be defined as success

TKA [4]. In general, a minimum of 90 degrees of knee flexion is required for functional recovery in daily activities, as 83 degrees of knee flexion is required for going up and down stairs and 93 degrees for sitting, which were demonstrated by a biomechanical study [5, 6]. Stiffness after TKA has variable incidence, ranging from 1.3 to 5.3 percent, but some literature proposed up to 60 percent of patients who suffered from stiff TKA [7]. These variables may cause by a variety of definitions as there was absolutely no consensus on degrees of knee flexion limitation defined as stiff TKA. The standardized definition by the TKA Complications Workgroup of The Knee Society described that limitation of ROM as reported by the patient with physical examination showed extension restriction to 15 degrees short of full extension or flexion less than 90 degrees were defined as stiffness. However, this definition could not be applicable if the preoperative arc of motion is less than 75 degrees [3].

2.1 Factors

The factors or etiologies related to stiff TKA could be categorized into three phases: preoperative, intraoperative, and postoperative periods [8]. Each period also has its specified causes and different management. Surgeons should evaluate the patients carefully for the proper treatment.

2.1.1 Preoperative period

Preoperative ROM limitation is the most important risk factor for postoperative stiffness [4, 9]. Patients with a greater degree of preoperative ROM had superior postoperative ROM and functional scores, with less complications. Only 71.4 percent of patients with preoperative ROM less than 90 degrees would achieve postoperative ROM at least 90 degrees, while more than 90 percent of patients with preoperative ROM greater than 90 degrees could perform ROM more than 90 degrees postoperatively [10]. Lee et al. demonstrated that 33 percent of patients with preoperative ROM less than 50 degrees developed either superficial or deep infection, as well as skin necrosis after the operation, whereas only 13 percent of patients with preoperative ROM between 50 and 90 degrees suffered from these complications [11]. The cause of stiffness before surgery is also one of the considerable factors for postoperative stiffness. The same study by Lee et al. showed patients with osteoarthritis or rheumatoid arthritis had greater postoperative ROM than patients with prior infectious arthritis or traumatic arthritis significantly [11]. Patients with younger age, absence of diabetes mellitus, and lower preoperative walking limitations were found to be the additional predictors with better postoperative ROM [12]. Moreover, obesity might be another factor influencing postoperative ROM. Järvenpää et al. proposed patients with body mass index (BMI) greater than 30 kg/m^2 had poorer postoperative ROM at 1-year follow-up approximately 6 degrees than patients with less BMI [13].

2.1.2 Intraoperative period

At the time of surgery, technical errors during the bone cut, soft tissue procedure, and implantation, which relate to an imbalance in flexion and extension gaps, are the most frequent causes of postoperative stiffness. All of these conditions may result in limitation of motion both flexion and extension after TKA (**Table 1**) [4, 9].

Bone cut	Soft tissue procedure	Implantation
• Insufficient posterior tibial slope or creation of anterior tibial slope • Inaccurate joint line level which alters the joint line and the patella, either patella alta or patella baja • Inadequate osteophytes resection • Insufficient bone cut, either proximal tibia or distal femur, especially the posterior condyle	• Inappropriate tension of posterior cruciate ligament (in case of cruciate-retaining prosthesis) • Inadequate soft tissue release, especially deep medial collateral ligament (MCL) for varus knee and iliotibial band for valgus knee	• Improper size of the prosthesis, especially incorrect choice of larger tibial insert • Malposition of the femoral component, either excessive hyperflexion or hyperextension • Malrotation of the prosthesis may also cause the problem of patellofemoral kinematics

Table 1.
The intraoperative conditions which result in stiff TKA.

2.1.3 Postoperative period

There are several factors causing stiffness following TKA in this period, including inadequate rehabilitation and poor patient motivation, deep infection, arthrofibrosis, complex regional pain syndrome (CRPS), associated stiffness or pain derived from the adjacent joints or spine that alters knee motion, and heterotropic ossification (HO) [14]. Adequate postoperative pain management is essential in improving functional recovery and achieving rehabilitation protocol, especially knee motion enhancement [15]. Deep infection or PJI is one of the conditions leading to difficulty in ROM with chronic dull pain. It should be considered, especially in patients who developed stiffness after achieving adequate ROM [4, 14]. The details of this condition are described later in this chapter.

Arthrofibrosis after TKA is the most common cause of stiffness with an incidence ranging from 1.2 to 17 percent [9]. The etiology is multifactorial and the exact pathophysiology is unclear. Patients with poor preoperative ROM, higher complexity surgery, and a history of previous knee surgery increase the risk of excessive fibrous tissue formation after TKA. The theory of developing arthrofibrosis is disruption of cytokines and growth factors signaling cell growth, differentiation, and death, resulting in uncontrolled proliferation of fibroconnective tissue [16]. The histology is characterized by metaplasia of calcified tissue, myofibroblasts, and excessive fibrosis, with the increasing number of macrophages and lymphocytes in the periarticular tissue [17, 18]. The clinical manifestation is broad spectrum, from a localized lesion to a generalized involvement of the entire joint, and results in the formation of extensive extra-articular fibrous tissue.

Recently, there is no gold standard for diagnosis of arthrofibrosis, and also no effective method to prevent the idiopathic arthrofibrosis after TKA, apart from patient education and early mobilization [4].

2.2 Treatment

Initial evaluation of stiff TKA to assess the causes is necessary before management. A correct diagnosis leads to correct treatment. The evaluation should review back to the preoperative status of the patient, especially the risk factors mentioned above. The radiological examination should perform in case of suspicious mechanical problems from surgical errors of bone cut and implantation. Do not hesitate to work up for PJI if infection or wound-related complications that predispose the patient to infection are suspected [4, 9].

There are various treatment options for stiff TKA: manipulation under anesthesia (MUA), arthroscopic arthrolysis, open arthrolysis, and revision surgery [4].

2.2.1 Manipulation under anesthesia (MUA)

The purpose of MUA is to break immature adhesions within the knee in patients who disadvantage of self-training or regular rehabilitation programs and accelerate the initial rehabilitation process [19]. This procedure should be performed within 6–8 weeks after initial TKA before the development of mature adhesions which increases the likelihood of complications after MUA, especially periprosthetic fractures or rupture of the extensor mechanism [20]. Aggressive rehabilitation is necessary to prevent further and recurrent stiffness. A systematic review by Fitzsimmons et al. showed a mean gain in knee motion from 30 to 47 degrees after MUA [7].

2.2.2 Arthroscopic arthrolysis

Arthroscopic arthrolysis is a minimal invasive surgery that resects fibrosis directly in the suprapatellar pouch, medial and lateral gutters, and also in the intercondylar groove [4]. The indication of this operative procedure is painless, stiff TKA after non-progression of conservative treatment for 3 months. Disadvantage is inadequate arthrolysis because of poor access to the posterior structure and the area above the suprapatellar pouch [9]. A systematic review demonstrated improvement of overall ROM between 18.5 and 60 degrees, which also achieved 30.8–42 degrees even performing arthroscopic arthrolysis after 1 year of index TKA [7].

2.2.3 Open arthrolysis

Open lysis of adhesions is recommended in case of severe ROM limitation which impedes the use of arthroscope without component malposition and after the failure of conservative treatment. This operative procedure can provide a broad assessment of the knee joint and fibrosis resection should be performed meticulously. However, exposure to the joint may be difficult from adhesions and need further operative technique, for example, tibial tubercle osteotomy, quadriceps snip, or VY-plasty [4, 9]. A systematic review by Fitzsimmons et al. showed an average increasing of ROM between 19 and 31 degrees after open arthrolysis [7].

2.2.4 Revision surgery

This is the final treatment option reserved for stiffness from surgical errors that need to be corrected. Accurate analysis of the errors is required for planning the revision correctly to meet the patient's satisfaction [4].

3. Periprosthetic joint infection (PJI)

PJI is a serious complication and is considered one of the most common causes of revision surgery following the failure of primary TKA [21]. The incidence of PJI after primary knee replacement is ranging from 0.85 to 2.2 percent [22], with a higher rate up to 9 percent in revision cases [23]. Despite a small incidence of infection following TKA, the trend of revision due to PJI was rising by 2.5-fold in the past decade [22].

This problem illustrates an increasing and substantial treatment burden to both orthopedic surgeons and the patients, as well as the health service system.

A systematic review and meta-analysis by Kunutsor et al. showed patients with smoking, BMI >30 kg/m^2, diabetes, depression, steroid use, previous joint surgery, and frailty were the significant risk factors associated with the long-term developing PJI [24]. A study by Rosteius et al. demonstrated the most common pathogen found in PJI after TKA was methicillin-susceptible *Staphylococcus aureus* (MSSA) which occurred in 28.2 percent of patients, followed by coagulase-negative *Staphylococcus* (CoNS), methicillin-resistant *Staphylococcus epidermidis* (MRSE), *Streptococcus*, ampicillin-susceptible *Enterococcus faecalis*, and methicillin-resistant *Staphylococcus aureus* (MRSA) with the frequency of 16.4, 13.2, 9.1, 7.1, and 6.6 percent, respectively. However, up to 17.8 percent of patients could not identify any pathogens [25].

3.1 Diagnosis

Recently, there is no gold standard for the diagnosis of PJI [21]. The Musculoskeletal Infection Society (MSIS) and the Infectious Diseases Society of America (IDSA) have previously developed criteria to standardize the definition of PJI in 2011 and 2013 [26, 27], together with an International Consensus Meeting on PJI in 2013 [28]. The latest consensus in 2018 proposed a new scoring-based definition for PJI after emerging of new diagnostic tests. Two positive cultures of the same organism or the presence of a sinus tract were considered as major criteria and a definite diagnosis of PJI. The minor criteria consisted of laboratory tests either serum or synovial fluid which were weighted differently. An elevated serum C-reactive protein (CRP) or D-dimer received 2 points, whereas an elevation of erythrocyte sedimentation rate (ESR) weighted 1 point. Furthermore, an elevated synovial white blood cell (WBC) count or leukocyte esterase (LE) was considered 3 points. The other diagnostic tests for synovial fluid were a positive alpha-defensin, an elevated synovial polymorphonuclear (PMN) percentage, and synovial CRP which took 3, 2, and 1 point, respectively. Patients with a total score of equal or greater than 6 were suggested infected, while a score between 2 and 5 was classified as inconclusive and required further intraoperative diagnostic score to fulfill the definition, and a score of 0 to 1 was defined as no infection.

The intraoperative diagnostic score consisted of positive histology, purulence, and a single positive culture which scored 3, 3, and 2 points, respectively. In combination with the inconclusive preoperative diagnostic score, patients with an overall score of equal or greater than 6 were considered infected, whereas a score between 4 and 5 was inconclusive and need further molecular findings, and a score of 3 or less was defined as aseptic (**Table 2**). The threshold of each laboratory test is detailed in **Table 3**. The sensitivity and specificity of this new scoring system are 97.7 and 99.5 percent, respectively, which is higher sensitivity than the previous diagnostic criteria [29].

3.2 Treatment

Management of PJI includes surgical intervention and medical treatment, especially antibiotics therapy, with the goals of eradicating the infection, minimizing pain by restoring the function of the infected joint before performing the revision arthroplasty, as well as reducing morbidity and mortality of the patients [30]. Tsukayama et al. classified characteristics of infection after TKA into four types with the guidance of surgical options among these scenarios (**Table 4**) [31].

Major criteria (at least one of the following)		Decision
1. Two positive cultures of the same organism		Infected
2. Sinus tract with evidence of communication to the joint or visualization of the prosthesis		
Minor criteria (Preoperative diagnosis)	**Score**	**Decision**
Serum		
1. Elevated CRP or D-dimer	2	
2. Elevated ESR	1	≥6 Infected 2–5 Inconclusive (possibly infected)* 0–1 Not infected
Synovial		
1. Elevated synovial WBC count or LE	3	
2. Positive alpha-defensin	3	
3. Elevated synovial PMN percentage	2	
4. Elevated synovial CRP	1	
Intraoperative diagnosis	**Score**	**Decision**
Inconclusive preoperative score* or dry tap with		
1. Positive histology	3	≥6 Infected 4–5 Inconclusive ≤3 Not infected
2. Positive purulence	3	
3. Single positive culture	2	

Modified from Parvizi et al. The 2018 Definition of Periprosthetic Hip and Knee Infection: An Evidence-Based and Validated Criteria. J Arthroplasty. 2018;33(5):1309–14.e2.

Table 2.
The 2018 International Consensus Meeting on Musculoskeletal Infection scoring-based definition for PJI.

Laboratory test	Acute (<90 days)	Chronic (>90 days)
1. Serum CRP (mg/L)	100	10
2. Serum D-dimer (ng/mL)	860	860
3. Serum ESR (mm/h)	—	30
4. Synovial WBC count (cells/μL)	10,000	3,000
5. Synovial alpha-defensin (signal-to-cutoff ratio)	1	1
6. Synovial PMN (%)	90	80
7. Synovial CRP (mg/L)	6.9	6.9

Modified from Parvizi et al. The 2018 Definition of Periprosthetic Hip and Knee Infection: An Evidence-Based and Validated Criteria. J Arthroplasty. 2018;33(5):1309–14.e2.

Table 3.
The threshold of laboratory test of the minor criteria.

4. Periprosthetic fracture

Periprosthetic fracture after TKA is found increasingly in recent years due to a large number of performed TKAs and growing of geriatric population. This serious complication is impact to the quality of life and functional recovery of the patients, which is recognized to develop high morbidity and mortality [32]. The incidence

Type and definition	Characteristics	Treatment options
I: Positive intraoperative culture	• A positive culture of an intraoperative specimen during a revision arthroplasty for aseptic loosening	• Antibiotics alone, without further operation
II: Early postoperative infection		
• Superficial	• Occurs within 1 month after joint replacement • Local inflammation of acute onset • No sinus tract • No extension through capsule	• Cultures of the tissues or drainage fluid • Débridement of the soft tissue • Wound closure/antibiotic beads (remove after 2 weeks) • 2–6 weeks of antibiotic therapy
• Deep	• Occurs within 1 month after joint replacement • Local inflammation of acute onset • No sinus tract • Extension through capsule	• Cultures of the tissues or drainage fluid • Arthrotomy, synovectomy, and débridement of all infected soft tissue • Exchange of polyethylene insert • Wound closure/antibiotic beads (remove after 2 weeks) • 4–6 weeks of antibiotic therapy
III: Acute hematogenous	• Occurs more than 1 month after joint replacement • Local inflammation of acute onset • No sinus tract • Extension through capsule • Represents hematogenous seeding of the joint from another primary site of infection	• Cultures of the tissues or drainage fluid • Arthrotomy, synovectomy, and débridement of all infected soft tissue • Exchange of polyethylene insert • Wound closure/antibiotic beads (remove after 2 weeks) • 6 weeks of antibiotic therapy
IV: Late chronic	• Occurs more than 1 month after joint replacement • Insidious onset, usually no fever or leukocytosis • Sinus tract may be observed • Extension through capsule	• Cultures of the tissues or drainage fluid • Débridement and removal of all prosthetic components and bone cement • Applying an antibiotic cement spacer • 6 weeks of antibiotic therapy

Table 4.
Tsukayama classification and treatment options.

of fracture following TKA varies from 0.3 to 5.5 percent in primary knee replacement and has been reported as high as 30 percent in revision knee surgery [33, 34]. The most common site of fracture is a supracondylar area of the distal femur which occurs ranging from 0.3 to 2.5 percent [32, 35], followed by patellar periprosthetic fracture, especially in the resurfaced patella, with an incidence around 0.68 percent. However, the true incidence of this type of fracture may be obscured from undetected and asymptomatic patients [36]. The least common pattern is a proximal tibial fracture which affected approximately 0.3 to 0.5 percent [37]. Most frequently, periprosthetic fracture results from low-energy trauma, and osteoporosis is considered a significant predictor of fracture risk [38]. The other predisposing factors are any causes that affected bone quality, for example, prolonged corticosteroid use, inflammatory joint diseases, especially rheumatoid arthritis, and patients with neurological and musculoskeletal problems, which have a high risk of falls [32, 35]. Iatrogenic causes from surgical procedure including anterior femoral notching, or alteration of anterior femoral cortex during bone preparation of distal femur is theorized to be an association of supracondylar femoral fracture after TKA [35]. A biomechanical study by Lesh et al. revealed a reduction of torsional strength and bending strength of the distal femur by 39.2 and 18 percent, respectively, after the full-thickness cortical defect was created [39]. However, the clinical outcome is still controversial [32, 40, 41]. The risk factors of periprosthetic tibial fractures in TKA are the use of long tibial stems, cementless press-fit fixation, malalignment of tibial component, and previous osteotomy of the tibia [37]. All other predisposing factors are detailed in **Table** 5 [42].

Medical factors	Surgical factors		
	Femur	Tibia	Patella
• Osteoporosis • Prolonged corticosteroid use • Inflammatory joint diseases e.g., rheumatoid arthritis • Neurological and musculoskeletal problems e.g., epilepsy, parkinsonism, myasthenia gravis, poliomyelitis, cerebral palsy	• Anterior femoral notching • Component malposition • Poorly reamed bone • Stress shielding • Box cut for posterior stabilized (PS) implants	• Use of long tibial stems • Cementless press-fit fixation • Intramedullary referencing • Malalignment • Osteolysis • Sclerosing subchondral bone • Tibial tubercle osteotomy	• Excessive bony resection • Central peg • Press-fit implants • Lateral release • Fat pad excision • Maltracking • Cement heat necrosis

Table 5.
Predisposing factors associated with periprosthetic fractures after TKA.

4.1 Classification

4.1.1 Femur

There were several classification systems described for supracondylar periprosthetic fracture of femur. Rorabeck et al. developed a classification that described fracture configuration and integrity of prosthesis to guide appropriate management of each fracture pattern. The key factors considered in the classification were the fracture displacement and the prosthesis stability [43, 44]. This classification later was widely known as "Lewis and Rorabeck classification" (**Table 6**).

The Lewis and Rorabeck classification recommended nonoperative treatment for type I classification [44]. However, Su et al. suggested surgical management in any type of fracture because of the high complication rate and further displacement in case of conservative treatment. An alternative classification was developed and proposed to characterize the fracture line in relation to the component for help in choosing among surgical options (**Figure 1**; **Table** 7) [45].

Type	Characteristics
I	Undisplaced fracture; prosthesis intact
II	Displaced fracture; prosthesis intact
III	Displaced or undisplaced fracture; prosthesis loosening or failing e.g., significant instability or polyethylene wear

Table 6.
Lewis and Rorabeck classification.

Type	Characteristics
I	Fractures are proximal to the femoral component
II	Fractures originate at the proximal end of the component and extend proximally
III	Any part of the fracture line is distal to the upper edge of the component's anterior flange

Table 7.
Su classification.

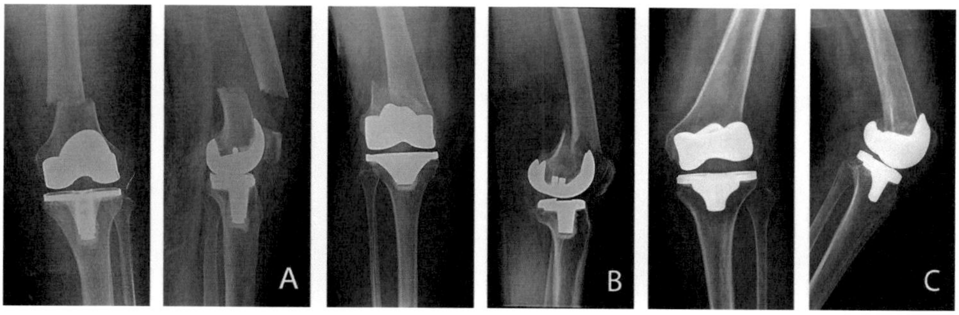

Figure 1.
Anteroposterior and lateral radiographs showing periprosthetic fracture of TKA (A) Su classification type I; Lewis and Rorabeck classification type II (B) Su classification type II; Lewis and Rorabeck classification type II (C) Su classification type III; Lewis and Rorabeck classification type III.

4.1.2 Tibia

The Mayo classification described by Felix et al. (also known as Felix classification) is widely recognized to assess periprosthetic tibial fractures following TKA [46]. Fractures are classified into four types based on location and proximity to the prosthesis and each type is subcategorized by stability and whether the fracture occurred intraoperatively or postoperatively. The details are described in **Table 8**.

4.1.3 Patella

The widely used classification for periprosthetic patellar fractures is the classification proposed by Goldberg et al. which is characterized by fracture configuration, stability of patellar component, and integrity of extensor mechanism [47]. The newer classification described by Ortiguera and Berry focused similarly on the stability of patellar components and integrity of extensor mechanism but differently on the quality of residual bone stock (**Tables 9** and **10**) [36].

Type	Characteristics
I	Fractures are located at the tibial plateau
II	Fractures occur inferior to the tibial plateau adjacent to the prosthetic stem
III	Fractures occur distal to the tibial stem
IV	Fractures involve the tibial tubercle
Additional subtype	**Characteristics**
A	A fracture with a stable prosthesis on radiographs
B	Fractures with radiographic evidence of component loosening
C	Intraoperative fractures

Table 8.
Mayo (Felix) classification.

Type	Characteristics
I	Fractures are located in the periphery of the patella and do not involve the patellar component and the extensor mechanism
II	Fractures disrupt the implant-bone composite or the extensor mechanism
III • IIIA • IIIB	Fractures involve the inferior pole of the patella • With ruptured patellar ligament • Intact patellar ligament
IV	Patellar fractures accompanied by patellofemoral dislocation

Table 9.
Goldberg classification.

Type	Characteristics
I	A stable implant and intact extensor mechanism
II	A stable implant with disruption of the extensor mechanism
III • IIIA • IIIB	Loose patellar component • With reasonable bone stock • With poor bone stock (<10 mm thickness or marked comminution)

Table 10.
Ortiguera and Berry classification.

4.2 Treatment

Fracture treatment options in each component are related on their classified types. For supracondylar femoral fracture, Lewis and Rorabeck classification recommended nonsurgical treatment in type I, whereas treatment options either closed reduction and fixation with an intramedullary nail or open reduction and internal fixation with a plate could be performed in type II. Type III fracture requires revision of the prosthesis using a long stem or structural allograft [44]. Su et al. suggested reduction with antegrade or retrograde intramedullary nail, or sometimes a fixed-angle device for Su classification type I fracture. Su classification type II requires management with either a fixed-angle device or retrograde supracondylar nail, and type III fracture may be managed with either a fixed-angle device or revision arthroplasty with a stemmed femoral component. However, if loosening is identified in any classification types, revision TKA with a femoral stem is recommended [45].

Felix et al. proposed a treatment algorithm for periprosthetic tibial fractures related to their classification. For type IA, nondisplaced IIA, and IIIA fracture, nonoperative treatment with protected weight-bearing is required. If displacement is observed in type IIA and IIIA fracture, closed reduction with casting or open reduction with internal fixation is recommended. Any loosening types (IB, IIB, and IIIB) should be treated with revision arthroplasty. In case of intraoperative fracture (subcategory C), bracing with protected weight-bearing can be treated in any type if the fracture is stable and nondisplaced. However, in unstable fracture pattern or displaced fracture, further surgical management is required. Type IC fracture may be treated by screw fixation and/or a long-stemmed tibial prosthesis to bypass the fracture site. Type IIC fracture can be managed with bone grafting at the cortical defect and bypassing the fracture site with a long tibial stem. Type IIIC fracture can be treated with either closed reduction and casting or open reduction with internal fixation [46].

For treatment of patellar periprosthetic fracture, Ortiguera and Berry suggested nonoperative treatment for type I fracture. If patients developed extensor mechanism disruption with a well-fixed implant (type II), open reduction with internal fixation of the displaced fragment, or alternatively, patellectomy with advancement and repair of the extensor mechanism is recommended. Operative treatment for type IIIA fracture required revision of the patellar component or component resection with patelloplasty, whereas implant removal with patellectomy is recommended for type IIIB fracture [36].

In the elderly, physiologic changes of bone, especially a high rate of bone resorption, result in diminishing bone mass and strength [48]. Osteoporosis workup and treatment are necessary in addition to fracture management in patients with periprosthetic fracture after TKA.

5. Conclusions

This chapter concludes with the principle, classification, and management of three typical conditions, which are considered serious and unsatisfied results after TKA. Causes of stiff TKA divide into three different periods and each period needs specific management, but the most important risk factor for postoperative stiffness is the limitation of preoperative ROM. Patient education and motivation either before or after surgery are necessary to prevent further problems and meet the patient's satisfaction. An exploration of new diagnostic tests enhances the accuracy of PJI diagnosis and the latest scoring-based definition achieved more sensitivity than the previous criteria. Major criteria of two positive cultures of a similar pathogen or the presence of a sinus tract to the knee joint can diagnose PJI. If a diagnosis has not been made, the further investigation of minor criteria, including serum and synovial laboratory tests, would have been collected preoperatively. An inconclusive diagnosis from the minor criteria needs furthermore investigation from intraoperative findings. Periprosthetic fractures are principally classified from the anatomy of fracture site. The most common is a femoral supracondylar fracture and the surgical options depend on fracture location and configuration. Finally, the goal of treatment among these three conditions is return to ambulation with a well-function knee prosthesis.

Conflict of interest

The authors declare no conflict of interest.

Author details

Atthakorn Jarusriwanna[1*] and Chaturong Pornrattanamaneewong[2]

1 Department of Orthopaedics, Faculty of Medicine, Naresuan University, Phitsanulok, Thailand

2 Department of Orthopaedic Surgery, Faculty of Medicine Siriraj Hospital, Mahidol University, Bangkok, Thailand

*Address all correspondence to: atthakorn.ton@gmail.com

References

[1] Carr AJ, Robertsson O, Graves S, Price AJ, Arden NK, Judge A, et al. Knee replacement. Lancet. 2012;**379**(9823):1331-1340

[2] Gunaratne R, Pratt DN, Banda J, Fick DP, Khan RJK, Robertson BW. Patient dissatisfaction following total knee arthroplasty: A systematic review of the literature. The Journal of Arthroplasty. 2017;**32**(12):3854-3860

[3] Healy WL, Della Valle CJ, Iorio R, Berend KR, Cushner FD, Dalury DF, et al. Complications of total knee arthroplasty: Standardized list and definitions of the Knee Society. Clinical Orthopaedics and Related Research. 2013;**471**(1):215-220

[4] Manrique J, Gomez MM, Parvizi J. Stiffness after total knee arthroplasty. The Journal of Knee Surgery. 2015;**28**(2):119-126

[5] Choi HR, Siliski J, Malchau H, Freiberg A, Rubash H, Kwon YM. How often is functional range of motion obtained by manipulation for stiff total knee arthroplasty? International Orthopaedics. 2014;**38**(8):1641-1645

[6] Laubenthal KN, Smidt GL, Kettelkamp DB. A quantitative analysis of knee motion during activities of daily living. Physical Therapy. 1972;**52**:34-43

[7] Fitzsimmons SE, Vazquez EA, Bronson MJ. How to treat the stiff total knee arthroplasty?: A systematic review. Clinical Orthopaedics and Related Research. 2010;**468**(4):1096-1106

[8] Chareoncholvanich K. Complications after Total Knee Arthroplasty. In: Charoencholvanich K, editor. Reconstructive Surgery of the Osteoarthritic Knee. Bangkok: Faculty of Medicine Siriraj Hospital, Mahidol University; 2016. pp. 283-319

[9] Schiavone Panni A, Cerciello S, Vasso M, Tartarone M. Stiffness in total knee arthroplasty. Journal of Orthopaedics and Traumatology. 2009;**10**(3):111-118

[10] Lizaur A, Marco L, Cebrian R. Preoperative factors influencing the range of movement after total knee arthroplasty for severe osteoarthritis. The Journal of Bone and Joint Surgery. British Volume (London). 1997;**79**(4):626-629

[11] Lee SA, Kang SB, Chang CB, Chang MJ, Kim YJ, Song MK, et al. Does the severity or cause of preoperative stiffness affect the clinical results and range of motion after total knee arthroplasty? PLoS One. 2018;**13**(10):e0205168

[12] Pua YH, Poon CL, Seah FJ, Thumboo J, Clark RA, Tan MH, et al. Predicting individual knee range of motion, knee pain, and walking limitation outcomes following total knee arthroplasty. Acta Orthopaedica. 2019;**90**(2):179-186

[13] Järvenpää J, Kettunen J, Soininvaara T, Miettinen H, Kröger H. Obesity has a negative impact on clinical outcome after total knee arthroplasty. Scandinavian Journal of Surgery. 2012;**101**(3):198-203

[14] Bong MR, Di Cesare PE. Stiffness after total knee arthroplasty. The Journal of the American Academy of Orthopaedic Surgeons. 2004;**12**(3):164-171

[15] Laoruengthana A, Jarusriwanna A, Rattanaprichavej P, Rasamimongkol S,

Varakornpipat P, Pongpirul K. Timing of periarticular injection has no effect on postoperative pain and functional recovery in simultaneous bilateral total knee arthroplasty: A prospective randomized, double-blinded trial. BMC Musculoskeletal Disorders. 2019;**20**(1):162

[16] Cheuy VA, Foran JRH, Paxton RJ, Bade MJ, Zeni JA, Stevens-Lapsley JE. Arthrofibrosis associated with total knee arthroplasty. The Journal of Arthroplasty. 2017;**32**(8):2604-2611

[17] Freeman TA, Parvizi J, Dela Valle CJ, Steinbeck MJ. Mast cells and hypoxia drive tissue metaplasia and heterotopic ossification in idiopathic arthrofibrosis after total knee arthroplasty. Fibrogenesis & Tissue Repair. 2010;**3**:17

[18] Freeman TA, Parvizi J, Della Valle CJ, Steinbeck MJ. Reactive oxygen and nitrogen species induce protein and DNA modifications driving arthrofibrosis following total knee arthroplasty. Fibrogenesis & Tissue Repair. 2009;**2**(1):5

[19] Maloney WJ. The stiff total knee arthroplasty: Evaluation and management. The Journal of Arthroplasty. 2002;**17**(4 Suppl. 1):71-73

[20] Stamos VP, Bono JV. Management of the stiff total knee arthroplasty. In: Bono JV, Scott RD, editors. Revision Total Knee Arthroplasty. New York: Springer; 2005. pp. 251-257

[21] Goswami K, Parvizi J, Maxwell CP. Current recommendations for the diagnosis of acute and chronic PJI for hip and knee-cell counts, alpha-defensin, leukocyte esterase, next-generation sequencing. Current Review Musculoskeletal Medicine. 2018;**11**(3):428-438

[22] Lenguerrand E, Whitehouse MR, Beswick AD, Toms AD, Porter ML, Blom AW, et al. Description of the rates, trends and surgical burden associated with revision for prosthetic joint infection following primary and revision knee replacements in England and Wales: An analysis of the National Joint Registry for England, Wales, Northern Ireland and the Isle of Man. BMJ Open. 2017;**7**(7):e014056

[23] Mortazavi SM, Schwartzenberger J, Austin MS, Purtill JJ, Parvizi J. Revision total knee arthroplasty infection: Incidence and predictors. Clinical Orthopaedics and Related Research. 2010;**468**(8):2052-2059

[24] Kunutsor SK, Whitehouse MR, Blom AW, Beswick AD. INFORM Team. Patient-related risk factors for periprosthetic joint infection after total joint arthroplasty: A systematic review and meta-analysis. PLoS One. 2016;**11**(3):e0150866

[25] Rosteius T, Jansen O, Fehmer T, Baecker H, Citak M, Schildhauer TA, et al. Evaluating the microbial pattern of periprosthetic joint infections of the hip and knee. Journal of Medical Microbiology. 2018;**67**(11):1608-1613

[26] Parvizi J, Zmistowski B, Berbari EF, Bauer TW, Springer BD, Della Valle CJ, et al. New definition for periprosthetic joint infection: From the Workgroup of the Musculoskeletal Infection Society. Clinical Orthopaedics and Related Research. 2011;**469**(11):2992-2994

[27] Osmon DR, Berbari EF, Berendt AR, Lew D, Zimmerli W, Steckelberg JM, et al. Executive summary: Diagnosis and management of prosthetic joint infection: Clinical practice guidelines by the Infectious Diseases Society of America. Clinical Infectious Diseases. 2013;**56**(1):1-10

[28] Parvizi J, Gehrke T, Chen AF. Proceedings of the international consensus on periprosthetic joint infection. Bone Joint Journal. 2013;**95**(11):1450-1452

[29] Parvizi J, Tan TL, Goswami K, Higuera C, Della Valle C, Chen AF, et al. The 2018 definition of periprosthetic hip and knee infection: An evidence-based and validated criteria. The Journal of Arthroplasty. 2018;**33**(5):1309-14.e2

[30] Tande AJ, Patel R. Prosthetic joint infection. Clinical Microbiology Reviews. 2014;**27**(2):302-345

[31] Tsukayama DT, Goldberg VM, Kyle R. Diagnosis and management of infection after total knee arthroplasty. The Journal of Bone and Joint Surgery. American Volume. 2003;**85-A**:S75-S80

[32] Whitehouse MR, Mehendale S. Periprosthetic fractures around the knee: Current concepts and advances in management. Current Reviews in Musculoskeletal Medicine. 2014;7(2):136-144

[33] Capone A, Congia S, Civinini R, Marongiu G. Periprosthetic fractures: Epidemiology and current treatment. Clinical Cases in Mineral and Bone Metabolism. 2017;**14**(2):189-196

[34] Della Rocca GJ, Leung KS, Pape HC. Periprosthetic fractures: Epidemiology and future projections. Journal of Orthopaedic Trauma. 2011;**25**(Suppl. 2):S66-S70

[35] Yoo JD, Kim NK. Periprosthetic fractures following total knee arthroplasty. Knee Surgery Related Research. 2015;**27**(1):1-9

[36] Ortiguera CJ, Berry DJ. Patellar fracture after total knee arthroplasty. The Journal of Bone and Joint Surgery. American Volume 2002;**84**(4):532-540

[37] Schreiner AJ, Schmidutz F, Ateschrang A, Ihle C, Stöckle U, Ochs BG, et al. Periprosthetic tibial fractures in total knee arthroplasty - an outcome analysis of a challenging and underreported surgical issue. BMC Musculoskeletal Disorders. 2018;**19**(1):323

[38] Rhee SJ, Cho JY, Choi YY, Sawaguchi T, Suh JT. Femoral periprosthetic fractures after total knee arthroplasty: New surgically oriented classification with a review of current treatments. Knee Surgery Related Research. 2018;**30**(4):284-292

[39] Lesh ML, Schneider DJ, Deol G, Davis B, Jacobs CR, Pellegrini VD Jr. The consequences of anterior femoral notching in total knee arthroplasty. A biomechanical study. The Journal of Bone and Joint Surgery. American Volume. 2000;**82**(8):1096-1101

[40] Ritter MA, Thong AE, Keating EM, Faris PM, Meding JB, Berend ME, et al. The effect of femoral notching during total knee arthroplasty on the prevalence of postoperative femoral fractures and on clinical outcome. The Journal of Bone and Joint Surgery. American Volume. 2005;**87**(11):2411-2414

[41] Gujarathi N, Putti AB, Abboud RJ, MacLean JG, Espley AJ, Kellett CF. Risk of periprosthetic fracture after anterior femoral notching. Acta Orthopaedica. 2009;**80**(5):553-556

[42] Sarmah SS, Patel S, Reading G, El-Husseiny M, Douglas S, Haddad FS. Periprosthetic fractures around total knee arthroplasty. Annals of the Royal College of Surgeons of England. 2012;**94**(5):302-307

[43] Rorabeck CH, Angliss RD, Lewis PL. Fractures of the femur, tibia, and patella after total knee arthroplasty: Decision

making and principles of management. Instructional Course Lectures. 1998;**47**:449-458

[44] Rorabeck CH, Taylor JW. Classification of periprosthetic fractures complicating total knee arthroplasty. The Orthopedic Clinics of North America. 1999;**30**(2):209-214

[45] Su ET, DeWal H, Di Cesare PE. Periprosthetic femoral fractures above total knee replacements. The Journal of the American Academy of Orthopaedic Surgeons. 2004;**12**(1):12-20

[46] Felix NA, Stuart MJ, Hanssen AD. Periprosthetic fractures of the tibia associated with total knee arthroplasty. Clinical Orthopaedics and Related Research. 1997;**345**:113-124

[47] Goldberg VM, Figgie HE 3rd, Inglis AE, Figgie MP, Sobel M, Kelly M, et al. Patellar fracture type and prognosis in condylar total knee arthroplasty. Clinical Orthopaedics and Related Research. 1988;**236**:115-122

[48] Unnanuntana A, Jarusriwanna A, Vanitcharoenkul E. Bone physiology and age-related bone changes. In: Unnanuntana A, editor. Textbook of Hip Fracture in The Elderly. Bangkok: Faculty of Medicine Siriraj Hospital, Mahidol University; 2019. pp. 18-39

Chapter 9

Modern Coatings in Knee Arthroplasty

Jörg Lützner, Brigitte Altermann, Ana Laura Puente Reyna and Thomas M. Grupp

Abstract

All metal implants in human bodies corrode, which results in metal ion release. This is not necessarily a problem and represents for most patients no hazard. However, both local and systemic effects are possible, including hypersensitivity. To avoid this, coatings on standard implants (mono- or multi-layer) and surface modifications have been developed and are in use. This chapter explains the background of metal ion release, biological reactions, coating technologies, biotribological and biomechanical properties, as well as the clinical results of modern knee arthroplasty implant coatings. There is no general concern about metal ion release from CoCrMo standard implants for most patients. If patients present with a confirmed metal allergy, a multilayer-coated or oxidized zirconium implant is currently the best option for these patients.

Keywords: metal ion release, hypersensitivity, coating, multilayer, biological effects

1. Introduction

Total knee arthroplasty (TKA) is a very effective treatment option for advanced osteoarthritis of the knee with overall low revision rates [1]. However, not all patients benefit from the surgery and not all problems have been solved. One issue is the biological reaction to implanted materials. Knee arthroplasty implants are usually made of cobalt-chromium alloys. Material from implants is always released after implantation, either as a result of mechanical (wear) or electrochemical processes (corrosion). Biological reactions in patients, caused by the release of metal particles and metal ions, have been reported (allergy, inflammatory response). Furthermore, cobalt, a relevant part of the implant alloy, has recently been listed as a potentially carcinogenic and mutagenic category 1B hazard by the European Commission. To overcome these potential issues, the surface of knee arthroplasty implants has been coated or ceramised. Besides a reduction in the release of metal ions and metallo-organic complexes, this results additionally in better wear performance. Unfortunately, there have been reports about less favorable results with such hypoallergenic materials [2–4]. In a retrieval study, 21% of the TKAs demonstrated coating delamination, which might affect the performance of the coating [4].

This chapter explains the background of metal ion release, current coating technologies being used in modern knee arthroplasty implants, their biomechanical properties, biological reactions and clinical results.

2. Biological reactions

2.1 Metal ion release

All metal implants in human bodies corrode which results in metal ion release. This represents for most patients no problem. However, if a critical metal ion concentration is exceeded, local or rarely systemic problems can occur. The released metal particles may accumulate in and around affected joints as well as in body fluids, lymph nodes, bone marrow and internal organs. As a result, both local and systemic reactions are possible. Local tissue reactions to metal particles around joint arthroplasties have been described in the past by the generic term "metallosis". Natu et al. [5] introduced the term "adverse reactions to metal debris" (ARMD) which is the most widely used description for local tissue reactions.

Potential systemic adverse effects of metal particles include toxicity-related organ damage, mutagenic effects (carcinogenesis) and teratogenicity. Discussions have primarily focused on the potential damage of cobalt and chromium. While chromium particles may be significant in terms of their mutagenic potential, cobalt has been described to cause organ toxicity. In a review, Leyssens et al. [6] described the potential damage from cobalt exposure with special reference to different routes of exposure (including metallic bearings). The highest concentrations of cobalt in the body were seen in oral uptake and failed metal implants. The clinically possible sequelae of cobalt intoxication include mainly neurological effects (particularly impaired hearing and eyesight) as well as cardiovascular and endocrine effects. In general, it is assumed that such cobalt-related effects on organs require concentrations higher than 300 μg/l, which have not been described in patients with standard knee arthroplasty implants [7, 8].

Another potential effect of metal ions may be chromosomal aberrations. Therefore, the potential carcinogenic effects of metal implants have been discussed. However, in two extensive meta-analysis, no evidence of an increase in systemic tumor incidence was found. Considering the available clinical data including large registry studies, there is no evidence that metal-containing arthroplasty implants increase the risk of cancer or mortality in patient [9]. The same applies to potential teratogenic effects, which have not been reported.

Both, local and systemic effects are mostly a problem of metal-on-metal (MoM) hip arthroplasties or dual taper modular hip stems [10–14] but rarely seen in knee arthroplasties. Only large knee arthroplasty implants (tumor implants, hinged TKA, MoM) have the potential to cause relevant metal ion release and therefore local or systemic effects [15]. In standard TKA implants, this is not a matter of concern. Several studies have investigated metal ion concentrations in standard and coated TKA [16]. Although a relevant reduction of metal ion release has been reported in-vitro [17], there have been no relevant differences in-vivo. However, there are reports about the relevant increase in large hinged TKA which is a matter of concern [15] and needs to be observed.

2.2 Hypersensitivity and immunological reactions

There is a debate if patients with skin allergies to implant materials may react to metal implants, resulting in incompatibility reactions including persistent swelling, pain and early loosening. Moreover, there is still a controversy if hypoallergenic implants may be advantageous for these patients [18–22]. Despite these controversies, the prevalence of contact allergies against implant materials is high (especially nickel), and affected patients usually ask for hypoallergenic implants [23].

It has been demonstrated that patients with metal implants have more often skin allergies against implant materials than patients without such implants [24]. It has been discussed that the long contact time to the metal implant may result in a hypersensitization. However, only very few patients present with symptoms. There are reports about the improvement of symptoms after the revision of standard TKA to coated TKA implants [25]. On the contrary, it has also been reported that there is no increased risk of failure when implanting a standard TKA in skin-sensitive patients [19, 26]. However, functional outcome after TKA is worse in patients with reported metal allergies [27], which might be explained by psychological aspects [28]. Even if there is to date no clear evidence that patients with reported metal allergies need hypoallergenic implants, this psychological advantage might be helpful for patient satisfaction.

Several proinflammatory cytokines have been reported to play a role in healing and pain after TKA [29, 30]. It has been demonstrated that an increased inflammatory reaction after TKA results in less favorable results [31] and that cytokines were lower after being coated compared to standard TKA [32]. Surface modification of TKA may therefore result in less inflammation and better results.

3. Coating technologies in total knee arthroplasty

Coating of metallic components, mostly applied by the physical vaporing deposition (PVD) process, was first conceived as a solution for patients with hypersensitivity reactions to cobalt and nickel, as it prevented the release of such ions from the substrate material. There are currently different coating technologies for TKA implants in use. Historically, single-layer coatings, also known as monolayer coatings, came first in clinical application. Monolayers are in clinical use in two versions: composed of titanium nitride (TiN) and titanium niobium nitride (TiNbN). TiN and TiNbN monolayer coatings are in clinical use for hip, knee, and ankle arthroplasty since the early 1990s. They are applied by means of PVD on typical orthopedic implant materials such as titanium alloy (Ti6Al4V) or cobalt chromium molybdenum alloy (CoCrMo).

Another option is the oxidized zirconium (OxZr), which is not considered as a coating technology but more a surface modification of a ZrNb2 base material [28] driven by thermal oxidation at 500°C [33]. The resulting zirconium oxide (ZrO2) is a ceramic surface with good wear characteristics and reduced release of metal ions. This material has been in clinical use for knee arthroplasty since the 1980s [34].

Further development is represented by a zirconium nitride multilayer coating, which is composed of seven layers applied via PVD and has been in clinical use since 2006. The ceramic surface is composed of zirconium nitride as the top layer, chromium nitride and chromium carbon nitride as transition layers and a bonding layer of chromium, which integrates with the base material of the implant.

4. Biocompatibility, biotribology and biomechanics

TKA was originally conceived as a procedure for elderly patients with low to moderate activity levels. As the survival rates increased to more than 90% after 10 years due to advances in the bearing materials [35–37], this procedure was expanded to younger and more active patients. However, register data has shown a decrease in the survival rate during the second and third decades of clinical performance [38–40], particularly in younger patients [38].

The most common causes for revision surgery in TKA are aseptic loosening including wear-induced osteolysis and periprosthetic infection. Aseptic loosening is a direct consequence of wear particles (metallic and polyethylene) released by the articulating surfaces, which are phagocytized by macrophages and giant cells that induce the liberation of proinflammatory cytokines (interleukins IL-1ß, IL-6, and the TNF-α), which, in turn, stimulate the osteoclasts and reduce the activity of the osteoblasts. As a result, an osteolytic activity at the implant-bone interface occurs, resulting in a loosening of the implant components. This inflammatory response is dependent on the amount of wear particles, as well as their type, size and shape [16, 22, 41–45]. For this reason, younger and more active patients that generate more wear particles during a longer period of time, are at a higher risk of revision due to aseptic loosening and wear [46].

One important requirement for the coatings is that they should be able to generate the same amount of wear or less as their uncoated versions and the coating should be able to withstand the whole clinical lifespan of the implant. In order to evaluate and compare the wear behavior of different knee implants, the standardized wear test ISO 14243 is performed. During this test, the knee implants are subjected to a serum-based test medium at 37°C to the motion and loading profiles of the level walking activity of a 75 kg person for a total of 5 million cycles.

Another important aspect regarding the wear behavior of the coated implants is the analysis of the metal ion and particle release, as a relationship between cobalt and chromium blood levels and failure of implants has been demonstrated [47–50]. Retrieval and in vitro studies have shown that the CoCrMo femoral components develop scratches through their articulation with the ultra-high molecular weight polyethylene (UHMWPE) gliding surface and thus release metal ions [17, 51–55].

4.1 Biocompatibility

Zirconium material and Titanium-based coatings are considered as very biocompatible surfaces [56]. Several cell-culture and animal laboratory studies have shown that TiN coatings do not increase cell activity, show no difference to Ti6Al4V and have lower adhesion and proliferation over 24 hours of bacteria cultures than other uncoated metals [3]. Furthermore, in biocompatibility tests, TiN-coated test specimens made out of cobalt-chromium and titanium alloys did not cause any biotoxic damage [57].

Regarding ZrN multilayer coating Thomas et al. [48] performed patch tests on patients with and without metal ion hypersensitivity and showed no allergic reaction to the ZrN multilayer coated probes. Moreover, implanted multilayer-coated sticks in rabbits showed no adverse reactions to bone or tissues. Finally, a laboratory test with bacterial contamination showed 45% less biofilm formation on the ZrN multilayer coated surface in comparison to CoCrMo [58].

4.2 Biotribology and biomechanics of OxZr and TiN/TiNbN monolayers

One of the main goals of the oxidized zirconium is wear reduction, which has been tested in several wear simulation tests. The wear reduction compared to a standard CoCrMo femur against UHMWPE inserts ranges between 42% and 89%, depending on the wear simulation method, implant design and measurement protocol [59]. It also shows better scratch resistance than CoCrMo [60], as the nano-hardness of the zirconia layer ranges from 12 to 14 GPa, which is significantly harder compared to the 2–4 GPa from the CoCrMo standard material [56]. This has been demonstrated in three out of six OxZr retrieval studies from 1 to 5 years in-situ, which showed significantly less roughness of the femur component or less damage in the UHMWPE insert compared to CoCrMo implants. However, the other three retrieval studies showed no difference in the component analysis for femur and polyethylene insert damage [59].

A review of the literature on the effects of TiN coatings showed that TiN coatings have a positive effect on the biocompatibility and tribological properties of implant surfaces. TiN-coated implants showed also a high scratch resistance and less polyethylene wear. Nevertheless, several reports of third body wear due to delamination and cohesive failure also show negative effects of the TiN-coating [3]. The hardness of TiN and TiNbN coatings are with 24 GPa much higher than oxidized zirconium and supports the findings for lower polyethylene wear and high scratch resistance.

The metal ion release analysis of TiN and TiNbN coatings during an immersion study showed a reduction of cobalt ions of 80% and 76%, respectively, compared to an uncoated CoCrMo implant [61]. Similarly, another immersion study found a reduction of 80% for cobalt, 63% for chromium and 48% for molybdenum ion using a TiNbN coated implant in comparison to its uncoated CoCrMo version [62].

4.3 Biotribology and biomechanics of the ZrN multilayer coating

4.3.1 Wear articulating against UHMWPE

Studies have shown a UHMWPE wear reduction of more than 50% (**Figure 1**) by using the ZrN multilayer coated femur and tibial components in comparison to their uncoated versions [17, 63]. A limitation of the standardized ISO 14243 test is that it only simulates the short-term performance of an implant, as it reproduces only about 3 years of in vivo service [64]. Based on in vivo measurements performed on eight patients with instrumented implants [65], a new highly demanding activities (HDA) knee wear simulation protocol was developed, which reproduces 15–30 years of in vivo service, depending on the activity level of the patient [66]. In the HDA wear protocol, the load and motion profiles of the high flexion activities of stairs ascending, stairs descending, chair raising, deep squatting and normal level walking are simulated. Moreover, the loading profiles were normalized to represent a patient weight of 100 kg. A wear test study performed with the HDA wear simulation protocol also demonstrated a 2.8-fold lower UHMWPE wear rate when articulated with ZrN multilayer coated implants compared to the uncoated version (**Figure 1**) [52].

Regarding the metal ion release, in vitro studies have shown that the ZrN multilayer coating (with a hardness of 25 GPa) is not impaired by failure modes such as delamination, surface disruption or flaking [17, 52, 53], even under third body particle contamination [17]. This has been confirmed by analysis of the metal ion concentration analysis performed on the test medium, where the metal ion release of the substrate material is several orders of magnitude lower than in the uncoated

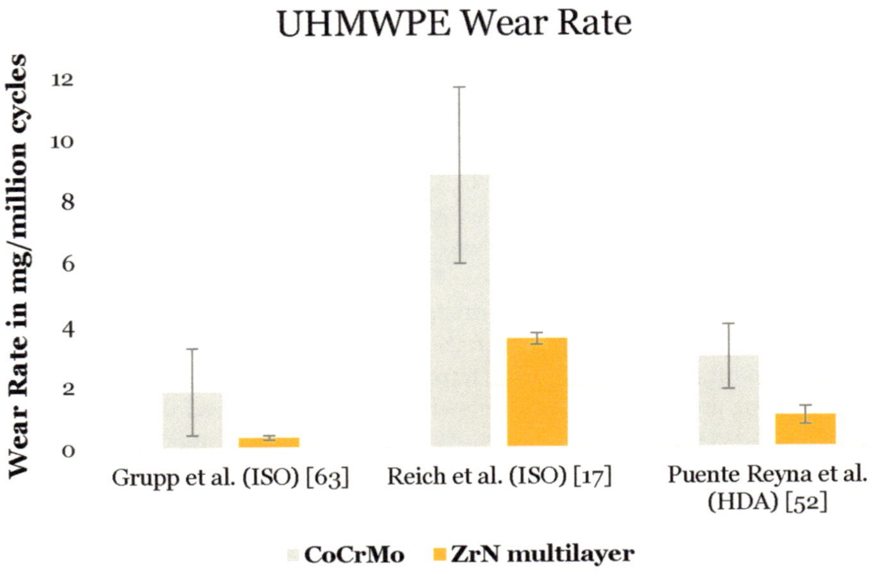

Figure 1.
UHMWPE wear rates comparison between uncoated CoCrMo and ZrN multilayer coated knee implants after ISO and HDA knee wear simulation protocols. Note: Reference [63] contains the results of the ZrN group only.

components (**Figure 2**). Moreover, it can be seen that the use of an HDA knee wear simulation increased the metal ion release in the uncoated components (both studies were performed on Columbus CR, Aesculap AG, Tuttlingen), whereas the ion release of the ZrN multilayer components remained in substantially a lower level.

4.3.2 Wear against CFR-PEEK

Besides UHMWPE, the ZrN multilayer coating also articulates against carbon-fiber-reinforced poly-ether-ether-ketone (CFR-PEEK) components from a rotating hinged total knee prosthesis used in complex revision cases (EnduRo, Aesculap AG, Tuttlingen, Germany). The selection of CFR-PEEK as an articulation surface was selected, as it showed superior wear factors compared with polyethylene [67, 68] and favorable creep behavior. In an in vitro wear study, the ZrN multilayer coating was able to reduce the amount of CFR-PEEK wear particles produced from the flanges and flexion axis in comparison to the uncoated CoCrMo version of the implant by more than 90% [53]. A study on retrievals with an in vivo service between 12 and 60 months has confirmed the wear patterns on the CFR-PEEK components seen during the in vitro wear simulation test [69].

4.3.3 Bone cement fixation

The modified surface could result different behavior for cement fixation, which was, therefore, investigated. A study comparing the implant-cement-bone fixation strength between uncoated and ZrN multilayer coated tibial components by means of a push-out test and cementation in polyurethane blocks using different bone cement and cementation times was performed [70]. There were no statistical differences in the bone-cement fixation strength between the uncoated and the ZrN multilayer

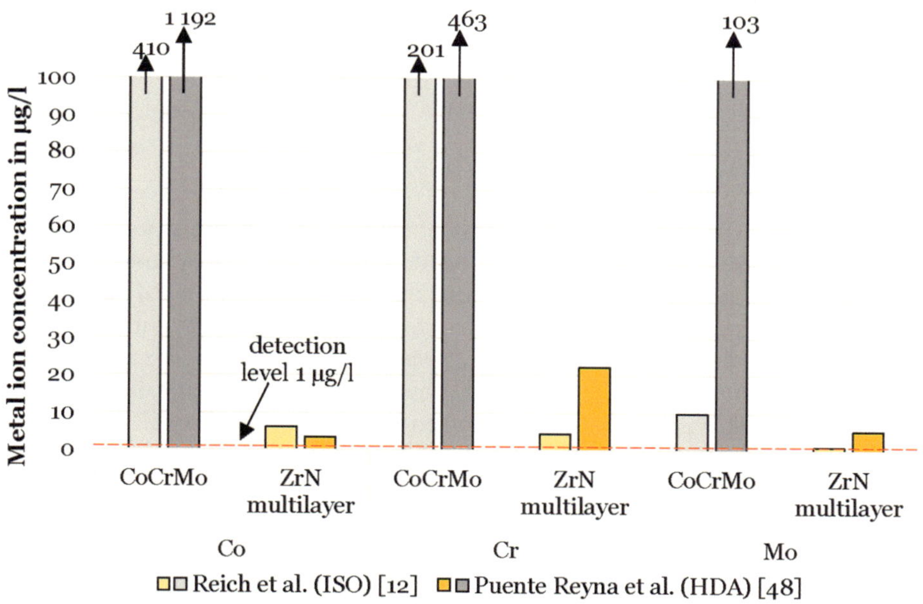

Figure 2.
Metal ion concentrations measured after 1 million cycles for the uncoated and ZrN coated version of Columbus CR/DD.

coated tibial components, and mixed failure modes at implant-cement and the cement-foam interface occurred.

Moreover, the fixation strength of the ZrN multilayer coated tibia components was statistically higher than that of a clinically long-term successful implant, whose failure mode was at the implant-cement interface.

4.3.4 Oxidation

Oxidation of the ZrN multilayer coating is normal behavior, as every metal in contact with biological systems will undergo a process of bio-corrosion [54, 71], and has been reported on in vitro studies before [52]. During the oxidation process, oxygen ions are exchanged with the nitrogen ions of the ZrN layer. This oxidation is visible in the ZrN layer because the color of zirconium alloys varies depending on the amount of oxygen and nitrogen, they contain [72–76]. It has, however, no influence on the biomechanical properties of the coating.

5. Clinical results and register data

The theoretical advantages of these improved implant surfaces need to be confirmed in patients. There are several clinical studies and several implants are monitored in arthroplasty registries. Because coated and standard implants are often used in different patient populations, a direct comparison of the implant performance is difficult. The more expensive implants with a surface modification or coating are more often used in patients with metal allergies. These patients have a high level of psychological distress when undergoing a TKA surgery [77], and it has been suggested that anxiety is the main reason for less favorable results in these patients [28]. It is therefore likely that patients with allergies to implant materials have a higher overall risk for revision because of an unsatisfactory result after TKA. This needs to be considered when looking at arthroplasty registry data.

5.1 Clinical studies

There are only a few studies comparing coated and standard implants. **Table 1** summarizes studies with a minimum 5-year follow-up. If the performance of the implant is the outcome of interest, coated and standard implants should be tested in similar patient populations. As it is difficult to randomize patients with allergies against implant materials, in most studies only patients without known allergies were included. This is not the target population for hypoallergenic implants, but investigation of the mechanical properties of implants in these patients is reasonable.

Studies are not available for all implants on the market. Published studies demonstrated no relevant differences between coated and standard TKA and overall good survival rates. Based on that data, modern coatings which have been tested in clinical studies seem to work well and there is no reason for concern. Because technologies are different, the published results cannot be transformed into different implants or coating technologies without additional clinical studies.

5.2 Arthroplasty registry results

The results of arthroplasty registries provide "real-world" information and are therefore an important source of data. However, it needs to be considered that, in most countries, patients who receive a coated TKA are somehow different from patients who receive a standard TKA, which results in patient groups with a different probability of revision. Therefore, as always with registry data, revision rates of an implant or implant group are not entirely be caused by the implant, but might also be influenced by the patient population.

There is a significant difference in the hazard ratio (HR) of revision between all the alternative surfaces (coatings and surface modifications) and standard CoCrMo femoral components in the Australian Arthroplasty Registry (AOANJRR). After 15 years, the CoCrMo implants have a revision rate of 6.3%, whereas the alternative surfaces have a revision rate of 9.4%. However, there are differences between the alternative surfaces. ZrN has lower revision rates than OxZr and TiN implants. After 5 years, the revision rate for the ZrN is 2.1% and for the uncoated components is 3.1%.

A review of more than 17,000 cases out of the AOANJRR evaluated outcomes of up to 12 years for the OxZr [88]. They found no significant difference for the 12-year cumulative percent revision (CPR) due to all causes (4.8% for CoCr and 7.7% for OxZr); non-septic causes, or osteolysis or loosening (0.6% for CoCr and 1.1% for OxZr). The only age-related difference was found with patients who were > 75 years old, for whom OxZr TKA had an increased CPR due to osteolysis or loosening.

In the National Joint Registry (NJR) of the United Kingdom, OxZr and ZrN have similar results in both versions [39]. AS Columbus (ZrN) had a cumulative revision rate of 2.42 compared to 2.05 of its uncoated version after 5 years. Genesis II Oxinium (OxZr) had a cumulative revision rate of 3.57 at 5 years and 7.67 at 15 years compared to the standard CoCr implants (2.05 at 5 years, 3.49 at 15 years). Both designs have a remarkably lower patient median age at primary TKA (AS Columbus 5 years lower, Genesis II

Author	Technology	Study design	Number of knees	follow-up (y)	Results
Lützner et al. 2022 [31]	ZrN	RCT ZrN vs. CoCrMo	120	5	No differences in cytokines
Postler et al. 2021 [78]	TiNbN	RCT TiNbN vs. CoCrMo	118	5	No difference in serum metal ion concentrations
Law et al. 2020 [79]	TNbN	Retrospective series TiNbN	346	5	90% survival
Hauer et al. 2020 [80]	TiN	Retrospective series TiN cementless mobile vs. CoCrMo fixed cemented	520	10.1 to 14.9	TAS was sign. Better for coated, KSF sign. Better for the uncoated group.
Louwerens et al. 2020 [81]	TiN	RCT TiN cementless vs. CoCrMo	101	10	Survival uncoated 92% coated 94%.
Thomas et al. 2018 [32]	ZrN	Retrospective series ZrN vs. CoCrMo	196	5	Survival 98% coated vs. 97% uncoated; significant difference in proinflammatory cytokines with higher values in CoCrMo
Beyer et al. 2016 [82]	ZrN	RCT ZrN vs. CoCrMo	120	5	100% survival of coated, 98.1% of uncoated group.
Hofer et al. 2014 [83]	OxZr	Retrospective series	109	5.9 (5–10)	Mean KSS 92, mean KSF 81
Innocenti et al. 2014 [84]	OxZr	Retrospective series	98	11.3 (10–12.6)	Mean KSS 84, Mean KSF 83, 97.8% survival at 10Y. Two loosenings
Mohammend et al. 2014 [85]	TiN	Retrospective series TiN cementless	305	6.5 (3–10)	95.1% survival
Kim et al. 2012 [86]	OxZr	RCT in bilateral TKA OxZr vs. CoCrMo	662	7.5 (6–8)	100% survival at 7.5 Y in both groups
Hui et al. 2011 [87]	OxZr	RCT in bilateral TKA OxZr vs. CoCrMo	80	5	Mean KSS OxZr 89 vs. CoCrMo 92

RCT = randomized controlled trial; TAS = Tegner activity scale; KSS = knee society score; and KSF = knee society function score.

Table 1.
Clinical studies involving monolayer and multilayer coatings as well as the OxZr surface modification.

Oxinium 12 years lower). The younger age in TKA is a higher risk for earlier revision, which could explain the slightly higher revision rates of both designs in the register [38].

Hypoallergenic implants demonstrated higher overall revision rates in the German Arthroplasty Registry after 3 years [89]. In this report, the main differences between coated and standard implant groups were the higher rate of metal allergies in female patients in the coated TKA group. Looking at the data in detail, it was recognized that for the most often used coated implants (Columbus, Vanguard, e.motion), there were no differences between coated and standard implants and that for these implants, revision rates were favorably lower than all implants. It seems that the higher revision rates are caused by less frequently used implants and that a general revision rate for "coated implants" is not sufficient. Each implant needs to be looked at separately.

An analysis of 62,177 primary TKAs from the Total Joint Replacement Registry in the USA compared OxZr to traditional CoCr TKA implants and showed no statistically significant higher risk for revision after a mean follow-up time of 2.8 years [90].

6. Practical approach for the use of coated implants

In all patients with suspected or confirmed allergy against implant materials, informed consent and shared decision-making are crucial to avoid negative psychological effects.

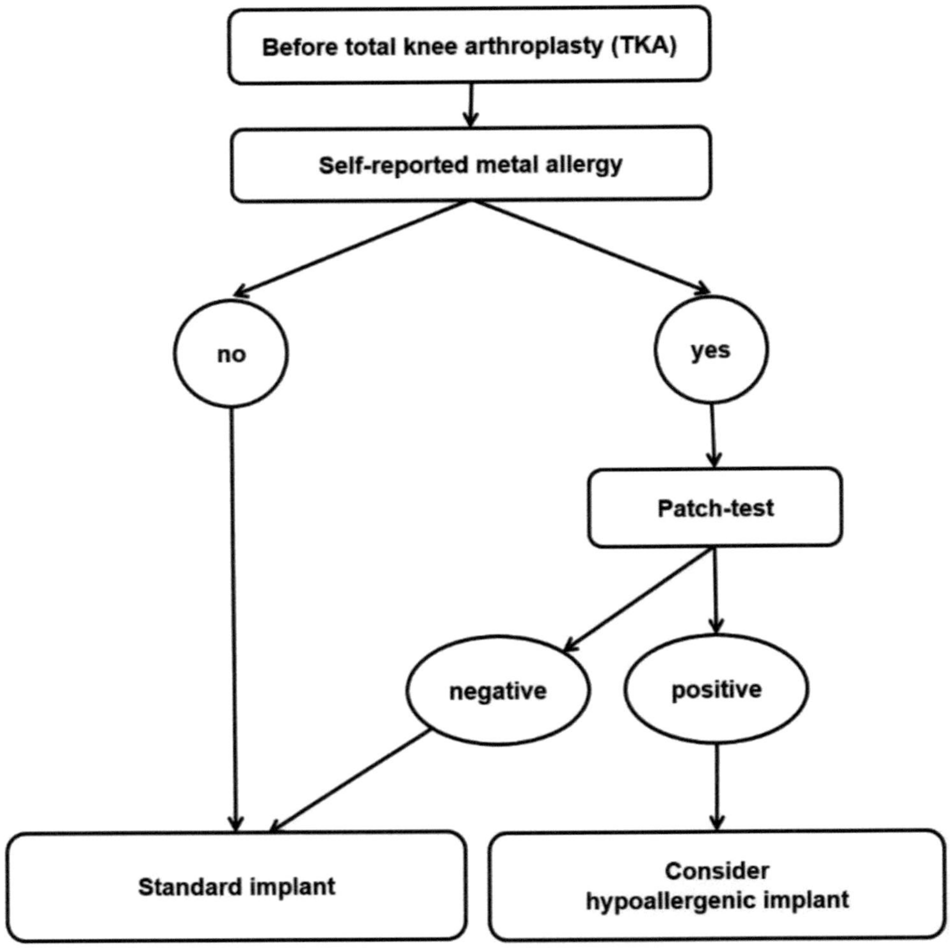

Figure 3.
A suggested algorithm for primary TKA [18, 50].

In primary TKA (**Figure 3**), all patients should be asked about allergies against implant materials before surgery. If an allergy is only self-reported, a test should be performed (usually a skin patch test). If the allergy is confirmed, pros and cons of different implants should be discussed with the patient, and a hypoallergenic implant should be considered. A multilayer-coated or oxidized zirconium implant is the best evaluated option in clinical studies and will probably have the best performance regarding the long-term reduction of metal ion release and wear.

In case of revision TKA (**Figure 4**) and suspected allergy against implant materials, additionally to the rule-out of other causes (especially periprosthetic joint infection), a histopathological evaluation (arthroscopic or open during two-stage revision) should be performed. If there is a confirmed allergy (Krenn type 6), a hypoallergenic implant should be considered as in primary TKA.

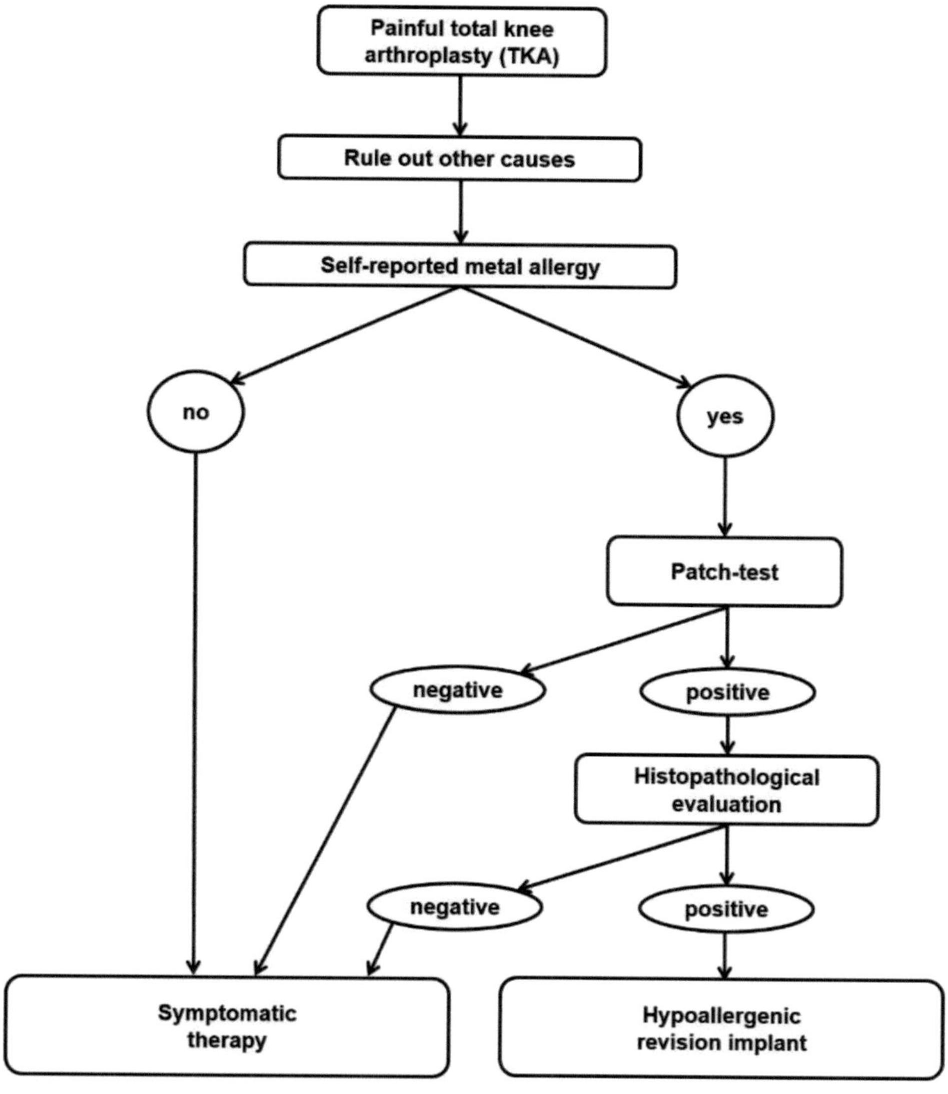

Figure 4.
A suggested algorithm for revision TKA [18, 50].

7. Conclusion

Modern coatings are safe and provide in numerous pre-clinical studies advantages compared to standard implants regarding wear and metal ion release. They are, however, more expensive in many countries and can therefore often not be used routinely. Therefore, advantages and disadvantages need to be balanced to choose the patients who will benefit most. There is no general concern about metal ion release from CoCrMo standard implants for most patients. If patients present with a confirmed metal allergy, a multilayer-coated or oxidized zirconium implant is currently the best option for these patients.

Conflict of interest

Jörg Lützner has received research grants from Aesculap, Link, Mathys, Smith & Nepehw and ZimmerBiomet and honoraria for lectures from Aesculap, Mathys, and Pfizer. Ana Laura Puente Reyna, Brigitte Altermann and Thomas M. Grupp are employees of Aesculap AG, Tuttlingen, a manufacturer of orthopedic implants.

Author details

Jörg Lützner[1*], Brigitte Altermann[2], Ana Laura Puente Reyna[2] and Thomas M. Grupp[2,3]

1 University Hospital Carl Gustav Carus, TU Dresden, Germany

2 Aesculap AG Research and Development, Tuttlingen, Germany

3 Ludwig Maximilians University Munich, Department of Orthopaedic and Trauma Surgery, Musculoskeletal University Center Munich (MUM), Munich, Germany

*Address all correspondence to: joerg.luetzner@ukdd.de

References

[1] Evans JT, Walker RW, Evans JP, Blom AW, Sayers A, Whitehouse MR. How long does a knee replacement last? A systematic review and meta-analysis of case series and national registry reports with more than 15 years of follow-up. The Lancet. 2019;**393**:655-663. DOI: 10.1016/S0140-6736(18)32531-5

[2] Galetz MC, Fleischmann EW, Konrad CH, Schuetz A, Glatzel U. Abrasion resistance of oxidized zirconium in comparison with CoCrMo and titanium nitride coatings for artificial knee joints. Journal of Biomedical Materials Research. Part B, Applied Biomaterials. 2010;**93**:244-251. DOI: 10.1002/jbm.b.31581

[3] van Hove RP, Sierevelt IN, van Royen BJ, Nolte PA. Titanium-nitride coating of orthopaedic implants: A review of the literature. BioMed Research International. 2015;**2015**:485975. DOI: 10.1155/2015/485975

[4] Herbster M, Döring J, Nohava J, Lohmann CH, Halle T, Bertrand J. Retrieval study of commercially available knee implant coatings TiN, TiNbN and ZrN on TiAl6V4 and CoCr28Mo6. Journal of the Mechanical Behavior of Biomedical Materials. 2020;**112**:104034. DOI: 10.1016/j.jmbbm.2020.104034

[5] Natu S, Sidaginamale RP, Gandhi J, Langton DJ, Nargol AV. Adverse reactions to metal debris: Histopathological features of periprosthetic soft tissue reactions seen in association with failed metal on metal hip arthroplasties. Journal of Clinical Pathology. 2012;**65**:409-418. DOI: 10.1136/jclinpath-2011-200398

[6] Leyssens L, Vinck B, van der Straeten C, Wuyts F, Maes L. Cobalt toxicity in humans-A review of the potential sources and systemic health effects. Toxicology. 2017;**387**:43-56. DOI: 10.1016/j.tox.2017.05.015

[7] Christian WV, Oliver LD, Paustenbach DJ, Kreider ML, Finley BL. Toxicology-based cancer causation analysis of CoCr-containing hip implants: A quantitative assessment of genotoxicity and tumorigenicity studies. Journal of Applied Toxicology: JAT. 2014;**34**:939-967. DOI: 10.1002/jat.3039

[8] Kovochich M, Monnot A, Kougias DG, More SL, Wilsey JT, Qiu Q-Q, et al. Carcinogenic hazard assessment of cobalt-containing alloys in medical devices: Review of in vivo studies. Regulatory Toxicology and Pharmacology. 2021;**122**:104910. DOI: 10.1016/j.yrtph.2021.104910

[9] Lützner J, Günther K-P, Postler A, Morlock M. Metallionenfreisetzung nach Hüft- und Kniegelenkendoprothetik – Mechanismen, biologische Wirkungen und notwendige Diagnostik. [Metal Ion Release after Hip and Knee Arthroplasty—Causes, Biological Effects and Diagnostics]. Zeitschrift für Orthopädie und Unfallchirurgie. 2020;**158**:369-382. DOI: 10.1055/a-0929-8121

[10] Grupp TM, Baxmann M, Jansson V, Windhagen H, Heller KD, Morlock MM, Knaebel HP. How to proceed with asymptomatic modular dual taper hip stems in the case of acetabular revision. Materials (Basel). 2 Mar 2020;**13**(5):1098. DOI: 10.3390/ma1305109

[11] Bernstein DT, Meftah M, Paranilam J, Incavo SJ. Eighty-six percent failure rate of a modular-neck femoral stem design at 3 to 5 years: Lessons learned. The Journal

of Bone and Joint Surgery. 2016;**98**:e49. DOI: 10.2106/JBJS.15.01082

[12] Dimitriou D, Liow MHL, Tsai T-Y, Leone WA, Li G, Kwon Y-M. Early outcomes of revision surgery for taper corrosion of dual taper total hip arthroplasty in 187 patients. The Journal of Arthroplasty. 2016;**31**:1549-1554. DOI: 10.1016/j.arth.2016.01.015

[13] Ghanem E, Ward DM, Robbins CE, Nandi S, Bono JV, Talmo CT. Corrosion and adverse local tissue reaction in one type of modular neck stem. The Journal of Arthroplasty. 2015;**30**:1787-1793. DOI: 10.1016/j.arth.2015.04.039

[14] Meftah M, Haleem AM, Burn MB, Smith KM, Incavo SJ. Early corrosion-related failure of the rejuvenate modular total hip replacement. The Journal of Bone and Joint Surgery. American Volume. 2014;**96**:481-487. DOI: 10.2106/JBJS.M.00979

[15] Gramlich Y, Hofmann L, Kress S, Ruckes C, Kemmerer M, Klug A, et al. Critically high metal ion levels found in metal-on-metal modular hinged knee arthroplasty: A comparison of two different systems. Bone Joint Journal. 2020;**104-B**:376-385. DOI: 10.1302/0301-620X.104B3.BJJ-2021-0492.R2

[16] Kellens J, Berger P, Vandenneucker H. Metal wear debris generation in primary total knee arthroplasty: Is it an issue? Acta Orthopaedica Belgica. 2021;**87**:681-695. DOI: 10.52628/87.4.13

[17] Reich J, Hovy L, Lindenmaier H-L, Zeller R, Schwiesau J, Thomas P, et al. Preclinical evaluation of coated knee implants for allergic patients. Orthopade. 2010;**39**:495-502. DOI: 10.1007/s00132-009-1581-9

[18] Matar HE, Porter PJ, Porter ML. Metal allergy in primary and revision total knee arthroplasty: A scoping review and evidence-based practical approach. Bone Jt Open. 2021;**2**:785-795. DOI: 10.1302/2633-1462.210.BJO-2021-0098.R1

[19] Bravo D, Wagner ER, Larson DR, Davis MP, Pagnano MW, Sierra RJ. No increased risk of knee arthroplasty failure in patients with positive skin patch testing for metal hypersensitivity: A Matched Cohort study. The Journal of Arthroplasty. 2016;**31**:1717-1721. DOI: 10.1016/j.arth.2016.01.024

[20] Middleton STA. Allergy in total knee arthroplasty: A review of the facts. Bone Joint Journal. 2016;**98-B**:437-441

[21] Guenther D, Thomas P, Kendoff D, Omar M, Gehrke T, Haasper C. Allergic reactions in arthroplasty: Myth or serious problem? International Orthopaedics. 2016;**40**:239-244. DOI: 10.1007/s00264-015-3001-6

[22] Münch HJ, Jacobsen SS, Olesen JT, Menné T, Søballe K, Johansen JD, et al. The association between metal allergy, total knee arthroplasty, and revision: Study based on the Danish knee arthroplasty register. Acta Orthopaedica. 2015;**86**:378-383. DOI: 10.3109/17453674.2014.999614

[23] Schäfer T, Böhler E, Ruhdorfer S, Weigl L, Wessner D, Filipiak B, et al. Epidemiology of contact allergy in adults. Allergy. 2001;**56**:1192-1196. DOI: 10.1034/j.1398-9995.2001.00086.x

[24] Granchi D, Cenni E, Giunti A, Baldini N. Metal hypersensitivity testing in patients undergoing joint replacement: A systematic review. Journal of Bone and Joint Surgery. British Volume (London). 2012;**94**:1126-1134. DOI: 10.1302/0301-620X.94B8.28135

[25] Basko-Plluska JL, Thyssen JP, Schalock P. Cutaneous and systemic

hypersensitivity reactions to metallic implants. Dermatitis. 2011;**22**:65-79

[26] Thienpont E, Berger Y. No allergic reaction after TKA in a chrome-cobalt-nickel-sensitive patient: Case report and review of the literature. Knee Surgery, Sports Traumatology, Arthroscopy. 2013;**21**:636-640. DOI: 10.1007/s00167-012-2000-z

[27] Nam D, Li K, Riegler V, Barrack RL. Patient-reported metal allergy: A risk factor for poor outcomes after total joint arthroplasty? The Journal of Arthroplasty. 2016;**31**:1910-1915. DOI: 10.1016/j.arth.2016.02.016

[28] Ferrer T, Hinarejos P, Goicoechea N, Leal-Blanquet J, Sanchez-Soler J, Torres-Claramunt R, et al. Anxiety is the cause of the worse outcomes of allergic patients after total knee arthroplasty. Knee Surgery, Sports Traumatology, Arthroscopy. 2020;**28**:3135-3141. DOI: 10.1007/s00167-019-05780-0

[29] Shah K, Mohammed A, Patil S, McFadyen A, Meek RMD. Circulating cytokines after hip and knee arthroplasty: A preliminary study. Clinical Orthopaedics and Related Research. 2009;**467**:946-951. DOI: 10.1007/s11999-008-0562-3

[30] Langkilde A, Jakobsen TL, Bandholm TQ, Eugen-Olsen J, Blauenfeldt T, Petersen J, et al. Inflammation and post-operative recovery in patients undergoing total knee arthroplasty-secondary analysis of a randomized controlled trial. Osteoarthritis and Cartilage. 2017;**25**:1265-1273. DOI: 10.1016/j.joca.2017.03.008

[31] Lützner J, Beyer F, Lützner C, Thomas P, Summer B. Increased inflammatory response is associated with less favorable functional results 5 years after total knee arthroplasty. Knee Surgery, Sports Traumatology, Arthroscopy. 11 Feb 2022. DOI: 10.1007/s00167-021-06836-w

[32] Thomas P, Hisgen P, Kiefer H, Schmerwitz U, Ottersbach A, Albrecht D, et al. Blood cytokine pattern and clinical outcome in knee arthroplasty patients: Comparative analysis 5 years after standard versus "hypoallergenic" surface coated prosthesis implantation. Acta Orthopaedica. 2018;**89**:646-651. DOI: 10.1080/17453674.2018.1518802

[33] Spector BM, Ries MD, Bourne RB, Sauer WS, Long M, Hunter G. Wear performance of ultra-high molecular weight polyethylene on oxidized zirconium total knee femoral components. The Journal of Bone and Joint Surgery. American Volume. 2001;**83-A**(Suppl. 2 Pt. 2):80-86. DOI: 10.2106/00004623-200100022-00004

[34] Kore L, Bates T, Mills G, Lybeck D. Oxidized zirconium total knee arthroplasty implant failure in a patient with knee instability. Arthroplast Today. 2020;**6**:552-555. DOI: 10.1016/j.artd.2020.06.015

[35] Bayliss LE, Culliford D, Monk AP, Glyn-Jones S, Prieto-Alhambra D, Judge A, et al. The effect of patient age at intervention on risk of implant revision after total replacement of the hip or knee: A population-based cohort study. The Lancet. 2017;**389**:1424-1430. DOI: 10.1016/S0140-6736(17)30059-4

[36] Civinini R, Carulli C, Matassi F, Lepri AC, Sirleo L, Innocenti M. The survival of total knee arthroplasty: Current data from registries on tribology: Review Article. HSS Journal. 2017;**13**:28-31. DOI: 10.1007/s11420-016-9513-9

[37] Pabinger C, Berghold A, Boehler N, Labek G. Revision rates

after knee replacement. Cumulative results from worldwide clinical studies versus joint registers. Osteoarthritis and Cartilage. 2013;**21**:263-268. DOI: 10.1016/j.joca.2012.11.014

[38] Graves S, de Steiger R, Lewis P, Harris I. Australian orthopaedic association national joint replacement registry (AOANJRR). Hip, Knee & Shoulder Arthroplasty. 2021:186-286

[39] Reed M, Brittain R, Howard P, Lawrence S, Stonadge J, Wilkinson M, Wilton T. National Joint Registry England, Wales, Northern Ireland & Isle of Man. 18th Annual Report 2021. 2021: 135-212

[40] Long WJ, Bryce CD, Hollenbeak CS, Benner RW, Scott WN. Total knee replacement in young, active patients: Long-term follow-up and functional outcome: A concise follow-up of a previous report. The Journal of Bone and Joint Surgery. 2014;**96**:e159. DOI: 10.2106/JBJS.M.01259

[41] Hallab NJ, Jacobs JJ. Biologic effects of implant debris. Bulletin of the NYU Hospital for Joint Diseases. 2009;**67**:182-188

[42] Ingham E, Fisher J. The role of macrophages in osteolysis of total joint replacement. Biomaterials. 2005;**26**:1271-1286. DOI: 10.1016/j.biomaterials.2004.04.035

[43] Catelas I, Wimmer MA, Utzschneider S. Polyethylene and metal wear particles: Characteristics and biological effects. Seminars in Immunopathology. 2011;**33**:257-271. DOI: 10.1007/s00281-011-0242-3

[44] Cadosch D, Chan E, Gautschi OP, Filgueira L. Metal is not inert: Role of metal ions released by biocorrosion in aseptic loosening—Current concepts. Journal of Biomedical Materials Research. Part A. 2009;**91**:1252-1262. DOI: 10.1002/jbm.a.32625

[45] Magone K, Luckenbill D, Goswami T. Metal ions as inflammatory initiators of osteolysis. Archives of Orthopaedic and Trauma Surgery. 2015;**135**:683-695. DOI: 10.1007/s00402-015-2196-8

[46] Ackerman IN, Busija L, Lorimer M, de Steiger R, Graves SE. Monitoring the lifetime risk of revision knee arthroplasty over a decade: A population-level analysis of Australian national registry data. Bone Joint Journal. 2022;**104-B**:613-619. DOI: 10.1302/0301-620X.104B5.BJJ-2021-1219.R1

[47] Luetzner J, Krummenauer F, Lengel AM, Ziegler J, Witzleb W-C. Serum metal ion exposure after total knee arthroplasty. Clinical Orthopaedics and Related Research. 2007;**461**:136-142. DOI: 10.1097/BLO.0b013e31806450ef

[48] Thomas P, Weik T, Roider G, Summer B, Thomsen M. Influence of surface coating on metal ion release: Evaluation in patients with metal allergy. Orthopedics. 2016;**39**:S24-S30. DOI: 10.3928/01477447-20160509-08

[49] Thomsen M, Rozak M, Thomas P. Pain in a chromium-allergic patient with total knee arthroplasty: Disappearance of symptoms after revision with a special surface-coated TKA—A case report. Acta Orthopaedica. 2011;**82**:386-388. DOI: 10.3109/17453674.2011.579521

[50] Mitchelson AJ, Wilson CJ, Mihalko WM, Grupp TM, Manning BT, Dennis DA, et al. Biomaterial hypersensitivity: Is it real? Supportive evidence and approach considerations for metal allergic patients following total knee arthroplasty. BioMed Research International. 2015;**2015**:137287. DOI: 10.1155/2015/137287

[51] Roy ME, Whiteside LA, Ly KK, Gauvain MJ. Cobalt-chromium femoral components developed scratches and released metal debris in simulated wear whereas ceramic femoral components did not. Bone Joint J. 2021;**103**:94-101

[52] Puente Reyna AL, Fritz B, Schwiesau J, Schilling C, Summer B, Thomas P, et al. Metal ion release barrier function and biotribological evaluation of a zirconium nitride multilayer coated knee implant under highly demanding activities wear simulation. Journal of Biomechanics. 2018;**79**:88-96. DOI: 10.1016/j.jbiomech.2018.07.043

[53] Grupp TM, Giurea A, Miehlke RK, Hintner M, Gaisser M, Schilling C, et al. Biotribology of a new bearing material combination in a rotating hinge knee articulation. Acta Biomaterialia. 2013;**9**:7054-7063. DOI: 10.1016/j.actbio.2013.02.030

[54] Kretzer JP, Reinders J, Sonntag R, Hagmann S, Streit M, Jeager S, et al. Wear in total knee arthroplasty-just a question of polyethylene? Metal ion release in total knee arthroplasty. International Orthopaedics (SICOT). 2014;**38**:335-340. DOI: 10.1007/s00264-013-2162-4

[55] Malikian R, Maruthainar K, Stammers J, Cannon SR, Carrington R, Skinner JA, et al. In vivo roughening of retrieved total knee arthroplasty femoral components. The Knee. 2014;**21**:278-282. DOI: 10.1016/j.knee.2012.09.008

[56] Davidson JA. Characteristics of metal and ceramic total hip bearing surfaces and their effect on long-term ultra high molecular weight polyethylene wear. Clinical Orthopaedics and Related Research. 1993;**294**:361-378

[57] Paschoal AL, Vanancio EC, Canale LC, da Silva OL, Huerta-Vilca D, Motheo AJ. Metallic biomaterials TiN-coated: Corrosion analysis and biocompatibility. Artificial Organs. 2003;**27**:461-464. DOI: 10.1046/j.1525-1594.2003.07241.x

[58] Pilz M, Staats K, Tobudic S, Assadian O, Presterl E, Windhager R, et al. Zirconium nitride coating reduced staphylococcus epidermidis biofilm formation on orthopaedic implant surfaces: An In Vitro Study. Clinical Orthopaedics and Related Research. 2019;**477**:461-466. DOI: 10.1097/CORR.0000000000000568

[59] Schüttler KF, Efe T, Heyse TJ, Haas SB. Oxidized zirconium bearing surfaces in total knee arthroplasty: Lessons learned. The Journal of Knee Surgery. 2015;**28**:376-381. DOI: 10.1055/s-0035-1551836

[60] Lee JKL, Maruthainar K, Wardle N, Haddad F, Blunn GW. Increased force simulator wear testing of a zirconium oxide total knee arthroplasty. The Knee. 2009;**16**:269-274. DOI: 10.1016/j.knee.2008.12.010

[61] Bader R, Bergschmidt P, Fritsche A, Ansorge S, Thomas P, Mittelmeier W. Alternative Werkstoffe und Lösungen in der Knieendoprothetik für Patienten mit Metallallergie. [Alternative materials and solutions in total knee arthroplasty for patients with metal allergy]. Der Orthopäde. 2008;**37**:136-142. DOI: 10.1007/s00132-007-1189-x

[62] Ragone V, Canciani E, Biffi CA, D'Ambrosi R, Sanvito R, Dellavia C, et al. CoCrMo alloys ions release behavior by TiNbN coating: An in vitro study. Biomedical Microdevices. 2019;**21**:61. DOI: 10.1007/s10544-019-0417-6

[63] Grupp TM, Schroeder C, Kyun Kim T, Miehlke RK, Fritz B, Jansson V, et al. Biotribology of a mobile bearing posterior stabilised knee design—Effect

of motion restraint on wear, tibio-femoral kinematics and particles. Journal of Biomechanics. 2014;**47**:2415-2423. DOI: 10.1016/j.jbiomech.2014.04.020

[64] Schwiesau J, Schilling C, Kaddick C, Utzschneider S, Jansson V, Fritz B, et al. Definition and evaluation of testing scenarios for knee wear simulation under conditions of highly demanding daily activities. Medical Engineering & Physics. 2013;**35**:591-600. DOI: 10.1016/j.medengphy.2012.07.003

[65] Bergmann G, Bender A, Graichen F, Dymke J, Rohlmann A, Trepczynski A, et al. Standardized loads acting in knee implants. PLoS One. 2014;**9**:e86035. DOI: 10.1371/journal.pone.0086035

[66] Schwiesau J, Fritz B, Kutzner I, Bergmann G, Grupp TM. CR TKA UHMWPE wear tested after artificial aging of the vitamin E treated gliding component by simulating daily patient activities. BioMed Research International. 2014;**2014**:567374. DOI: 10.1155/2014/567374

[67] Kurtz SM, Devine JN. PEEK biomaterials in trauma, orthopedic, and spinal implants. Biomaterials. 2007;**28**:4845-4869. DOI: 10.1016/j.biomaterials.2007.07.013

[68] Scholes SC, Unsworth A. Wear studies on the likely performance of CFR-PEEK/CoCrMo for use as artificial joint bearing materials. Journal of Materials Science: Materials in Medicine. 2009;**20**:163-170. DOI: 10.1007/s10856-008-3558-3

[69] Schierjott RA, Giurea A, Neuhaus HJ, Schwiesau J, Pfaff AM, Utzschneider S, Tozzi G, Grupp TM. Analysis of Carbon Fiber Reinforced PEEK Hinge Mechanism Articulation Components in a Rotating Hinge Knee Design: A Comparison of In Vitro and Retrieval Findings. Biomed Research International. 2016;**2016**:7032830. DOI: 10.1155/2016/7032830

[70] Grupp TM, Schilling C, Schwiesau J, Pfaff A, Altermann B, Mihalko WM. Tibial implant fixation behavior in total knee arthroplasty: A study with five different bone cements. The Journal of Arthroplasty. 2020;**35**:579-587. DOI: 10.1016/j.arth.2019.09.019

[71] Jacobs JJ, Gilbert JL, Urban RM. Corrosion of metal orthopaedic implants. The Journal of Bone and Joint Surgery. 1998;**80**:268-282. DOI: 10.2106/00004623-199802000-00015

[72] Brown R, Alias MN, Fontana R. Effect of composition and thickness on corrosion behavior of TiN and ZrN thin films. Surface and Coating Technology. 1993;**62**:467-473. DOI: 10.1016/0257-8972(93)90285-V

[73] Cheng Y, Zheng YF. A study of ZrN/Zr coatings deposited on NiTi alloy by PIIID technique. IEEE Transactions on Plasma Science. 2006;**34**:1105-1108. DOI: 10.1109/TPS.2006.877502

[74] Ferreira SC, Ariza E, Rocha LA, Gomes JR, Carvalho P, Vaz F, et al. Tribocorrosion behaviour of ZrOxNy thin films for decorative applications. Surface and Coatings Technology. 2006;**200**:6634-6639

[75] Milošev I, Strehblow H-H, Navinseka B. Comparison of TiN, ZrN and CrN hard nitride coatings: Electrochemical and thermal oxidation. Thin Solid Films. 1997;**303**:246-254. DOI: 10.1016/S0040-6090(97)00069-2

[76] Reddy G, Ramana JV, Kumar S, Kumar SV, Raju VS. Investigations on the oxidation of zirconium nitride films in air by nuclear reaction analysis and backscattering spectrometry. Applied

Surface Science. 2007;**253**:7230-7237. DOI: 10.1016/j.apsusc.2007.03.004

[77] Peña P, Ortega MA, Buján J, De la Torre B. Influence of Psychological Distress in Patients with hypoallergenic total knee arthroplasty. Treatment algorithm for patients with metal allergy and knee osteoarthritis. International Journal of Environmental Research and Public Health. 3 Jun 2021;**18**(11):5997. DOI: 10.3390/ijerph18115997

[78] Postler A, Beyer F, Lützner C, Tille E, Lützner J. Die Anwendung antiallergisch beschichteter Knieendoprothesen ist mittelfristig sicher: Eine randomisierte kontrollierte Studie [The use of knee prostheses with a hypoallergenic coating is safe in the medium term: A randomized controlled study]. Orthopade (German). 3 Nov 2021. DOI: 10.1007/s00132-021-04186-6

[79] Law JI, Morris MJ, Hurst JM, Berend KR, Lombardi AV, Crawford DA. Early outcomes of an alternative bearing surface in primary total knee arthroplasty in patients with self-reported metal allergy. Arthroplast Today. 2020;**6**:639-643. DOI: 10.1016/j.artd.2020.07.021

[80] Hauer G, Leitner L, Ackerl MC, Klim S, Vielgut I, Ehall R, et al. Titanium-nitride coating does not result in a better clinical outcome compared to conventional cobalt-chromium Total Knee Arthroplasty after a Long-Term Follow-Up: A Propensity Score Matching Analysis. Coatings. 2020;**10**:442. DOI: 10.3390/coatings10050442

[81] Louwerens JKG, Hockers N, Achten G, Sierevelt IN, Nolte PA, van Hove RP. No clinical difference between TiN-coated versus uncoated cementless CoCrMo mobile-bearing total knee arthroplasty; 10-year follow-up of a randomized controlled trial. Knee Surgery, Sports Traumatology, Arthroscopy. 2021;**29**:750-756. DOI: 10.1007/s00167-020-05997-4

[82] Beyer F, Lützner C, Kirschner S, Lützner J. Midterm results after coated and uncoated TKA: A randomized controlled study. Orthopedics. 2016;**39**:S13-S17. DOI: 10.3928/01477447-20160509-10

[83] Hofer JK, Ezzet KA. A minimum 5-year follow-up of an oxidized zirconium femoral prosthesis used for total knee arthroplasty. The Knee. 2014;**21**:168-171. DOI: 10.1016/j.knee.2013.08.015

[84] Innocenti M, Carulli C, Matassi F, Carossino AM, Brandi ML, Civinini R. Total knee arthroplasty in patients with hypersensitivity to metals. International Orthopaedics. 2014;**38**:329-333. DOI: 10.1007/s00264-013-2229-2

[85] Mohammed A, Metcalfe A, Woodnutt D. Medium-term outcome of titanium nitride, mobile bearing total knee replacement. Acta Orthopaedica Belgica. Jun 2014;**80**:269-275

[86] Kim YH, Park JW, Kim JS. Comparison of the Genesis II total knee replacement with oxidised zirconium and cobalt-chromium femoral components in the same patients: A prospective, double-blind, randomised controlled study. Journal of Bone and Joint Surgery. British Volume (London). 2012;**94**:1221-1227

[87] Hui C, Salmon L, Maeno S, Roe J, Walsh W, Pinczewski L. Five-year comparison of oxidized zirconium and cobalt-chromium femoral components in total knee arthroplasty: A randomized controlled trial. The Journal of Bone and Joint Surgery. 2011;**93**:624-630. DOI: 10.2106/JBJS.I.01753

[88] Vertullo CJ, Lewis PL, Graves S, Kelly L, Lorimer M, Myers P. Twelve-year

outcomes of an oxinium total knee replacement compared with the same cobalt-chromium design: An analysis of 17,577 prostheses from the australian orthopaedic association national joint replacement registry. The Journal of Bone and Joint Surgery. American Volume. 2017;**99**:275-283. DOI: 10.2106/JBJS.16.00092

[89] Grimberg AW, Grupp TM, Elliott J, Melsheimer O, Jansson V, Steinbrück A. Ceramic coating in cemented primary total knee arthroplasty is not associated with decreased risk of revision due to early prosthetic joint infection. The Journal of Arthroplasty. 2021;**36**:991-997. DOI: 10.1016/j.arth.2020.09.011

[90] Inacio MCS, Cafri G, Paxton EW, Kurtz SM, Namba RS. Alternative bearings in total knee arthroplasty: Risk of early revision compared to traditional bearings: an analysis of 62,177 primary cases. Acta Orthopaedica. 2013;**84**:145-152. DOI: 10.3109/17453674.2013.784660

Chapter 10

Motor Imagery as Adjunct Therapy for Rehabilitation of Total Knee Arthroplasty Patients: The State-of-the-Art Umbrella Review with Meta-Analysis

Armin H. Paravlic

Abstract

One of the most common causes of disability in older adults is osteoarthritis (OA), which often affects the knee. When conventional treatments fail to produce positive changes in patients' physical function, pain relief, and quality of life, replacement of the degenerated and/or malformed joint is recommended. Total knee arthroplasty (TKA) has been shown to be beneficial in improving aforementioned factors in patients with OA. However, despite comprehensive surgical methods and postoperative rehabilitation approaches, knee extensor weakness persists over a long period of time and may not reach the preoperative level of the non-OA leg for up to 6 months after surgery. Therefore, current rehabilitation programs do not seem to be sufficient to counteract these negative changes after TKA. When overt movement is limited due to various factors, several cognitive strategies have been shown to be useful in improving neuromuscular function without mechanically loading the muscles. One of the most studied strategies is motor imagery (MI). While there is some preliminary evidence supporting the use of MI in TKA rehabilitation practice, an umbrella review with meta-analysis is needed to summarize these findings and draw a clear conclusion about the efficacy of MI in terms of physical function and pain relief in TKA patients.

Keywords: cognitive practice, total knee replacement, pain relief, physical function, functional performance, strength, range of motion

1. Introduction

Aging is a progressive deterioration at the cellular, tissue and organ levels, resulting in a loss of homeostasis, a reduced ability to adapt to internal and/or external stimuli and an increased susceptibility to disease. Structural changes in various tissues are usually accompanied by negative changes in the functionality of all systems in the human body. With increasing age, there is an increased incidence of various diseases, which further accelerates disability and independence. One of the most frequent occurring causes of disability among older adults is osteoarthritis (OA), which commonly affects a knee due to high mechanical forces stressing the joint. When more conventional, i.e. nonsurgical treatments do not produce positive changes in physical function, pain relief and quality of life, the replacement of the degenerated and/or malformed joint is recommended for OA patients. Depending on the extent of the degenerated tissue, surgical replacement can be either total (e.g., when OA affects both compartments of the knee, TKA) or partial (e.g. when OA is limited to only one compartment of the knee; UKA). However, TKA is preferably performed as surgical treatment in almost 90% of all patients diagnosed with end-stage OA [1]. Since both, the incidence and prevalence of OA increase with age [2, 3], the longer life expectancy that is being faced globally will result in an increase of primary TKA rates which, by the year 2030, are anticipated to grow for more than 6 folds [4].

TKA has been shown as beneficial in improving physical function, pain relief and improving QoL of OA patients. However, despite using comprehensive surgical methods and post-operative rehabilitation approaches, the knee extensors muscle weakness persists over a long period, and might not achieve preoperative levels of the OA unaffected leg for up to 6 months post-surgery [5, 6]. Current rehabilitation practice after TKA consists of a more conventional approach to exercises that mechanically stresses the musculoskeletal system. Such exercise programs include joint mobility exercises to improve range of motion, gait relearning, weight-bearing exercises, neuromuscular function and proprioception training and strength and endurance exercises, using both voluntary and electrically triggered actions [7, 8]. A finding from a recent review and meta-analysis showed that outpatients professionally guided rehabilitation practice group had a consistently lower decline of the OA-affected knee extensors strength in the early periods following TKA when compared to usual care group. However, the authors suggested that strategies focused on preserving neural circuits of motor control must be considered for achieving optimal rehabilitation outcomes.

In the first days after TKA, patients are hardly physically active due to the pain caused by the surgical trauma. Therefore, inpatient rehabilitation is usually performed by passive exercises provided by physical therapists, continuous passive motion devices and transcutaneous electrical stimulation of the lower limb muscles. When overt movement is limited due to various factors (e.g. pain, opioids, cast, etc.), various cognitive strategies have been shown to be beneficial in improving neuromuscular function without mechanically stressing the muscles. One of the most studied strategies is motor imagery (MI). Recently, Paravlic and colleagues published the first systematic review paper with a meta-analysis that examined the effects of mental simulation strategies on physical function in TKA patients [9]. The authors showed a promising result favoring cognitive interventions over routine physical therapy alone, taking into account overall physical function, maximal strength of the affected leg, fast walking speed, timed up-to-go test and active knee joint flexion. Two other reviews were published in last 2 years that examined a similar question [10, 11]. These studies focused exclusively on MI practice only and included several different measures, such as range of motion of the affected knee joint and pain intensity. Currently, there is a substantial body of evidence regarding the effects of MI in the rehabilitation of TKA patients, warranting a collective assessment of their effects in the context of a review and representing a summary effect of MI in this specific patient population.

The purpose of this study was to examine the effects of the MI practice intervention in TKA patients on several measures of physical function and pain intensity using the umbrella review.

2. Methods

This umbrella review with meta-analysis was performed according to guidelines provided by the working group of Aromataris et al. [12], whereas the Preferred Reporting Items for Systematic Reviews and Meta-Analysis (PRISMA) updated statement guidelines were followed [13].

2.1 Search strategy

The main author (AP) performed a literature search on the PubMed, SPORTDiscus and Web of Science online-based databases. The search syntaxes (including keywords) were as follows:

Search: (motor imagery OR mental simulation OR imagery) AND (total knee replacement OR total knee arthroplasty) AND (physical function OR strength OR rehabilitation outcomes) AND (systematic review OR literature review OR meta-analysis).

((("motor"[All Fields] OR "motor s"[All Fields] OR "motoric"[All Fields] OR "motorically"[All Fields] OR "motorics"[All Fields] OR "motoring"[All Fields] OR "motorisation"[All Fields] OR "motorized"[All Fields] OR "motorization"[All Fields] OR "motorized"[All Fields] OR "motors"[All Fields]) AND ("imageries"[All Fields] OR "imagery, psychotherapy"[MeSH Terms] OR ("imagery"[All Fields] AND "psychotherapy"[All Fields]) OR "psychotherapy imagery"[All Fields] OR "imagery"[All Fields])) OR (("mental"[All Fields] OR "mentalities"[All Fields] OR "mentality"[All Fields] OR "mentalization"[MeSH Terms] OR "mentalization"[All Fields] OR "mentalizing"[All Fields] OR "mentalize"[All Fields] OR "mentalized"[All Fields] OR "mentally"[All Fields]) AND ("computer simulation"[MeSH Terms] OR ("computer"[All Fields] AND "simulation"[All Fields]) OR "computer simulation"[All Fields] OR "simulation"[All Fields] OR "simul"[All Fields] OR "simulate"[All Fields] OR "simulated"[All Fields] OR "simulates"[All Fields] OR "simulating"[All Fields] OR "simulation s"[All Fields] OR "simulational"[All Fields] OR "simulations"[All Fields] OR "simulative"[All Fields] OR "simulator"[All Fields] OR "simulator s"[All Fields] OR "simulators"[All Fields])) OR ("imageries"[All Fields] OR "imagery, psychotherapy"[MeSH Terms] OR ("imagery"[All Fields] AND "psychotherapy"[All Fields]) OR "psychotherapy imagery"[All Fields] OR "imagery"[All Fields])) AND ("arthroplasty, replacement, knee"[MeSH Terms] OR ("arthroplasty"[All Fields] AND "replacement"[All Fields] AND "knee"[All Fields]) OR "knee replacement arthroplasty"[All Fields] OR ("total"[All Fields] AND "knee"[All Fields] AND "replacement"[All Fields]) OR "total knee replacement"[All Fields] OR ("arthroplasty, replacement, knee"[MeSH Terms] OR ("arthroplasty"[All Fields] AND "replacement"[All Fields] AND "knee"[All Fields]) OR "knee replacement arthroplasty"[All Fields] OR ("total"[All Fields] AND "knee"[All Fields] AND "arthroplasty"[All Fields]) OR "total knee arthroplasty"[All Fields])) AND ((("physical examination"[MeSH Terms] OR ("physical"[All Fields] AND "examination"[All Fields]) OR "physical examination"[All Fields] OR "physical"[All Fields] OR "physically"[All Fields] OR "physicals"[All Fields]) AND ("functional"[All Fields]

OR "functional s"[All Fields] OR "functionalities"[All Fields] OR "functionality"[All Fields] OR "functionalization"[All Fields] OR "functionalizations"[All Fields] OR "functionalize"[All Fields] OR "functionalized"[All Fields] OR "functionalizes"[All Fields] OR "functionalizing"[All Fields] OR "functionally"[All Fields] OR "functionals"[All Fields] OR "functioned"[All Fields] OR "functioning"[All Fields] OR "functionings"[All Fields] OR "functions"[All Fields] OR "physiology"[MeSH Subheading] OR "physiology"[All Fields] OR "function"[All Fields] OR "physiology"[MeSH Terms])) OR ("strength"[All Fields] OR "strengths"[All Fields]) OR (("rehabilitant"[All Fields] OR "rehabilitants"[All Fields] OR "rehabilitate"[All Fields] OR "rehabilitated"[All Fields] OR "rehabilitates"[All Fields] OR "rehabilitating"[All Fields] OR "rehabilitation"[MeSH Terms] OR "rehabilitation"[All Fields] OR "rehabilitations"[All Fields] OR "rehabilitative"[All Fields] OR "rehabilitation"[MeSH Subheading] OR "rehabilitation s"[All Fields] OR "rehabilitational"[All Fields] OR "rehabilitator"[All Fields] OR "rehabilitators"[All Fields]) AND ("outcome"[All Fields] OR "outcomes"[All Fields]))) AND ("systematic review"[Publication Type] OR "systematic reviews as topic"[MeSH Terms] OR "systematic review"[All Fields] OR ("review"[Publication Type] OR "review literature as topic"[MeSH Terms] OR "literature review"[All Fields]) OR ("meta analysis"[Publication Type] OR "meta analysis as topic"[MeSH Terms] OR "meta analysis"[All Fields]))

2.2 Translations

Motor: "motor"[All Fields] OR "motor's"[All Fields] OR "motoric"[All Fields] OR "motorically"[All Fields] OR "motorics"[All Fields] OR "motoring"[All Fields] OR "motorisation"[All Fields] OR "motorized"[All Fields] OR "motorization"[All Fields] OR "motorized"[All Fields] OR "motors"[All Fields].

Imagery: "imageries"[All Fields] OR "imagery, psychotherapy"[MeSH Terms] OR ("imagery"[All Fields] AND "psychotherapy"[All Fields]) OR "psychotherapy imagery"[All Fields] OR "imagery"[All Fields].

Mental: "mental"[All Fields] OR "mentalities"[All Fields] OR "mentality"[All Fields] OR "mentalization"[MeSH Terms] OR "mentalization"[All Fields] OR "mentalizing"[All Fields] OR "mentalize"[All Fields] OR "mentalized"[All Fields] OR "mentally"[All Fields].

Simulation: "computer simulation"[MeSH Terms] OR ("computer"[All Fields] AND "simulation"[All Fields]) OR "computer simulation"[All Fields] OR "simulation"[All Fields] OR "simul"[All Fields] OR "simulate"[All Fields] OR "simulated"[All Fields] OR "simulates"[All Fields] OR "simulating"[All Fields] OR "simulation's"[All Fields] OR "simulational"[All Fields] OR "simulations"[All Fields] OR "simulative"[All Fields] OR "simulator"[All Fields] OR "simulator's"[All Fields] OR "simulators"[All Fields].

Imagery: "imageries"[All Fields] OR "imagery, psychotherapy"[MeSH Terms] OR ("imagery"[All Fields] AND "psychotherapy"[All Fields]) OR "psychotherapy imagery"[All Fields] OR "imagery"[All Fields].

Total knee replacement: "arthroplasty, replacement, knee"[MeSH Terms] OR ("arthroplasty"[All Fields] AND "replacement"[All Fields] AND "knee"[All Fields]) OR "knee replacement arthroplasty"[All Fields] OR ("total"[All Fields] AND "knee"[All Fields] AND "replacement"[All Fields]) OR "total knee replacement"[All Fields].

Total knee arthroplasty: "arthroplasty, replacement, knee"[MeSH Terms] OR ("arthroplasty"[All Fields] AND "replacement"[All Fields] AND "knee"[All Fields]) OR "knee replacement arthroplasty"[All Fields] OR ("total"[All Fields] AND "knee"[All Fields] AND "arthroplasty"[All Fields]) OR "total knee arthroplasty"[All Fields].

Physical: "physical examination"[MeSH Terms] OR ("physical"[All Fields] AND "examination"[All Fields]) OR "physical examination"[All Fields] OR "physical"[All Fields] OR "physically"[All Fields] OR "physicals"[All Fields].

Function: "functional"[All Fields] OR "functional's"[All Fields] OR "functionalities"[All Fields] OR "functionality"[All Fields] OR "functionalization"[All Fields] OR "functionalizations"[All Fields] OR "functionalize"[All Fields] OR "functionalized"[All Fields] OR "functionalizes"[All Fields] OR "functionalizing"[All Fields] OR "functionally"[All Fields] OR "functionals"[All Fields] OR "functioned"[All Fields] OR "functioning"[All Fields] OR "functionings"[All Fields] OR "functions"[All Fields] OR "physiology"[Subheading] OR "physiology"[All Fields] OR "function"[All Fields] OR "physiology"[MeSH Terms].

Strength: "strength"[All Fields] OR "strengths"[All Fields].

Rehabilitation: "rehabilitant"[All Fields] OR "rehabilitant's"[All Fields] OR "rehabilitants"[All Fields] OR "rehabilitate"[All Fields] OR "rehabilitated"[All Fields] OR "rehabilitates"[All Fields] OR "rehabilitating"[All Fields] OR "rehabilitation"[MeSH Terms] OR "rehabilitation"[All Fields] OR "rehabilitations"[All Fields] OR "rehabilitative"[All Fields] OR "rehabilitation"[Subheading] OR "rehabilitation's"[All Fields] OR "rehabilitational"[All Fields] OR "rehabilitator"[All Fields] OR "rehabilitators"[All Fields].

Outcomes: "outcome"[All Fields] OR "outcomes"[All Fields].

Systematic review: "systematic review"[Publication Type] .or. "systematic reviews as topic"[MeSH Terms] .or. "systematic review"[All Fields].

Literature review: "review"[Publication Type] .or. "review literature as topic"[MeSH Terms] .or. "literature review"[All Fields].

Meta-analysis: "meta-analysis"[Publication Type] .or. "meta-analysis as topic"[MeSH Terms] .or. "meta-analysis"[All Fields] A several additional strategies were used to find any additional reference relevant to this topic as follows:

- Google scholar alerts with inception on September 2017;
- reading a reference list of the full text articles included
- ResearchGate recommendations;
- Two online pages i.e. www.elicite.com research assistant and www.connectedpapers.com were utilized, respectively.

Duplicates were identified and removed by two reviewers separately (AP and KD). Two reviewers (AP and KD) independently screened titles and abstracts to identify articles that matched the eligibility criteria.

2.3 Inclusion criteria

The Assessing the Methodological Quality of Systematic Reviews 2 (AMSTAR – 2) rating system was applied to rate and classify all published systematic reviews and

Participants	Male and female patients of all ages who were scheduled for total knee arthroplasty
Interventions	For the MI intervention, studies on both visual and kinaesthetic types of imagery and both perspectives of movement representations such as from the first-person view or the third-person view were considered eligible.
Comparison group	The effectiveness of MI practice as an independent intervention or in combination with other cognitive interventions was compared to routine physical rehabilitation practice (i.e. physical therapy, exercise intervention) or with placebo intervention if applicable.
Outcome	Any measure of physical function such as strength, mobility, balance, self-reported physical function (questionnaires) and pain intensity was considered

Table 1.
Inclusion criteria.

meta-analyses into low quality (< 40% items satisfied), moderate quality (40–80% items satisfied) or high quality (>80% items satisfied) [14]. Only systematic reviews with meta-analysis of moderate- and high-quality were included in the present study. Published reviews were included regardless of the original language they were written. There were no restrictions considering a year of publication.

The Participant-Intervention-Comparison-Outcome process for evidence-based practice was followed to describe inclusion criteria **Table 1.**

2.4 Methodological quality and quality of evidence evaluation

The main author assessed the methodological quality of the included articles using the AMSTAR – 2 tool. If the assessment was unclear, the consensus was reached by the constructive discussion with a second reviewer (KD). The 16 items of the AMSTAR – 2 checklist were answered with either "yes" or "no", with each "yes" equaling one point and were classified as mentioned above. In addition, an adapted Grade of Recommendation, Assessment, Development and Evaluation (GRADE) quality of evidence checklist was applied in the included reviews, as it was used previously [15]. The reviews were classified into five GRADE categories: high, moderate, low, very low and no evidence from systematic review. A review was classified as high quality if it contained at least two high-quality studies. Reviews with at least one study of high quality or two studies of moderate quality were classified as moderate quality. If a review contained only primary studies of moderate quality and/or primary studies with inconsistent results, this review was classified as being of low quality. Reviews are classified as of very low quality if they do not contain studies of moderate to high quality. Finally, if the quality of the primary studies was not assessed by the reviewers, the GRADE system was not applied and the review was classified as no evidence from systematic review as recommended previously [15].

2.5 Data extraction

The following data were extracted from the reviews included (a) Study reference; (b) Type of study, number of original studies included, and number of subjects; (c) Objectives of the review; (d) Description of the population; (e) Description of the intervention and comparison group within the review; (f) Number of original studies included in meta-analysis per each outcome measure; (g) Outcome measures; and (h)

Main results. Data extraction was performed by the author (AP) and checked for accuracy by a second reviewer (KD).

2.6 Data synthesis and analysis

The meta-analyses were performed using Comprehensive Meta-analysis software (version 3.0). For all reported outcome measures, the standardized mean difference (SMD) along with 95% CIs were calculated. If at least two included studies reported the same outcome and were considered homogenous, then a meta-analysis was conducted and presented with a forest plot. Due to differences in outcomes assessed and measurement scales used between studies, general physical function assessments, self-reported physical function tests and evaluation of the pain intensity were treated separately. Therefore, composite ES (cES) and 95% CI were calculated for each study to overcome the problem of dependence from multiple outcomes and pre-post evaluation periods [16]. A random-effects model of the meta-analysis was used in all comparisons. However, to assess the sensitivity of each meta-analysis conducted, along with random effect, the fixed effect of the meta-analyses was presented. In addition, the publication bias was assessed by examining the asymmetry of the funnel plots using Egger's test, whereas a significant publication bias was considered if the p value was <0.10. The magnitude of the MI practice effects on outcome measures of interest was interpreted as changes using the following criteria: *trivial* (<0.20), *small* (0.21–0.60), *moderate* (0.61–1.20), *large* (1.21–2.00), *very large* (2.01–4.00) and *extremely large* (>4.00) [17]. The I^2 statistic was used to investigate between-study heterogeneity; where values of 25, 50, and 75% represent *low, moderate* and *high* statistical heterogeneity, respectively [18]. Statistical significance for all tests performed was set at the level of $p \leq 0.05$ [17].

3. Results

Figure 1 shows the search strategy process followed for the present review. Initially, NO articles were identified by using predefined search criteria. No additional articles were found by using other sources as mentioned above. Following the initial step, duplicate records were removed and reviews were excluded based on their titles and abstracts. Of this NO of full-text reviews were assessed with only three reviews with meta-analysis were included in this study.

3.1 Characteristics of the included systematic reviews

The characteristics of the included reviews are presented in **Table 2**. Current study included 3 systematic reviews with meta-analysis, amounting to 10 original studies (5 overlapping between reviews), 9 RCTs and one non RCT, with a total of 558 participants (Experimental group: 278; Control group: 280 patients). All studies included patients scheduled to total knee arthroplasty, both sexes and aged between 50 and 85 years. In all systematic reviews, the main intervention used MI as adjunct therapy, while two reviews included combination of MI with other cognitive interventions such as action observation and/or guided imagery [9, 11]. Included reviews differed in terms of outcomes assessed. Thus, all reviews assessed affected knee extension strength and timed up to go test. Two reviews assessed pain intensity assessed by Visual Analogue Scale (VAS) [10, 11], while two studies assessed

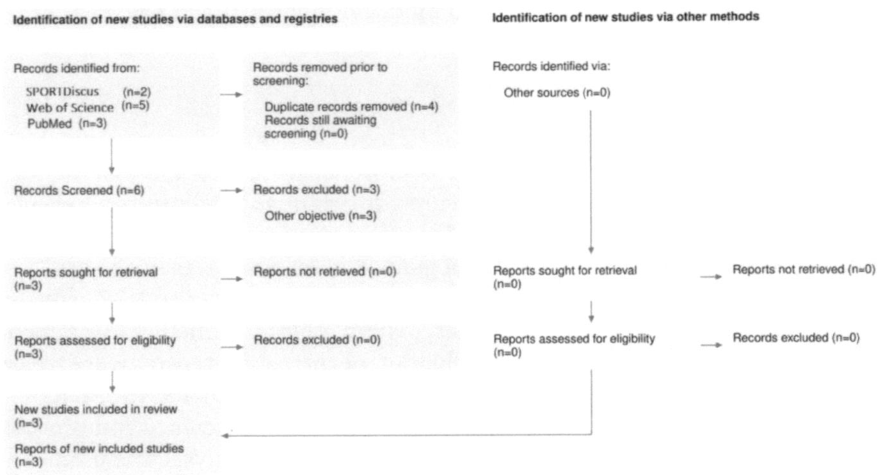

Figure 1.
Flow diagram of included studies.

self-perceived knee function [9, 10], and Paravlic et al. [9] self-selected and brisk walking speed under dual and single tasks.

3.2 Methodological quality assessment and quality of the evidence evaluation

The methodological quality of the included reviews is presented in **Table 3**. All three reviews were rated as of high quality using the AMSTAR-2 checklist. Reviews did not provide a list of excluded studies justifying the exclusion reasons (Item 7) and the report of sources of funding of the studies included in the review (Item 10). Only one review [10] did not perform sensitivity analysis considering publication bias (Item 15). The quality of evidence assessed by adopted GRADE principles showed that all three included studies were rated as of high quality.

3.3 Results of meta-analyses

The Egger's test was performed to provide statistical evidence of funnel plot asymmetry. Results indicated no publication bias for two meta-analyses only: strength ($p = 0.139$) and TUG ($p = 0.225$), respectively. For self-reported physical function and pain intensity, a publication bias analysis was not performed, due to low number of included studies.

Nine ESs from three included meta-analyses showed *small* effect (random effect: cES = 0.55, 95% CI 0.38 to 0.71, n = 9; $p < 0.001$; $I^2 = 32\%$; fixed effect: cES = 0.53, 95% CI 0.39 to 0.66, n = 9; $p < 0.001$; $I^2 = 32\%$;) on measures of physical function in general (**Figure 2A**). Three ESs from all three included reviews showed a *moderate* effect (random effect: ES = 0.85, 95% CI 0.58 to 1.11, n = 3; $p < 0.001$; $I^2 = 0\%$; fixed effect: –//–) on measures on maximal knee extension strength (**Figure 2B**). Furthermore, three ESs from all three included reviews showed *small* effect (random effect: ES = 0.49, 95% CI 0.25 to 0.73, n = 3; $p < 0.001$; $I^2 = 0\%$; fixed effect: –//–) on measures on timed-up and go test (**Figure 2C**). Summarized effect of MI intervention showed *small* effect (random effect: ES = 0.34, 95% CI 0.07 to 0.61, n = 2; $p = 0.015$;

Study	Data extracted	Description of extracted data
Paravlic et al. 2020 [9]	Type of study; N°, type of included studies (subjects)	Systematic review and meta-analysis; 7 RCTs, 1 nRCT (n = 228)
	Objectives	To determine the effectiveness of mental simulation practice (MSP) on measures of physical function recovery in patients who have undergone a joint replacement surgery of lower limbs.
	Population	Population: men and women who underwent primary unilateral joint arthroplasty.
	Intervention	*Intervention group:* Mental simulation intervention. Given the specificity of rehabilitation procedures and ethical issues, MSP was always delivered as an adjunct therapy to SPT and was compared with SPT intervention; *Comparison group:* Measures of interest were compared: (a) in general between MSP and SPT, (b) between different MSP practices, for example, MI versus AO versus guided imagery versus MI and AO and (c) between different rehabilitation phases such as (a) acute rehabilitation (up to 3wk after surgery), (b) early postacute rehabilitation (3-12wk) and (c) late postacute rehabilitation phase (from 12wk-12mo), respectively.
	N° of studies included in meta-analysis (subjects) per each outcome measure	Physical Function in general, 8 (n = 228); Affected knee extension strength, 2 (n = 46); Uninvolved knee extension strength, 2 (n = 46); Mobility Self-selected gait speed, 4 (n = 153); Self-selected gait speed DT, 2 (n = 47); Brisk walking speed, 2 (n = 47); Brisk walking speed DT, 2 (n = 47); Timed up to go test, 3 (n = 67); Active flexion, 4 (n = 101); Passive flexion, 3 (n = 81); Active knee extension, 2 (n = 57) and Self-reported physical function, 4 (n = 163);
	Outcome measures	General physical function; Strength; Mobility; ROM; Self-reported physical function
	Results	When compared with standard physical therapy (SPT), MSP showed an effect on physical function in general (effect size [ES], 0.67; 95% confidence interval [CI], 0.38–0.96; nZ7) and maximal voluntary strength of knee extensor muscles of the affected leg (ES, 1.41; 95% CI, 0.64–2.18; nZ2), brisk walking speed (ES, 1.20; 95% CI, 0.58–1.83; nZ2), brisk walking speed with dual task (ES, 1.02; 95% CI, 0.41–1.63; nZ2), timed up-to go test (ES, 0.96; 95% CI, 0.15–1.77; nZ3) and active flexion of the affected leg (ES, 0.70; 95% CI, 0.29–1.11; nZ4). Finally, meta-regression analysis revealed that the effects of MSP were significantly predicted only by the total number of training sessions per study.
Ferrer-Pena et al. 2022 [11]	Type of study; N°, type of included studies (subjects)	Systematic review and meta-analysis; 7 RCTs, (n = 186)
	Objectives	To assess the impact of MI on strength, active range of motion, pain intensity and physical function in patients with TKA.
	Population	Population: men and women who underwent primary unilateral joint arthroplasty.

Study	Data extracted	Description of extracted data
	Intervention	*Intervention group:* For the MI intervention, studies on both visual and kinaesthetic strategies and both perspectives of movement representations were considered eligible (first-person or third person). Kinaesthetic MI is performed by constructing an image of movement and, in turn, incorporates the ability to feel what is being imagined. Visual MI only constructs the image of movement. *Comparison:* the efficacy of MI as an independent intervention or in combination with other interventions compared to usual care or standard rehabilitation (i.e. physical therapy, exercise intervention) or with placebo interventions
	N° of studies included in meta-analysis (subjects) per each outcome measure	Affected knee extension strength, 4 (n = 104); Active ROM, 6 (n = 152); TUG, 4 (n = 118) and Pain intensity, 5 (n = 132)
	Outcome measures	Strength, mobility, ROM and pain
	Results	The addition of MI to standard therapy, based on low quality of evidence, showed a moderate increase in quadriceps strength (4 studies; SMD: 0.88; 95% CI: 0.42, 1.34) and a small reduction in pain intensity (SMD: 0.63; 95% CI: 0.08, 1.19). It is unclear whether MI can provide beneficial effects for active ROM and function.
Li et al. 2022 [10]	Type of study; N°, type of included studies (subjects)	Systematic review and meta-analysis; 6 RCTs, (n = 144)
	Objectives	The study aimed to investigate the effects of motor imagery on the functional performance improvement in patients scheduled for TKA.
	Population	Population: men and women who underwent unilateral total knee arthroplasty primarily due to osteoarthritis
	Intervention	*Intervention:* Motor imagery; *Comparison:* MI was compared to control group, which was without additional treatment or a corresponding placebo treatment; physical therapy was routinely used in both groups.
	N° of studies included in meta-analysis (subjects) per each outcome measure	Affected knee extension strength, 4 (n = 96); TUG, 4 (n = 94) and Self-reported physical function by Oxford Knee Score questionnaire, 2 (n = 46); Pain intensity, 4 (n = 98)
	Outcome measures	Strength, mobility, ROM and pain
	Results	The MI as adjunct intervention to standard physical therapy showed large effect on strength improvement (SMD = 0.90, 95% CI = [0.47]–[1.32], P < 0.001), reduced pain (SMD = – 0.91; 95% CI = [– 1.29]–[– 0.52], P < 0.001) and improved TUG performance (SMD = – 0.56, 95% CI = [– 0.94]–[– 0.19], P = 0.003) when compared to routine physical therapy alone. However, self-reported physical function by OKS questionnaire, even slightly increased (MD = 0.79-point, 95% CI = [– 0.31]–[1.88], P = 0.159), the observed changes were not significant.

Table 2.
Summary of reviews with meta-analysis that investigated the effects of motor imagery practice on physical rehabilitation outcomes following total knee arthroplasty (TKA).

Study	1	2	3	4	5	6	7	8	9	10	11	12	13	14	15	16	AMSTAR	GRADE
Paravlic et al. 2020 [9]	YES	YES	YES	YES	YES	YES	NO	YES	YES	NO	YES	YES	YES	YES	YES	YES	HIGH	HIGH
Ferrer-Pena et al. 2022 [11]	YES	YES	YES	YES	YES	YES	NO	YES	YES	NO	YES	YES	YES	YES	YES	YES	HIGH	HIGH
Li et al. 2022 [10]	YES	YES	YES	YES	YES	YES	NO	YES	YES	NO	YES	YES	YES	YES	NO	YES	HIGH	HIGH

Table 3.
Overall results of the Assessing the Methodological Quality of Systematic Reviews (AMSTAR-2) and adopted Grade of Recommendation, Assessment, Development and Evaluation (GRADE) quality of evidence checklist.

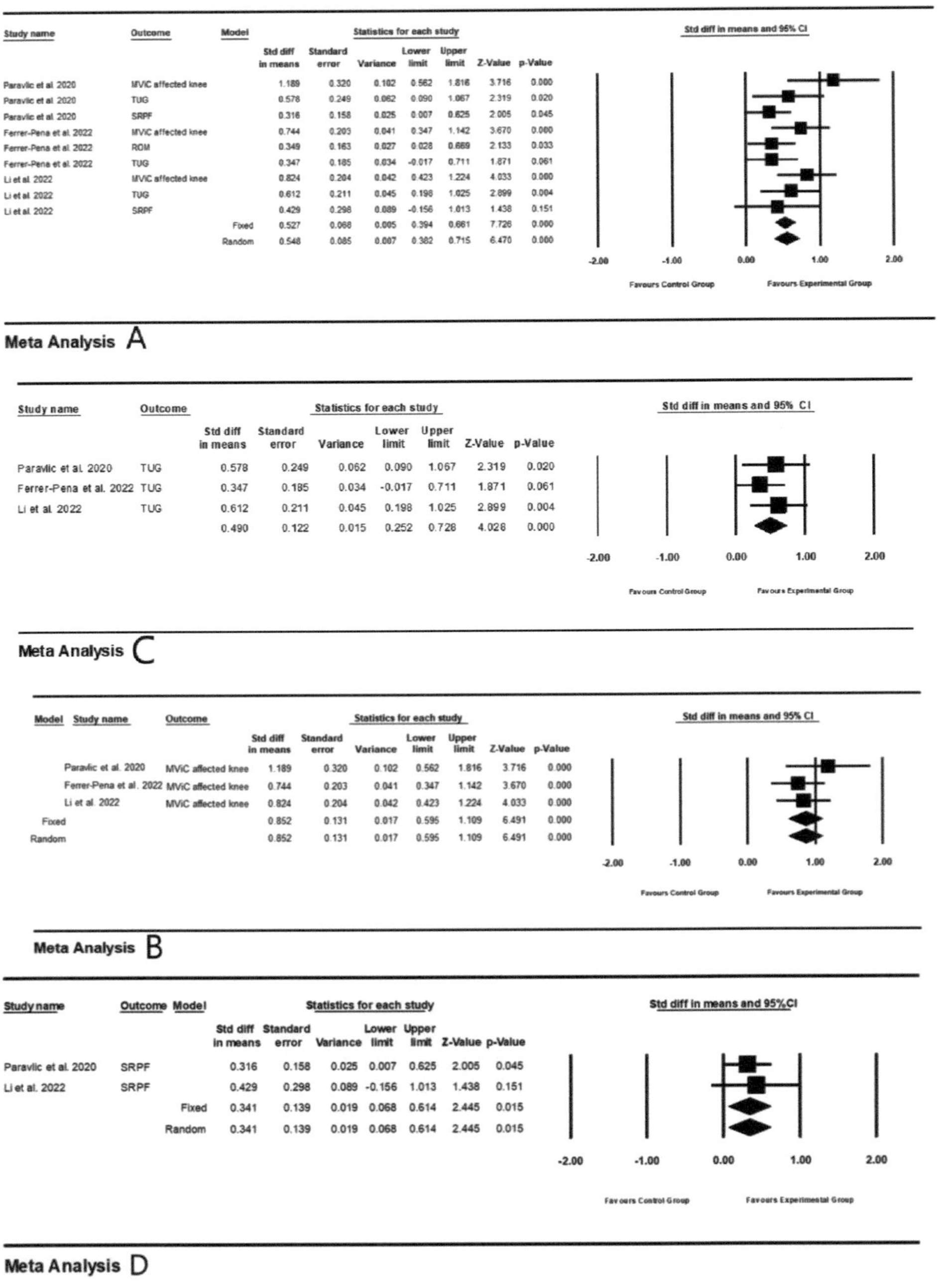

Figure 2.
Summarized effect of MI practice intervention on (A) physical function in general; (B) timed-up to go test; (C) knee extensors strength of the affected knee; and (D) self-reported physical function.

I^2 = 0%; fixed effect: —//—) on measures of self-reported physical function (**Figure 2D**). And finally, a *moderate* effect (random effect: ES = 0.67, 95% CI 0.16 to 1.18, n = 2; p = 0.010; I^2 = 72%, p = 0.058; fixed effect: ES = 0.64, 95% CI 0.37 to 0.90, n = 2; p < 0.001; I^2 = 72%, p = 0.058) was observed for pain intensity. Given there were no differences in the magnitude of the effects when random and fixed effects analyses were applied, these findings can be interpreted as robust (**Figure 3**).

Study name	Outcome	Model	Std diff in means	Standard error	Variance	Lower limit	Upper limit	Z-Value	p-Value
Ferrer-Pena et al. 2022	Pain		0.425	0.175	0.031	0.083	0.768	2.433	0.015
Li et al. 2022	Pain		0.948	0.213	0.045	0.530	1.365	4.449	0.000
		Fixed	0.635	0.135	0.018	0.370	0.900	4.702	0.000
		Random	0.672	0.261	0.068	0.161	1.184	2.576	0.010

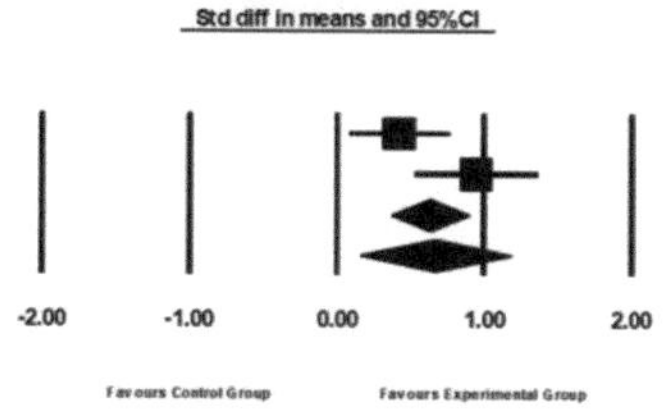

Meta Analysis

Figure 3.
Effect of MI practice intervention on the pain intensity of the affected knee.

4. Discussion

The aim of this study was to investigate the effectiveness of MI practice as adjunct intervention to routine physical therapy in patients after TKA on measures of physical function and pain.

A current umbrella review with a meta-analysis showed a positive effect of MI on physical function in general (small cES = 0.55), strength (moderate ES = 0.85), timed-up and go test (small ES = 0.49), self-reported physical function (small ES = 0.34), and pain intensity reduction (moderate ES = 0.67) in TKA patients. Given that both fixed and random meta-analysis models showed similar results, these findings can be interpreted as robust.

There are several review articles aimed to investigate the effects of psychological interventions on physical function measures in the apparently healthy [19, 20] and diseased populations [10, 11, 21, 22]. However, these investigations substantially differed in the primary aims, the population included and measures of interests, which consequently resulted in the overall methodology adopted. For example, Paravlic et al. [19] investigated the effects of MI practice on the measures of maximal strength in the healthy adults. Authors found positive effects of MI practice on maximal strength, favoring isometric imagined muscle actions over dynamic muscle actions, whereas a combination of MI with physical practice was found equally effective as physical practice alone [19]. In other reviews, authors investigated the effects of various cognitive strategies in athletes sustaining anterior cruciate injuries (ACL) [21], TKA and total hip arthroplasty patients [9, 22] or TKA patients in isolation [10, 11]. These studies were looking at different measures of interest such as functional mobility [9, 21, 23], balance [9–11, 23], maximal strength [10, 11, 19] or pain intensity [10, 11] and found equivocal results. Therefore, the current study with a rigorous methodological approach showed robust and positive findings supporting MI practice intervention use in rehabilitation of TKA patients when physical function and pain are primary rehabilitation goals.

Ample evidence suggests that the mechanism underlying effectiveness of imagined contractions relies on both neurophysiological and psychological factors [19, 24, 25]. There is an evidence that imagined movements are functionally equivalent to the physically executed movements in terms of intention, planning, execution duration and task difficulty [25, 26]. The present study found a positive effect of MI on maximal strength and other measures of physical function that are more complex in nature, such as walking and dynamic balance (assessed by TUG test). TUG test is a complex test that evaluates a several motor-related domains such as lower body strength (e.g. getting up from the chair), walking speed (e.g. walking from the chair to the first turning point at a distance of 4.5 m), agility (turning around a cone), and dynamic balance (e.g. all these tasks together). Paravlic et al. showed a positive transfer from simple MI task that focused only on strength to more complex motor tasks mentioned above. The authors also showed that strength improvements following MI practice in TKA patients were significantly and positively correlated with pre-to-post-intervention changes in patients' kineasthetic (high, $r = 0.741$) and internal (moderate, $r = 0.623$) ability to imagine given tasks. This supports previous findings in the literature that the effects of MI depend on the individual's ability to imagine a particular task as well as the MI type and MI perspective used by the subject [27]. It is suggested that someone who cannot visualize a given task will not benefit from the MI practice [27]. However, Paravlic et al. demonstrated that MI ability can be improved by the MI practice intervention exposure, providing those unfamiliar with MI with new knowledge about how to begin using MI and benefit from it.

In addition to improving physical function, this study showed a positive effect of MI on pain reduction in TKA patients. This finding is consistent with a recent review by Benjamin et al. [28], which showed that MI as adjunctive therapy is superior to standard physical therapy alone in terms of pain reduction and ROM improvements in patients with chronic musculoskeletal conditions. In contrast, the authors found no differences in efficacy between MI and routine therapies acute pain is considered. Because centrally driven mechanisms (e.g. neuroplastic changes and central sensations) [29] predominate in chronic pain, in contrast to acute pain conditions that are driven by peripheral factors (e.g. structural impairment at a peripheral site) [30], the efficacy of MI can be explained by the modulation of cortical areas associated with pain-related cortical reorganization, such as the primary somatosensory cortex, the anterior cingulate cortex and the insula [31]. Although the subsequent mechanisms behind the efficacy of MI in chronic pain are still controversial, MI actually allows activation of motor cortex without overt movement execution [19, 25], sending a motor-related cortical potential via efferents and consequently uncoupling movement from pain perception [28, 31]. Even preliminary data indicate that the MI practice may not be more effective than routine therapy alone, given its mechanism, it could serve to prevent further exacerbation of symptoms and avoid chronic pain events [28].

Considering MI practice programming, only one review with meta-analysis examined a MI practice dose–response relationship, suggesting that effects of cognitive training on outcomes in TKA patients were predicted by the total number of training sessions per study [9]. A recent review by Paravlic suggested recommendations for MI rehabilitation practice in the home setting [32]. In brief, there are some steps that should be followed to benefit from MI practice: (a) patients' imagery ability must be assessed to inform the therapist which MI perspective and which MI type should be used; (b) it is recommended to provide patients with audio instructions to follow during practice sessions [33]; (c) at the beginning of MI practice therapist should propose simple motor task that is easy to perform by patient and (d) the following motor imagery variables were associated with strength improvement: a training period of 4 weeks, a training frequency of three sessions per week, a training volume of two to three sets, 25 repetitions per set and a single session duration of 15 minutes [19]. While the latter recommendations were compiled from the published literature, the original studies aimed at investigating the effects of different MI practice volumes (training duration, weekly frequency, number of imagined contractions per set, and per single session) are justified.

5. Conclusion

In conclusion, this study provides strong evidence for the use of MI practice as an adjunct to standard rehabilitation treatment in improving physical function and reducing pain after TKA surgery.

Acknowledgements

The author would like to thank the IntechOpen publisher for supporting an open access publication of this article.

Funding

The open access publishing of this article was supported by the Slovenian Research Agency (ARRS) (project no. P5-0147 entitled "The kinesiology of mono-structured, poly-structured and conventional sports," project manager: Prof. Dr. Matej Supej).

Conflict of interest

The author declares no conflict of interest.

Author details

Armin H. Paravlic[1,2]

1 Faculty of Sport, University of Ljubljana, Ljubljana, Slovenia

2 Science and Research Centre Koper, Koper, Slovenia

*Address all correspondence to: armin.paravlic@hotmail.com

References

[1] Campi S, Tibrewal S, Cuthbert R, Tibrewal SB. Unicompartmental knee replacement – Current perspectives. Journal of Clinical Orthopedic Trauma. 2018;**9**(1):17-23

[2] Woolf AD, Pfleger B. Burden of major musculoskeletal conditions. Bulletin of the World Health Organization. 2003; **81**(9):646-656

[3] Srikanth VK, Fryer JL, Zhai G, Winzenberg TM, Hosmer D, Jones G. A meta-analysis of sex differences prevalence, incidence and severity of osteoarthritis. Osteoarthritis and Cartilage. 2005;**13**(9):769-781

[4] Kurtz S, Ong K, Lau E, Mowat F, Halpern M. Projections of primary and revision hip and knee arthroplasty in the United States from 2005 to 2030. Journal of Bone Joint Surgery. 2007;**89**(4):780-785

[5] Paravlic AH, Meulenberg CJ, Drole K. The time course of quadriceps strength recovery after Total knee arthroplasty is influenced by body mass index, sex, and age of patients: Systematic review and meta-analysis. Frontiers in Medicine. 2022;**9**:25

[6] Paravlic AH, Kovač S, Pisot R, Marusic U. Neurostructural correlates of strength decrease following total knee arthroplasty: A systematic review of the literature with meta-analysis. Bosnian Journal of Basic Medical Sciences. Feb 5, 2020;**20**(1):1-12

[7] Andrade R, Pereira R, Van Cingel R, Staal JB, Espregueira-Mendes J. How should clinicians rehabilitate patients after ACL reconstruction? A systematic review of clinical practice guidelines (CPGs) with a focus on quality appraisal (AGREE II). British Journal of Sports Medicine. 2020;**54**(9):512-519

[8] Kittelson SSK, Stevens-lapsley JE. Neuromuscular electrical stimulation after total joint arthroplasty: A critical review of recent controlled studies. European Journal of Physical and Rehabilitation Medicine. 2013;**49**(6):909-920

[9] Paravlic A, Tod D, Milanovic Z. Mental simulation practice has beneficial effects on patients' physical function following lower limb arthroplasty: A systematic review and Meta-analysis. Archives of Physical and Medical Rehabilitation. 2020;**101**(8):1447-1461

[10] Li R, Du J, Yang K, Wang X, Wang W. Effectiveness of motor imagery for improving functional performance after total knee arthroplasty: A systematic review with meta-analysis. Journal of Orthopedic Surgery and Research. 2022; **17**(1):1-12

[11] Ferrer-Peña R, Cuenca-Martínez F, Romero-Palau M, Flores-Román LM, Arce-Vázquez P, Varangot-Reille C, et al. Effects of motor imagery on strength, range of motion, physical function, and pain intensity in patients with total knee arthroplasty: A systematic review and meta-analysis. Brazilian Journal of Physical Therapy. Nov-Dec 2021;**25**(6):698-708

[12] Aromataris E, Fernandez R, Godfrey CM, Holly C, Khalil H, Tungpunkom P. Summarizing systematic reviews: Methodological development, conduct and reporting of an umbrella review approach. International Journal of Evidence-Based Healthcare. 2015;**13**(3):132-140

[13] Page MJ, McKenzie JE, Bossuyt PM, Boutron I, Hoffmann TC, Mulrow CD, et al. The PRISMA 2020 statement: An updated guideline for reporting

systematic reviews. International Journal of Surgery. 2021;**88**:1-11

[14] Shea BJ, Reeves BC, Wells G, Thuku M, Hamel C, Moran J, et al. AMSTAR 2: A critical appraisal tool for systematic reviews that include randomised or non-randomised studies of healthcare interventions, or both. BMJ. 2017;**358**:1-9

[15] Brunner R, Friesenbichler B, Casartelli NC, Bizzini M, Maffiuletti NA, Niedermann K. Effectiveness of multicomponent lower extremity injury prevention programmes in team-sport athletes: An umbrella review. British Journal of Sports Medicine. 2019;**53**(5): 282-288

[16] Scammacca N. Meta-analysis with complex research designs: Dealing with dependence from multiple measures and multiple group comparisons. Review of Educational Research. 2014;**84**(3):328-364

[17] Hopkins MSW, Batterham AM, Hanin J. Progressive statistics for studies in sports medicine and exercise science. Medicine and Science in Sports and Exercise. 2009;**41**(1):3-13

[18] Higgins JPT, Thompson SG, Deeks JJ, Altman DG. Measuring inconsistency in meta-analyses. BMJ [British Medical Journal]. 2003; **327**(7414):557-560

[19] Paravlic AH, Slimani M, Tod D, Marusic U, Milanovic Z, Pisot R. Effects and dose–response relationships of motor imagery practice on strength development in healthy adult populations: A systematic review and meta-analysis. Sports Medicine. May 2018;**48**(5):1165-1187

[20] Tod D, Iredale F, Gill N. "Psyching-Up" and muscular force production. Sports Medicine. 2003;**33**(1):47-58

[21] Zach S, Dobersek U, Filho E, Inglis V, Tenenbaum G. A meta-analysis of mental imagery effects on post-injury functional mobility, perceived pain, and self-efficacy. Psychology of Sport and Exercise. 2018;**34**:79-87

[22] Bay S, Kuster L, McLean N, Byrnes M, Kuster MS. A systematic review of psychological interventions in total hip and knee arthroplasty. BMC Musculoskeletal Disorders. 2018;**19**(1): 1-11

[23] Nicholson V, Watts N, Chani Y, Keogh JW. Motor imagery training improves balance and mobility outcomes in older adults: A systematic review. Journal of Physiotheraphy. 2019;**65**(4): 200-207

[24] Paravlic PR, Marusic U. Specific and general adaptations following motor imagery practice focused on muscle strength in total knee arthroplasty rehabilitation : A randomized controlled trial. PLoS One. 2019;**14**(8):1-19

[25] Munzert J, Lorey B, Zentgraf K. Cognitive motor processes: The role of motor imagery in the study of motor representations. Brain Research Reviews. 2009;**60**(2):306-326

[26] Jeannerod. The representing brain: Neural correlates of motor intention and imagery. The Behavioral and Brain Sciences. 1994;**17**(2):187-245

[27] Martin KA, Moritz SE, Hall CR. Imagery use in sport: A literature review and applied model. Sport Psychologist. 1999;**13**:245-268

[28] Yap BW, Lim ECW. The effects of motor imagery on pain and range of motion in musculoskeletal disorders. The Clinical Journal of Pain. 2019;**35**(1): 87-99

[29] Pelletier R, Higgins J, Bourbonnais D. Is neuroplasticity in the central nervous system the missing link to our understanding of chronic musculoskeletal disorders? BMC Musculoskeletal Disorders. 2015;**16**(1): 1-13

[30] Mackey S. The "Continuum of Pain" and the American academy of pain medicine. Pain Medicine (United States). 2015;**16**(3):413-415

[31] Moseley GL, Flor H. Targeting cortical representations in the treatment of chronic pain: A review. Neurorehabilitation and Neural Repair. 2012;**26**(6):646-652

[32] Paravlic AH. Motor imagery and action observation as appropriate strategies for home-based rehabilitation: A Mini-review focusing on improving physical function in Orthopedic patients. Frontiers in Psychology. 2022;**13** (March):1-9

[33] Paravlic A, Maffulli N, Kovac S, Pisot R. Home-based motor imagery intervention improves functional performance following total knee arthroplasty in the short term: A randomized controlled trial. Journal of Orthopaedic Surgery and Research. 2020;**15**(1):451

Section 4

Research and Advanced Clinical Practice in the Treatment of Osteoarthritis

Chapter 11

Mesenchymal Stem Cell-based Cytotherapy for Osteoarthritis Management: State of the Art

Leisheng Zhang, Zhihai Han, Zhongchao Han and Hui Cai

Abstract

Osteoarthritis (OA), a principal and challenging disorder of articular cartilage, has been regarded as the most frequent and prevalent chronic disease of degenerative joints, which is caused by multiple factors including aging, trauma, overweight, joint deformity and congenital abnormality, together with the increase in life expectancy. In spite of considerable improvements that have been obtained by conducting multidisciplinary therapies such as surgical procedures and anti-inflammatory drugs, the pathogenesis and efficacy of OA with functional losses and degeneration are still elusively complicated for ascertainment. Mesenchymal stem/stromal cells (MSCs), also termed as multipotent mesenchymal progenitor/precursor cells, skeletal stem cells, or medicinal signaling cells, are heterogeneous cell populations with hematopoietic-supporting and immunomodulatory properties, together with multilineage differentiation property. For decades, investigators have illuminated the application of the advantaged and promising sources with/without remarkable biomaterials for the treatment of recurrent and refractory disorders including OA. In this chapter, we mainly concentrate on the current progress of MSC-based cytotherapy in both preclinical study and clinical practice as well as the promising prospective and critical challenges in the field, which will conformably benefit the administration of OA in future.

Keywords: osteoarthritis, mesenchymal stem cells, cytotherapy, biomaterials, tissue engineering

1. Introduction

Osteoarthritis (OA) is a whole organ disease characterized by the destruction or degeneration of articular cartilage, which is one of the most widespread and frequent chronic diseases and public health issues worldwide [1, 2]. During the course of OA, inflammatory response is a pivotal factor resulting in cartilage destruction or exacerbation of symptoms [2–4]. As satisfactory osteochondral repair, it's of great importance for the zonal restoration of adjacent cartilage and the subchondral bone [5]. For the past decades, despite the significant number of progress have been achieved by multidisciplinary strategies such as surgeries (e.g., microfracture, mosaicplasty), autologous chondrocyte implantation (ACI), joint lubricants (e.g., hyaluronic acid), antiinflammatory drugs (e.g., NSAIDs) as well as cytotherapies (e.g., autologous chondrocyte implantation), the inherent limitations of regeneration and self-repair capacity in OA individuals still largely hinder the remission of the degeneration of articular cartilage [4, 6–8]. For example, even though joint replacement serves as an effective remedy for symptomatic end-stage disease including OA, most of the functional outcomes in patients are unsatisfactory and the lifespan of prosthesis is also largely limited [2, 9]. Distinguishing from the traditional remedies, cell-based strategies have emerged as an alternative with promising prospective in the treatment of OA and cartilage defects [10, 11].

State-of-the-art updates have turned to MSC-based cytotherapy for OA management both clinically and preclinically [5, 12]. The multifaceted superiorities of MSCs including multidirectional differentiation, high portability property, and low immunogenicity have made themselves ideal seed cells for OA treatment [3]. Meanwhile, MSCs or the derivatives are often encapsulated into natural or synthetic hydrogels, which can function by providing tunable biodegradability, and biocompatibility or enhancing cell vitality and functionality [10].

Herein, we mainly focus on the recent literatures relating to the application of MSCs for OA treatment based on the chondrogenic differentiation, and antiinflammatory and immunomodulatory effects of MSCs with or without biological scaffolds for cartilage regeneration. Meanwhile, we further discuss the promising prospective and formidable challenges of MSC-based cytotherapy in cartilage repair and regeneration as well.

2. MSCs and derivatives

MSCs are cell populations with unique immune-privileged and hematopoietic properties, which are capable of differentiating into a variety of functional cells such as adipocytes, osteoblasts and chondrocytes, which thus have garnered increased interest for clinical translation in the last few decades [13, 14]. Therewith, MSCs have been considered as the uppermost components in the bone marrow microenvironment as well as splendid sources for regenerative medicine [15, 16]. Not until the year of 2006, International Society for Cellular Therapy (ISCT) released the basic criteria for MSC definition including spindle-shaped morphology, high expression of mesenchymal-associated biomarkers (CD73, CD90, CD105) whereas minimal expression of hematopoietic-associated biomarkers (CD31, CD34, CD45), *in vitro* differentiation towards adipocytes, osteoblasts and chondrocytes [17].

Since the 1970s, MSCs have been isolated from various adult tissues including bone marrow, adipose tissues, synovial fluid, periosteum and dental tissues (e.g., dental pulp, periodontium) [18–20]. After that, perinatal or fetal tissues including umbilical cord, placenta, amniotic member and amniotic fluid have also been reported for MSC isolation [21]. Distinguish from those derived from adult tissues, MSCs isolated from the "discarded" perinatal tissues have been considered with preferable immunoregulatory properties and long-term *in vitro* proliferative capacity, and in particular, release from ethical risks, invasiveness and pathogenic contamination [14, 21–23]. Notably, current studies have also put forward the feasibility of generating large-scale MSCs from induced pluripotent stem cells (iPSCs) or embryonic stem cells (ESCs) as well [24–26]. To date, MSCs with different origins have been involved in numerous refractory and relapse disease administration including acute-on-chronic liver failure (ACLF), acute myocardial infarction (AMI), aplastic anemia, premature ovarian failure (POF), fistulizing Crohn's disease, critical limb ischemia (CLI), cutaneous wounds, coronavirus disease 2019 (COVID-19)-induced acute lung injury and acute respiratory distress syndrome (ALI/ARDS) [26–32].

For decades, the derivatives generated from MSCs such as exosomes and relative microvesicles have been extensively investigated and regarded as the dominating factor during pathogenesis and disease treatment [20, 33]. Exosomes, also known as small extracellular vesicles (sEVs) or biological spherical lipid bilayer vesicles, are nano-sized extracellular vesicles secreted by various types of cells (e.g., MSCs, natural killer cells, T or B lymphocytes, epithelial cells, macrophages, dendritic cells, tumor cells) with partial sizes ranging from 20 to 200 nm according to the Minimal Information for Studies of Extracellular Vesicles 2018 (MISEV 2018) guidelines [34–36]. The plasma membrane-derived vesicles contain lipids, proteins (e.g., CD9, CD63, CD81, GTPases, HSP70, HSP90, Tsg101, Alix), nucleic acids (e.g., microRNAs, LncRNAs, mRNAs), and other bioactive substances, which thus play an important role in various physiological and pathological processes, and in particular, serving as intermediators for material exchange and intercellular communication via delivering a variety of the aforementioned bioactive substances [37, 38]. Numerous preclinical and clinical investigations including the International Society for Extracellular Vesicles (ISEV) have shown that MSC-derived extracellular vesicles (EVs) including exosomes and microvesicles (MV) are rich in growth factors, cytokines, mRNAs, signaling lipids and regulatory miRNAs, which are adequate to influence intercellular neighbors and tissue responses to infections, injuries, and diseases [39, 40]. However, the concomitant shortcomings of exosomes such as low purity, low yield, stability for storage and weak targeting collectively limit their preclinical investigation and clinical application. Therefore, there's still a long way to optimize the aforementioned problems and facilitate further exploration upon large-scale preparation (e.g., ultracentrifugation techniques, polymer precipitation, size-based isolation techniques, immunoaffinity chromatography, micro-vortex chips, commercial isolation kits) for translational purposes [41–43].

3. Biomaterials/MSC-based composites for osteoarthritis management

Biomaterials of different categories and characteristics have attracted great concerns of investigators in the field of MSC-based regenerative medicine, and thus allow the utilization of unique scaffolds to promote the expansion of MSCs and facilitate their differentiation into appropriate lineages [24, 44]. Biomaterials with highly biocompatible properties are adequate to act as splendid scaffolds for cell attachment and supply preferable microenvironment for the maintenance, differentiation, and biofunction of the encapsulated MSCs, which collectively benefit the *in situ* tissue engineering and translational medicine [45–47]. To date, a series of biomaterials with discrete advantages and disadvantages have been developed and combined with MSCs for regenerative purposes such as the highly biocompatible natural (e.g., collagen, chitosan) and synthetic (e.g., poly-ethylene-glycol, polycaprolactone) biomaterials [44, 46].

3.1 Hydrogel/MSC-based scaffolds for OA management

Hydrogels are splendid biomaterials with unique physical and chemical properties for both soft and hard tissue engineering and regenerative medicine, which largely attributes to the feasibility of orchestrating the critical properties (e.g., elasticity, water content, bioactivity, mechanical stiffness, degradation) rationally and conveniently [48–50]. For decades, hydrogels alone or in combination with appropriate biomaterials have been extensively investigated in various osteoarticular disorders such as OA and meniscus injury [51–53]. For example, our groups recently reported the reinforced efficacy upon OA rabbits by hyaluronic acid (HA) hydrogel and PSC-MSCs composite (HA/PSC-MSCs) compared to those with HA hydrogel or PSC-MSCs alone [24]. Instead, Chung and colleagues systematically compared the efficacy by implanting various hydrogels/UC-MSCs composites in rats such as alginate, chitosan, pluronic, hyaluronic acid (HA), and verified that HA/hUC-MSCs composites rather than relative hydrogels resulted in preferable cartilage repair and achieved collagen organization pattern and cellular arrangements much similar to the adjacent uninjured articular cartilage [54].

Recently, Yang and colleagues further reported the utilization of an injectable and biocompatible Diels-Alder crosslinked hyaluronic acid/PEG (DAHP) hydrogel for OA treatment, which was found with considerable improvement by controlling the release of MSC-derived small extracellular vesicles (MSC-sEVs) [55]. Similarly, Heirani-Tabasi et al. confirmed the enhanced chondrogenic differentiation capacity of adipose-derived MSCs (AD-MSCs) after incubation with an injectable chitosan-hyaluronic acid (CS-HA) hydrogel [56]. Additionally, Tang et al. demonstrated that sEVs derived from umbilical cord MSCs (UC-MSC-sEVs) revealed comparable therapeutic effects for OA but with upregulated proteins mostly involved in extracellular matrix (ECM) organization, immune effector process, PI3K-AKT and Rap1 signaling pathways [57]. Collectively, MSCs or derivatives (e.g., exosomes, sEVs) in combination with injectable hydrogels have attracted considerable attention in OA management for their advantaged chondrogenic differentiation capacity [51, 56, 58].

3.2 Hydroxyapatite (HAP)/MSCs scaffolds for OA management

State-of-the-art renewals have also highlighted the combination of HAP-based biomaterials with MSCs for OA administration and bone regeneration. For instance, Ji and colleagues recently took advantage of a novel hybrid scaffold composed of nano-hydroxyapatite (nHA)/poly ε-caprolactone (PCL) and thermosensitive hydroxypropyl chitin hydrogel (HPCH) for bone defect repair via a mechanism of enhancing vascularization and osteogenesis of encapsulated MSCs [59].

Instead, Shimomura et al. took advantage of a scaffold-free tissue-engineered construct (TEC) and a HAP artificial bone for the treatment of a rabbit osteochondral defect model, and found that osteochondral defects treated with the synovial MSC-derived TEC and HAP composite revealed more rapid and efficient subchondral bone repair coupled with cartilaginous tissues as well as good tissue integration to adjacent host cartilage. Moreover, the combined MSC-based implants significantly accelerated postoperative rehabilitation and sustained the longer-term durability of repaired osteochondral lesions in patients with OA [5]. Similarly, with the aid of bone marrow-derived MSCs (BM-MSCs) and an interconnected porous hydroxyapatite ceramic (IP-CHA), the large osteochondral defect of the knee in a 21-year-old man was effectively alleviated, and cartilage-like regeneration and bone formation were observed as well [12]. Additionally, we recently also reported the preferable outcomes of OA by conducting multidimensional optimization of MSC-based formulation in combination with the advantageous HA/PG biomaterials, which showed evaluated therapeutic efficacy over HA alone in ameliorating osteoarthritis progression [60, 61].

4. Molecular mechanism of MSC-based cytotherapy for OA management

Generally, MSCs function mainly via orchestrating a series of mode of action including compositional microenvironment, immunoregulation, autocrine, paracrine, and direct- or trans-differentiation into functional cells [15, 62, 63]. In particular, the unique immunomodulatory property and paracrine manner have prompted the enthusiasm for allogenic transplantation of the “off-the-shelf” MSC products in both preclinical and clinical practices in the field of regenerative medicine.

4.1 Compositional microenvironment

In the bone marrow microenvironment, MSCs function as dominating component and stromal cells for the homeostasis and regeneration of hematopoietic stem cells (HSCs) and the concomitant derived cells [30, 64, 65]. In the context of physiological hematogenesis, MSCs are competent for the maintenance or replenishment of the stem cell pool in damaged tissues, and thus help reconstruct the microenvironment for the subsequent hematopoietic reconstitution [22, 30]. As to OA, by conducting MSC infusion into the articular cavity, the hyperactivated inflammatory response caused by inflammatory cytokines is supposed to be effectively suppressed by the released anti-inflammatory factors, extracellular organelles, and vesicles in the microenvironment [24, 66]. As to OA, the roles of MSCs are to orchestrate the spatiotemporal balance between the inflammation and cartilage tissue reconstruction via providing the damaged tissues including bone tissue and cartilage tissue with a relatively desirable environment for tissue repair [24, 67].

4.2 Immunomodulatory effect

To date, extensive literatures have demonstrated the therapeutic or ameliorative effects of MSCs on refractory and recurrent diseases via a bidirectional immunomodulatory approach [14, 25]. Notably, a variety of antiinflammatory factors and cytokines have been reported to play a pivotal role during inflammatory reactions such as interleukins (e.g., IL-6, IL-8, IL-10), transforming growth factor (TGF), stromal cell-derived factor 1 (SDF-1), and vascular endothelial growth factor (VEGF) [22, 68, 69]. The underlying molecular mechanism lies in the sensitive response of MSCs toward the concentration gradient of inflammatory cytokines and chemokines [70]. As to OA, low-grade inflammation has been demonstrated critically in the pathogenesis, which therefore hinders the deposition of cartilage matrix at the damaged sites, delays the proliferation of osteoblast and chondrocytes, and thus resulting in low efficiency of articular cartilage repair [71, 72]. Currently, various kinds of immune cells have been observed in the synovium of OA, including the classically activated and proinflammatory macrophages (M1Mφ), antiinflammatory macrophages (M2Mφ), and T cells. For example, as the major counterparts of immune cells in the joints, Mφ can be hyperactivated by proinflammatory factors in OA patients such as tumor necrosis factor-α (TNF-α), interferon-γ (IFN-γ), and even the pathogen-associated molecular patterns [73]. Therefore, the efficient treatment of OA should also pay close attention to the regulation of the local inflammatory microenvironment. As mentioned above, MSC with multilineage differentiation potential and effective immunomodulatory properties have been supposed as an alternative remedy in the administration of cartilage degradation [74]. In detail, MSCs are purposefully recruited to the site of the damaged cartilage and initiate the therapeutic effects upon osteochondral defects, and thus accelerating the reconstruction of articular surface in OA patients [70]. MSCs have been demonstrated involved in the regulation of M1Mφ towards M2Mφ via releasing growth and angiogenic factors as well as down-regulating inflammation and accelerating the remodeling of damaged tissue in OA. Additionally, the immunoregulatory effect of MSCs or MSC-derived EVs upon T cell subsets has also been extensively and in-detail described during the Th1/Th2 cell transformation, Th17 cell and Treg cell generation, and the apoptosis of hyperactivated T cells [75–79]. Similarly, state-of-the-art renewal has also indicated the immunomodulatory effect of MSCs upon $CD24^{+}CD38^{+}$ B cells partially via soluble secreted factors. Interestingly, the role of MSC-derived EVs in mediating B-cell immunoregulation merit seems contradictory and still needs further investigation [67, 80].

4.3 Autocrine and paracrine

Autocrine and paracrine play a critical role in intercellular communications among MSCs and the adjacent osteochondral defects, which are at the cornerstone of regenerative medicine for MSC-based cytotherapy [81, 82]. The secreted substances such as cytokines and anti-inflammatory factors are responsible for the majority of the ascribed bioremediation via promoting the survival and proliferation of adjacent damaged cells and tissues. For example, mediators (e.g., VEGF, bFGF, IL-6, IL-8) in the conditioned media have been considered to play an important role in influencing the differentiation capacity of MSCs or cocultured cells through an autocrine loop [22, 23, 83]. Interestingly, Lee and colleagues have demonstrated that MSC-secreted PGE-2 plays a key role in the maintenance of self-renewal via EP2 receptor [84].

Of the indicated mode of action, the paracrine phenomenon has been widely recognized as the main benefit of MSC therapy based on the secreted factors acting on MSCs and the neighboring cells. Up to now, a variety of key factors have been isolated and verified including SDF-1, TGF, VEGF, prostaglandin E2 (PGE2), hepatocyte growth factor (HGF), and granulocyte-macrophage colony-stimulating factor (GM-CSF), and the diversity in the constitutive secretome has also been put forward by pioneering investigators in the field [23, 84–86]. As to OA, MSC-derived exosomes or sEVs are supposed to effectively avoid the inherent risks of MSCs and thus hold rosy prospects in clinical applications [87, 88]. However, the inherent disadvantages such as low efficacy in preparations, rapid degradation and clearance still need sustained efforts for further improvement [33, 80].

4.4 Direct- or trans-differentiation

For the past decades, the differentiation potential including direct-differentiation and tans-differentiation has been recognized as the key avenue for MSC-based repair [81]. Of note, the differentiation of MSCs into osteoblasts and chondrocytes has been extensively reported as achievable according to the ISCT guidelines [17]. However, current updates in the field indicate that it is likely that paracrine rather than the direct-differentiation or trans-differentiation play a core role in cartilage repair of OA after MSC delivery because intrathecal injection has presented limited MSC retention and engraftment. For example, aw we previously reviewed, initial attempts upon the molecular mechanisms for disease treatment with MSC transplantation focused on seeking direct evidence for generating functional cells during the rehabilitation of damaged tissues, whereas it was found to be difficult by most investigators when considering the insufficiency of effective retention rate (<5%) [89]. Instead, based on the unique homing property, MSCs mainly migrate to the damaged tissues and perform the restorative function through an orchestration of modulation, which is further verified with the aid of fluorescence *in situ* hybridization [90].

5. Clinical trials of MSC-based cytotherapy for OA management

In recent years, MSC-based cytotherapy has also aroused the intense interest of clinicians in OA treatment. According to the Clinicaltrials.gov database, a total number of 128 clinical trials have been registered worldwide to explore the safety and effectiveness of MSC-based remedies for OA treatment, and in particular, for knee OA and hip OA (**Figure 1**). Of the aforementioned clinical trials, 22 were respectively registered in China and the United States (USA) and followed by 10 in Korea and 9 in Iran (**Table 1**). Meanwhile, we noticed that most of the registered clinical trials were in Phase 1 and/or Phase 2 stage(s), and a total number 13 trials were in the Phase 3 stage instead (**Table 1**). For instance, by conducting a two-year follow-up visit (NCT number: NCT01183728), Orozco and colleagues reported a significant improvement in cartilage quality in 11 of the 12 enrolled knee OA patients with autologous MSC intervention according to the Visual Analogue Scale (VAS) measurements and the pain relief–versus–initial pain score plot [91, 92]. Furthermore, the pain improvement was maintained without significant modifications during the 2-year follow-up, and no serious adverse effects were observed in the aforementioned patients as they previously reported [93].

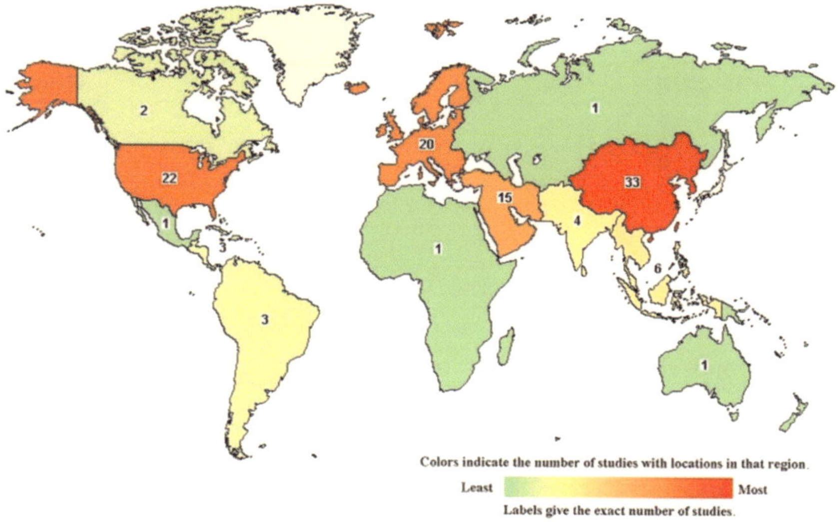

Figure 1.
Clinical trials upon MSC-based cytotherapy for OA administration.

Rank	NCT No.	Age	Phases	Enrollment	Location
1	NCT05160831	18–70	Not Applicable	50	
2	NCT03956719	15–65	Not Applicable	8	China
3	NCT01504464	18–65	Phase 2	40	Iran
4	NCT03383081	≤70	Phase 2	60	China
5	NCT04351932	18–70	Phase 3	54	Ecuador
6	NCT01459640	18–70	Phase 2	50	Malaysia
7	NCT03164083	25–65	Phase 2	0	Iran
8	NCT04130100	40–70	Early Phase 1	60	China
9	NCT03800810	30–80	Early Phase 1	9	Indonesia
10	NCT01809769	40–70	Phase 1, Phase 2	18	China
11	NCT01207661	18–65	Phase 1	6	Iran
12	NCT01499056	18–65	Phase 1	6	Iran
13	NCT02544802	50–70	Phase 1	4	China
14	NCT03357575	18–75	Not Applicable	14	
15	NCT02237846	18–80	Phase 1, Phase 2	0	Panama
16	NCT03166865	30–70	Phase 1, Phase 2	60	China
17	NCT04208646	40–75	Phase 2	108	China
18	NCT02963727	42–75	Phase 1	10	Jordan
19	NCT03869229	30–75	Phase 1, Phase 2	100	Poland
20	NCT02966951	42–75	Phase 1	10	Jordan
21	NCT01586312	18–75	Phase 1, Phase 2	30	Spain
22	NCT01985633	40–75	Phase 1, Phase 2	24	India
23	NCT02641860	18–70	Phase 1	22	China
24	NCT01183728	18–76	Phase 1, Phase 2	12	Spain
25	NCT03969680	40–70	Not Applicable	60	China
26	NCT04212728	40–70	Not Applicable	60	China
27	NCT04326985	18–65	Early Phase 1	20	China
28	NCT01453738	40–70	Phase 2	60	India
29	NCT02123368	50–80	Phase 1, Phase 2	30	Spain
30	NCT03602872	35–65	Phase 1	0	Mexico
31	NCT02365142	40–80	Phase 1, Phase 2	38	Spain
32	NCT03358654	18–75	Not Applicable	9	
33	NCT01448434	20–70	Phase 2	72	Malaysia
34	NCT01895413	25–65	Phase 1, Phase 2	10	Brazil
35	NCT01436058	18–65	Phase 1	6	Iran
36	NCT02162693	18–70	Phase 2	53	China
37	NCT03866330	30–75	Phase 1, Phase 2	100	Poland
38	NCT03477942	18–60	Phase 1	16	USA

Rank	NCT No.	Age	Phases	Enrollment	Location
39	NCT02003131	18–80	Phase 1, Phase 2	0	Panama
40	NCT04368806	≥18	Phase 2, Phase 3	140	USA
41	NCT04448106	≥18	Phase 2	300	USA
42	NCT02958267	40–70	Phase 2	32	USA
43	NCT05288725	18–80	Phase 1, Phase 2	120	USA
44	NCT04863183	30–75	Phase 1, Phase 2	30	
45	NCT05147675		Phase 1	20	Antigua and Barbuda
46	NCT04893174	40–90	Phase 1	6	China
47	NCT00850187	45–60	Phase 1	6	Iran
48	NCT04520945	30–70	Phase 2	100	Malaysia
49	NCT04314661	55–70	Phase 1, Phase 2	15	Indonesia
50	NCT01300598	18–75	Phase 1, Phase 2	18	Korea
51	NCT02776943	18–70	Phase 1, Phase 2	20	
52	NCT05016011	18–65	Phase 2	50	Malaysia
53	NCT03357770	18–75	Not Applicable	9	
54	NCT03589287	≥40	Phase 1, Phase 2	18	China
55	NCT05349565	41–70	Not Applicable	26	Pakistan
56	NCT01873625	10–65	Phase 2, Phase 3	60	Iran
57	NCT05086939	18–75	Phase 3	120	Spain
58	NCT04240873	20–80	Phase 1, Phase 2	24	Korea
59	NCT02291926	18–75	Phase 1	20	China
60	NCT03818737	40–70	Phase 3	480	USA
61	NCT05027581	40–80	Phase 2	70	China
62	NCT02118519	40–68	Phase 2	13	Jordan
63	NCT03955497	18–70	Phase 1, Phase 2	30	China
64	NCT01879046	≥18	Not Applicable	35	France
65	NCT03990805	20–100	Phase 3	260	Korea
66	NCT03000712	20–80	Not Applicable	26	Korea
67	NCT03509025	≥18	Phase 2	11	Korea
68	NCT03014037	18–70	Not Applicable	35	USA
69	NCT03337243	50–85	Not Applicable	60	USA
70	NCT02855073	18–70	Phase 2	28	China
71	NCT04037345	≥19	Phase 1	12	Korea
72	NCT05344157	40–75	Phase 1, Phase 2	54	Australia
73	NCT05182034	≥19	Phase 2	90	
74	NCT02674399	22–60	Phase 2	28	USA
75	NCT00891501	15–55	Phase 2, Phase 3	25	Egypt
76	NCT03028428	40–75	Phase 2	1	

Rank	NCT No.	Age	Phases	Enrollment	Location
77	NCT03943576	40–80	Phase 1, Phase 2	30	China
78	NCT04339504	≥19	Phase 1	12	Korea
79	NCT03648463		Not Applicable	20	
80	NCT01159899	30–75	Early Phase 1	50	France
81	NCT04427930	≥20	Phase 3	260	Korea
82	NCT04825730	≥20	Not Applicable	14	
83	NCT02468492	≥40	Early Phase 1	18	USA
84	NCT05280002	40–80	Phase 2	30	Bangladesh
85	NCT00557635	18–65	Phase 2	50	
86	NCT01931007	18–99	Phase 1	25	USA
87	NCT01041001	≥18	Phase 3	104	Korea
88	NCT03308006	45–65	Phase 2	18	Saudi Arabia
89	NCT02658344	≥18	Phase 2	24	Korea
90	NCT03379168	≥18	Not Applicable	100	USA
91	NCT02696876	16–55	Not Applicable	20	United Kingdom
92	NCT04230902	≥45	Phase 3	48	Lebanon
93	NCT05000593	30–75	Not Applicable	60	China
94	NCT04604288				USA
95	NCT02580695	18–70	Phase 1, Phase 2	30	Chile
96	NCT03790189	35–75	Not Applicable	25	Italy
97	NCT03067870	17–75	Phase 1	100	
98	NCT01626677	≥18	Phase 3	103	Korea
99	NCT04821102	≥20	Not Applicable	21	
100	NCT04716803	45–75	Not Applicable	10	USA
101	NCT01926327	18–65	Phase 3	150	Iran
102	NCT04234412	30–65	Not Applicable	10	
103	NCT03788265	≥18	Not Applicable	60	China
104	NCT02351011	40–65	Phase 1, Phase 2	12	Canada
105	NCT02582489	≥18	Not Applicable	100	USA
106	NCT01227694	18–65	Phase 1, Phase 2	15	Spain
107	NCT04990128	18–65	Phase 3	100	USA
108	NCT05276895	40–80	Phase 1, Phase 2	60	
109	NCT03048773	≥20	Not Applicable	40	China
110	NCT02964143	50–80	Not Applicable	306	
111	NCT04749758	≥18	Not Applicable	77	Andorra
112	NCT04310852	40–70		25	Italy
113	NCT05193877	55–85	Not Applicable	60	Iraq
114	NCT03410355	16–60	Not Applicable	6	Canada

Rank	NCT No.	Age	Phases	Enrollment	Location
115	NCT04453111	18–75	Phase 1, Phase 2	45	Ukraine
116	NCT04308213	35–75	Not Applicable	30	Italy
117	NCT05305833	18–65	Phase 1, Phase 2	20	Turkey
118	NCT04043819	18–80	Phase 1	125	USA
119	NCT05081921	40–70	Phase 1, Phase 2	200	Poland
120	NCT01739504	18–80	Not Applicable	10	USA
121	NCT01413061	18–80	Not Applicable	140	USA
122	NCT04222140	25–60	Not Applicable	40	USA
123	NCT04223622	≥18		24	Italy
124	NCT01585857	50–75	Phase 1	18	Germany
125	NCT03608579	18–65	Phase 1	24	USA
126	NCT02838069	45–75	Phase 2	153	France
127	NCT01038596	50–90		30	Germany
128	NCT01733186	≥18	Phase 1, Phase 2	12	USA

Table 1.
MSC-based clinical trials for OA management.

6. Conclusions

MSCs and concomitant derivatives have emerged as advantaged and alternative sources for OA administration and cartilage repair. MSC- or MSC-exo/sEVs- laden biomaterial systems have supplied overwhelming new tissue-engineering platforms to sequentially improve the osteochondral interface and alleviate the full-thickness articular cartilage defects, which collectively accelerates the reestablishment of osteochondral and cartilage tissues (**Table 2**). Of note, injecting MSCs into joints with

Cell type	Stage	Outcome	Ref.
UC-MSCs	Clinical trials	Safe and superior to active comparator in knee OA	Matas, et al. [94]
AD-MSC/BM-MSC/UC-MSC/AD-MSCs	Clinical trials	Subjective improvements in knee function and pain reduction	Buzaboon, et al. [95]
BM-MSCs/S-MSCs/AD-MSCs	Clinical trials	Pain relief and functional improvement	Cui, et al. [96]
HA hydrogel/ hPSC-MSCs	Preclinical study	Preferable restorative and ameliorative function on OA rabbits	Zhang, et al. [24]
HA hydrogel/UC-MSCs	Preclinical study	Significant gross and histological improvements in hyaline cartilage regeneration	Wu, et al. [97]
Hydrogel/MSCs	Preclinical study	The defects significantly better histologic scores with morphologic characteristics of hyaline cartilage	Zscharnack, et al. [98]
DAHP hydrogel/MSC-sEVs	Preclinical study	Enhanced efficacy for OA improvement	Yang, et al. [55]

Table 2.
Advances in MSC-based cytotherapy for OA.

an inflammatory environment may elevate the risk of ectopic calcification and osteoproliferation in patients with OA. Therefore, systematic and detailed investigations are urgently needed to ensure the maintenance of the intra-articular environment for cartilage repair before large-scale application in clinical practice. In spite of the tremendous progresses in the field of OA management and MSC-based regenerative medicine, it still remains challenging and there's a long way to go to efficiently and cost-effectively repair the full-thickness articular cartilage defects and osteochondral interface via achieving efficient osteogenesis and chondrogenesis.

Acknowledgements

The authors would like to thank the members of the Key Laboratory of Molecular Diagnostics and Precision Medicine for Surgical Oncology in Gansu Province & NHC Key Laboratory of Diagnosis and Therapy of Gastrointestinal Tumor, Gansu Provincial Hospital, and the Institute of Biology & Hefei Institute of Physical Science, Chinese Academy of Sciences for their kind suggestions. This study was supported by grants from the National Natural Science Foundation of China (82260031), the project Youth Fund funded by Shandong Provincial Natural Science Foundation (ZR2020QC097), the Non-profit Central Research Institute Fund of Chinese Academy of Medical Sciences (2019PT320005), Science and technology projects of Guizhou Province (QKH-J-ZK[2021]-107), The 2021 Central-Guided Local Science and Technology Development Fund (ZYYDDFFZZJ-1), Gansu Key Laboratory of molecular diagnosis and precision treatment of surgical tumors (18JR2RA033), Natural Science Foundation of Jiangxi Province (20212BAB216073), Key project funded by Department of Science and Technology of Shangrao City (2020AB002, 2020 K003, 2021F013, 2022AB003), Jiangxi Provincial Key New Product Incubation Program Funded by Technical Innovation Guidance Program of Shangrao (2020G002), Natural Science Foundation of Gansu Province (21JR11RA186, 20JR10RA415), Key talent project of Gansu Province of the Organization Department of Gansu provincial Party committee (2020RCXM076).

Conflict of interest

The authors declare no conflict of interest.

Notes/thanks/other declarations

Not applicable.

Appendix A: appendices and nomenclature

Abbreviation	Nomenclature
MSCs	mesenchymal stem/stromal cells
OA	osteoarthritis
POF	premature ovarian failure
AMI	acute myocardial infarction

ACLF	acute-on-chronic liver failure
P-MSCs	placental-derived MSCs
DPSCs	dental pulp-derived stem cells
UC-MSCs	umbilical cord-derived MSCs
AD-MSCs	adipose-derived MSCs
sEVs	small extracellular vesicles
PSC-MSCs	pluripotent stem cell-derived MSCs
ESCs	embryonic stem cells
iPSCs	induced pluripotent stem cells
ECM	extracellular matrix
TEC	tissue-engineered construct
PCL	poly ε-caprolactone
HA	hyaluronic acid
nHA	nano-hydroxyapatite
HAP	hydroxyapatite
BM-MSCs	bone marrow-derived MSCs
HPCH	hydroxypropyl chitin hydrogel
MV	microvesicles
MISEV	Minimal Information for Studies of Extracellular Vesicles
COVID-19	corona virus disease 2019
CLI	critical limb ischemia
ALI/ARDS	acute lung injury and acute respiratory distress syndrome
ACI	autologous chondrocyte implantation
ISCT	International Society for Cellular Therapy
CS-HA	chitosan-hyaluronic acid
BM-MSCs	bone marrow-derived MSCs
IP-CHA	interconnected porous hydroxyapatite ceramic
SDF-1	stromal cell-derived factor 1
TGF	transforming growth factor
HSCs	hematopoietic stem cells
VEGF	vascular endothelial growth factor
GM-CSF	granulocyte-macrophage colony-stimulating factor
Mφ	macrophages
PGE2	prostaglandin E2
HGF	hepatocyte growth factor

Author details

Leisheng Zhang[1,2,3,4,5,6]*, Zhihai Han[4], Zhongchao Han[4,5,6] and Hui Cai[1]

1 Key Laboratory of Molecular Diagnostics and Precision Medicine for Surgical Oncology in Gansu Province and NHC Key Laboratory of Diagnosis and Therapy of Gastrointestinal Tumor, Gansu Provincial Hospital, Lanzhou, China

2 CAS Key Laboratory of Radiation Technology and Biophysics in Institute of Biology and Hefei Institute of Physical Science, Chinese Academy of Sciences, Hefei, China

3 Center for Cellular Therapies, The First Affiliated Hospital of Shandong First Medical University, Ji-nan, China

4 Jiangxi Research Center of Stem Cell Engineering, Jiangxi Health-Biotech Stem Cell Technology Co., Ltd., Shangrao, China

5 Institute of Health-Biotech, Health-Biotech (Tianjin) Stem Cell Research Institute Co., Ltd, Tianjin, China

6 Stem Cell Bank of Guizhou Province, Guizhou Health-Biotech Biotechnology Co., Ltd., Guiyang, China

*Address all correspondence to: leisheng_zhang@163.com

References

[1] Barnett R. Osteoarthritis. Lancet. 2018;**391**(10134):1985

[2] Bijlsma JW, Berenbaum F, Lafeber FP. Osteoarthritis: An update with relevance for clinical practice. Lancet. 2011;**377**(9783): 2115-2126

[3] Ding N, Li E, Ouyang X, Guo J, Wei B. The therapeutic potential of bone marrow mesenchymal stem cells for articular cartilage regeneration in osteoarthritis. Current Stem Cell Research & Therapy. 2021;**16**(7): 840-847

[4] Xia B, Di C, Zhang J, Hu S, Jin H, Tong P. Osteoarthritis pathogenesis: A review of molecular mechanisms. Calcified Tissue International. 2014; **95**(6):495-505

[5] Shimomura K, Moriguchi Y, Ando W, Nansai R, Fujie H, Hart DA, et al. Osteochondral repair using a scaffold-free tissue-engineered construct derived from synovial mesenchymal stem cells and a hydroxyapatite-based artificial bone. Tissue Engineering. Part A. 2014; **20**(17–18):2291-2304

[6] Nelson AE. Osteoarthritis year in review 2017: Clinical. Osteoarthritis and Cartilage. 2018;**26**(3):319-325

[7] Appleton CT. Osteoarthritis year in review 2017: Biology. Osteoarthritis and Cartilage. 2018;**26**(3):296-303

[8] Pereira D, Ramos E, Branco J. Osteoarthritis. Acta Médica Portuguesa. 2015;**28**(1):99-106

[9] Glyn-Jones S, Palmer AJ, Agricola R, Price AJ, Vincent TL, Weinans H, et al. Osteoarthritis. Lancet. 2015;**386**(9991): 376-387

[10] Wagenbrenner M, Mayer-Wagner S, Rudert M, Holzapfel BM, Weissenberger M. Combinations of hydrogels and mesenchymal stromal cells (MSCs) for cartilage tissue engineering-A review of the literature. Gels. 2021;7(4):217

[11] Jo CH, Lee YG, Shin WH, Kim H, Chai JW, Jeong EC, et al. Intra-articular injection of mesenchymal stem cells for the treatment of osteoarthritis of the knee: A proof-of-concept clinical trial. Stem Cells. 2014;**32**(5):1254-1266

[12] Adachi N, Ochi M, Deie M, Ito Y. Transplant of mesenchymal stem cells and hydroxyapatite ceramics to treat severe osteochondral damage after septic arthritis of the knee. The Journal of Rheumatology. 2005;**32**(8):1615-1618

[13] Aitong W, Leisheng Z, Hao Y. Visualized analyses of investigations upon mesenchymal stem/stromal cell-based cytotherapy and underlying mechanisms for COVID-19 associated ARDS. Current Stem Cell Research & Therapy. 2022;**17**(1):2-12

[14] Zhao Q, Zhang L, Wei Y, Yu H, Zou L, Huo J, et al. Systematic comparison of hUC-MSCs at various passages reveals the variations of signatures and therapeutic effect on acute graft-versus-host disease. Stem Cell Research & Therapy. 2019;**10**(1):354

[15] Zhang L, Wang H, Liu C, Wu Q, Su P, Wu D, et al. MSX2 initiates and accelerates mesenchymal stem/stromal cell specification of hPSCs by regulating TWIST1 and PRAME. Stem Cell Reports. 2018;**11**(2):497-513

[16] Zhang X, Yang Y, Zhang L, Lu Y, Zhang Q, Fan D, et al. Mesenchymal

stromal cells as vehicles of tetravalent bispecific Tandab (CD3/CD19) for the treatment of B cell lymphoma combined with IDO pathway inhibitor D-1-methyl-tryptophan. Journal of Hematology & Oncology. 2017;**10**(1):56

[17] Horwitz EM, Le Blanc K, Dominici M, Mueller I, Slaper-Cortenbach I, Marini FC, et al. International society for cellular T: Clarification of the nomenclature for MSC: The international society for cellular therapy position statement. Cytotherapy. 2005;**7**(5):393-395

[18] Kim BS, Chun SY, Lee EH, Chung JW, Lee JN, Ha YS, et al. Efficacy of combination therapy with pentosan polysulfate sodium and adipose tissue-derived stem cells for the management of interstitial cystitis in a rat model. Stem Cell Research. 2020;**45**:101801

[19] Zhang L, Chi Y, Wei Y, Zhang W, Wang F, Zhang L, et al. Bone marrow-derived mesenchymal stem/stromal cells in patients with acute myeloid leukemia reveal transcriptome alterations and deficiency in cellular vitality. Stem Cell Research & Therapy. 2021;**12**(1):365

[20] Murphy MB, Moncivais K, Caplan AI. Mesenchymal stem cells: Environmentally responsive therapeutics for regenerative medicine. Experimental & Molecular Medicine. 2013;**45**:e54

[21] Dizaji Asl K, Shafaei H, Soleimani Rad J, Nozad HO. Comparison of characteristics of human amniotic membrane and human adipose tissue derived mesenchymal stem cells. World Journal of Plastic Surgery. 2017;**6**(1): 33-39

[22] Wei Y, Zhang L, Chi Y, Ren X, Gao Y, Song B, et al. High-efficient generation of VCAM-1(+) mesenchymal stem cells with multidimensional superiorities in signatures and efficacy on aplastic anaemia mice. Cell Proliferation. 2020;**53**(8):e12862

[23] Du W, Li X, Chi Y, Ma F, Li Z, Yang S, et al. VCAM-1+ placenta chorionic villi-derived mesenchymal stem cells display potent pro-angiogenic activity. Stem Cell Research & Therapy. 2016;**7**:49

[24] Zhang L, Wei Y, Chi Y, Liu D, Yang S, Han Z, et al. Two-step generation of mesenchymal stem/stromal cells from human pluripotent stem cells with reinforced efficacy upon osteoarthritis rabbits by HA hydrogel. Cell & Bioscience. 2021;**11**(1):6

[25] Kagia A, Tzetis M, Kanavakis E, Perrea D, Sfougataki I, Mertzanian A, et al. Therapeutic effects of mesenchymal stem cells derived from bone marrow, umbilical cord blood, and pluripotent stem cells in a mouse model of chemically induced inflammatory bowel disease. Inflammation. 2019; **42**(5):1730-1740

[26] Wei Y, Hou H, Zhang L, Zhao N, Li C, Huo J, et al. JNKi- and DAC-programmed mesenchymal stem/stromal cells from hESCs facilitate hematopoiesis and alleviate hind limb ischemia. Stem Cell Research & Therapy. 2019;**10**(1):186

[27] Zhang K, Zhao X, Chen X, Wei Y, Du W, Wang Y, et al. Enhanced therapeutic effects of mesenchymal stem cell-derived exosomes with an injectable hydrogel for hindlimb ischemia treatment. ACS Applied Materials & Interfaces. 2018;**10**(36):30081-30091

[28] Shi M, Zhang Z, Xu R, Lin H, Fu J, Zou Z, et al. Human mesenchymal stem cell transfusion is safe and improves liver function in acute-on-chronic liver failure

patients. Stem Cells Translational Medicine. 2012;**1**(10):725-731

[29] Lim M, Wang W, Liang L, Han ZB, Li Z, Geng J, et al. Intravenous injection of allogeneic umbilical cord-derived multipotent mesenchymal stromal cells reduces the infarct area and ameliorates cardiac function in a porcine model of acute myocardial infarction. Stem Cell Research & Therapy. 2018;**9**(1):129

[30] Huo J, Zhang L, Ren X, Li C, Li X, Dong P, et al. Multifaceted characterization of the signatures and efficacy of mesenchymal stem/stromal cells in acquired aplastic anemia. Stem Cell Research & Therapy. 2020;**11**(1):59

[31] He X, Ai S, Guo W, Yang Y, Wang Z, Jiang D, et al. Umbilical cord-derived mesenchymal stem (stromal) cells for treatment of severe sepsis: Aphase 1 clinical trial. Translational Research. 2018;**199**:52-61

[32] Hocking AM. Mesenchymal stem cell therapy for cutaneous wounds. Advances in Wound Care. 2012;**1**(4): 166-171

[33] Doyle LM, Wang MZ. Overview of extracellular vesicles, their origin, composition, purpose, and methods for exosome isolation and analysis. Cells. 2019;**8**(7):727

[34] Zhang Y, Bi J, Huang J, Tang Y, Du S, Li P. Exosome: A review of its classification, isolation techniques, storage, diagnostic and targeted therapy applications. International Journal of Nanomedicine. 2020;**15**:6917-6934

[35] Zhang H, Wang L, Li C, Yu Y, Yi Y, Wang J, et al. Exosome-induced regulation in inflammatory bowel disease. Frontiers in Immunology. 2019; **10**:1464

[36] Kalluri R, LeBleu VS. The biology, function, and biomedical applications of exosomes. Science. 2020;**367**(6478): eaau6977

[37] He C, Zheng S, Luo Y, Wang B. Exosome theranostics: Biology and translational medicine. Theranostics. 2018;**8**(1):237-255

[38] Wortzel I, Dror S, Kenific CM, Lyden D. Exosome-mediated metastasis: Communication from a distance. Developmental Cell. 2019;**49**(3):347-360

[39] Yang D, Zhang W, Zhang H, Zhang F, Chen L, Ma L, et al. Progress, opportunity, and perspective on exosome isolation - Efforts for efficient exosome-based theranostics. Theranostics. 2020;**10**(8):3684-3707

[40] Thery C, Witwer KW, Aikawa E, Alcaraz MJ, Anderson JD, Andriantsitohaina R, et al. Minimal information for studies of extracellular vesicles 2018 (MISEV2018): A position statement of the International Society for Extracellular Vesicles and update of the MISEV2014 guidelines. Journal of Extracellular Vesicles. 2018;**7**(1): 1535750

[41] Phinney DG, Pittenger MF. Concise review: MSC-derived exosomes for cell-free therapy. Stem Cells. 2017;**35**(4): 851-858

[42] Duan L, Xu L, Xu X, Qin Z, Zhou X, Xiao Y, et al. Exosome-mediated delivery of gene vectors for gene therapy. Nanoscale. 2021;**13**(3): 1387-1397

[43] Ludwig N, Whiteside TL, Reichert TE. Challenges in exosome isolation and analysis in health and disease. International Journal of Molecular Sciences. 2019;**20**(19):4684

[44] Nugud A, Alghfeli L, Elmasry M, El-Serafi I, El-Serafi AT. Biomaterials as a vital frontier for stem cell-based tissue regeneration. Frontiers in Cell and Development Biology. 2022;**10**:713934

[45] Abdulghani S, Mitchell GR. Biomaterials for in situ tissue regeneration: A review. Biomolecules. 2019;**9**(11):750

[46] Chaudhari AA, Vig K, Baganizi DR, Sahu R, Dixit S, Dennis V, et al. Future prospects for scaffolding methods and biomaterials in skin tissue engineering: A review. International Journal of Molecular Sciences. 2016;**17**(12):1974

[47] Naahidi S, Jafari M, Logan M, Wang Y, Yuan Y, Bae H, et al. Biocompatibility of hydrogel-based scaffolds for tissue engineering applications. Biotechnology Advances. 2017;**35**(5):530-544

[48] Yang J, Zhang YS, Yue K, Khademhosseini A. Cell-laden hydrogels for osteochondral and cartilage tissue engineering. Acta Biomaterialia. 2017;**57**: 1-25

[49] Ansari S, Chen C, Hasani-Sadrabadi MM, Yu B, Zadeh HH, Wu BM, et al. Hydrogel elasticity and microarchitecture regulate dental-derived mesenchymal stem cell-host immune system cross-talk. Acta Biomaterialia. 2017;**60**:181-189

[50] Ding Y, Zhao AS, Liu T, Wang YN, Gao Y, Li JA, et al. An Injectable nanocomposite hydrogel for potential application of vascularization and tissue repair. Annals of Biomedical Engineering. 2020;**48**(5):1511-1523

[51] Hasani-Sadrabadi MM, Sarrion P, Pouraghaei S, Chau Y, Ansari S, Li S, et al. An engineered cell-laden adhesive hydrogel promotes craniofacial bone tissue regeneration in rats. Science Translational Medicine. 2020;**12**(534): eaay6853

[52] Portron S, Merceron C, Gauthier O, Lesoeur J, Sourice S, Masson M, et al. Effects of in vitro low oxygen tension preconditioning of adipose stromal cells on their in vivo chondrogenic potential: application in cartilage tissue repair. PLoS One. 2013;**8**(4):e62368

[53] Merceron C, Portron S, Masson M, Lesoeur J, Fellah BH, Gauthier O, et al. The effect of two- and three-dimensional cell culture on the chondrogenic potential of human adipose-derived mesenchymal stem cells after subcutaneous transplantation with an injectable hydrogel. Cell Transplantation. 2011;**20**(10):1575-1588

[54] Chung JY, Song M, Ha CW, Kim JA, Lee CH, Park YB. Comparison of articular cartilage repair with different hydrogel-human umbilical cord blood-derived mesenchymal stem cell composites in a rat model. Stem Cell Research & Therapy. 2014;**5**(2):39

[55] Yang Y, Zhu Z, Gao R, Yuan J, Zhang J, Li H, et al. Controlled release of MSC-derived small extracellular vesicles by an injectable Diels-Alder crosslinked hyaluronic acid/PEG hydrogel for osteoarthritis improvement. Acta Biomaterialia. 2021;**128**:163-174

[56] Heirani-Tabasi A, Hosseinzadeh S, Rabbani S, Ahmadi Tafti SH, Jamshidi K, Soufizomorrod M, et al. Cartilage tissue engineering by co-transplantation of chondrocyte extracellular vesicles and mesenchymal stem cells, entrapped in chitosan-hyaluronic acid hydrogel. Biomedical Materials. 2021;**16**(5)

[57] Tang S, Chen P, Zhang H, Weng H, Fang Z, Chen C, et al. Comparison of

curative effect of human umbilical cord-derived mesenchymal stem cells and their small extracellular vesicles in treating osteoarthritis. International Journal of Nanomedicine. 2021;**16**: 8185-8202

[58] Zhang S, Liu Y, Zhang X, Zhu D, Qi X, Cao X, et al. Prostaglandin E2 hydrogel improves cutaneous wound healing via M2 macrophages polarization. Theranostics. 2018;**8**(19):5348-5361

[59] Ji X, Yuan X, Ma L, Bi B, Zhu H, Lei Z, et al. Mesenchymal stem cell-loaded thermosensitive hydroxypropyl chitin hydrogel combined with a three-dimensional-printed poly(epsilon-caprolactone) /nano-hydroxyapatite scaffold to repair bone defects via osteogenesis, angiogenesis and immunomodulation. Theranostics. 2020; **10**(2):725-740

[60] Brewer K, Gundsambuu B, Facal Marina P, Barry SC, Blencowe A. Thermoresponsive poly(ε-Caprolactone)-poly(ethylene/propylene glycol) copolymers as injectable hydrogels for cell therapies. Polymers. 2020;**12**(2):367

[61] Das S, Sharma DK, Chakrabarty S, Chowdhury A, Sen Gupta S. Bioactive polymersomes self-assembled from amphiphilic PPO-glycopolypeptides: Synthesis, characterization, and dual-dye encapsulation. Langmuir. 2015; **31**(11):3402-3412

[62] Nombela-Arrieta C, Ritz J, Silberstein LE. The elusive nature and function of mesenchymal stem cells. Nature Reviews. Molecular Cell Biology. 2011;**12**(2):126-131

[63] Shi Y, Wang Y, Li Q, Liu K, Hou J, Shao C, et al. Immunoregulatory mechanisms of mesenchymal stem and stromal cells in inflammatory diseases. Nature Reviews. Nephrology. 2018; **14**(8):493-507

[64] Sagaradze GD, Basalova NA, Efimenko AY, Tkachuk VA. Mesenchymal stromal cells as critical contributors to tissue regeneration. Frontiers in Cell and Development Biology. 2020;**8**:576176

[65] Wang L, Zhang L, Liang X, Zou J, Liu N, Liu T, et al. Adipose tissue-derived stem cells from type 2 diabetics reveal conservative alterations in multidimensional characteristics. International Journal of Stem Cells. 2020;**13**(2):268-278

[66] Jeyaraman M, Muthu S, Ganie PA. Does the source of mesenchymal stem cell have an effect in the management of osteoarthritis of the Knee? Meta-analysis of randomized controlled trials. Cartilage. 2021;**13**(1_suppl):1532S-1547S

[67] Cosenza S, Toupet K, Maumus M, Luz-Crawford P, Blanc-Brude O, Jorgensen C, et al. Mesenchymal stem cells-derived exosomes are more immunosuppressive than microparticles in inflammatory arthritis. Theranostics. 2018;**8**(5):1399-1410

[68] Ahn SY, Park WS, Kim YE, Sung DK, Sung SI, Ahn JY, et al. Vascular endothelial growth factor mediates the therapeutic efficacy of mesenchymal stem cell-derived extracellular vesicles against neonatal hyperoxic lung injury. Experimental & Molecular Medicine. 2018;**50**(4):26

[69] Zhang LS, Yu Y, Yu H, Han ZC. Therapeutic prospects of mesenchymal stem/stromal cells in COVID-19 associated pulmonary diseases: From bench to bedside. World Journal of Stem Cells. 2021;**13**(8):1058-1071

[70] Huh JW, Kim SY, Lee JH, Lee JS, Van Ta Q, Kim M, et al. Bone marrow cells repair cigarette smoke-induced emphysema in rats. American Journal of Physiology. Lung Cellular and Molecular Physiology. 2011;**301**(3):L255-L266

[71] Chow YY, Chin KY. The role of inflammation in the pathogenesis of osteoarthritis. Mediators of Inflammation. 2020;**2020**:8293921

[72] Hedbom E, Hauselmann HJ. Molecular aspects of pathogenesis in osteoarthritis: The role of inflammation. Cellular and Molecular Life Sciences. 2002;**59**(1):45-53

[73] Zhao X, Zhao Y, Sun X, Xing Y, Wang X, Yang Q. Immunomodulation of MSCs and MSC-derived extracellular vesicles in osteoarthritis. Frontiers in Bioengineering and Biotechnology. 2020;**8**:575057

[74] Fernandez-Pernas P, Barrachina L, Marquina M, Rodellar C, Arufe MC, Costa C. Mesenchymal stromal cells for articular cartilage repair: Preclinical studies. European Cells & Materials. 2020;**40**:88-114

[75] Ha DH, Kim HK, Lee J, Kwon HH, Park GH, Yang SH, et al. Mesenchymal stem/stromal cell-derived exosomes for immunomodulatory therapeutics and skin regeneration. Cells. 2020;**9**(5):1157

[76] Harrell CR, Jovicic N, Djonov V, Arsenijevic N, Volarevic V. Mesenchymal stem cell-derived exosomes and other extracellular vesicles as new remedies in the therapy of inflammatory diseases. Cells. 2019;**8**(12):1605

[77] Liu H, Li R, Liu T, Yang L, Yin G, Xie Q. Immunomodulatory effects of mesenchymal stem cells and mesenchymal stem cell-derived extracellular vesicles in rheumatoid arthritis. Frontiers in Immunology. 1912; **2020**:11

[78] Arabpour M, Saghazadeh A, Rezaei N. Anti-inflammatory and M2 macrophage polarization-promoting effect of mesenchymal stem cell-derived exosomes. International Immunopharmacology. 2021;**97**:107823

[79] Behm C, Blufstein A, Gahn J, Nemec M, Moritz A, Rausch-Fan X, et al. Cytokines differently define the immunomodulation of mesenchymal stem cells from the periodontal ligament. Cells. 2020;**9**(5):1222

[80] Carreras-Planella L, Monguio-Tortajada M, Borras FE, Franquesa M. Immunomodulatory effect of MSC on B cells is independent of secreted extracellular vesicles. Frontiers in Immunology. 2019;**10**:1288

[81] Sid-Otmane C, Perrault LP, Ly HQ. Mesenchymal stem cell mediates cardiac repair through autocrine, paracrine and endocrine axes. Journal of Translational Medicine. 2020;**18**(1):336

[82] Hou H, Zhang L, Duan L, Liu Y, Han Z, Li Z, et al. Spatio-temporal metabolokinetics and efficacy of human placenta-derived mesenchymal stem/stromal cells on mice with refractory crohn's-like enterocutaneous fistula. Stem Cell Reviews and Reports. 2020; **16**(6):1292-1304

[83] Hemmingsen M, Vedel S, Skafte-Pedersen P, Sabourin D, Collas P, Bruus H, et al. The role of paracrine and autocrine signaling in the early phase of adipogenic differentiation of adipose-derived stem cells. PLoS One. 2013;**8**(5):e63638

[84] Lee BC, Kim HS, Shin TH, Kang I, Lee JY, Kim JJ, et al. PGE2 maintains

self-renewal of human adult stem cells via EP2-mediated autocrine signaling and its production is regulated by cell-to-cell contact. Scientific Reports. 2016;**6**: 26298

[85] Nakagami H, Maeda K, Morishita R, Iguchi S, Nishikawa T, Takami Y, et al. Novel autologous cell therapy in ischemic limb disease through growth factor secretion by cultured adipose tissue-derived stromal cells. Arteriosclerosis, Thrombosis, and Vascular Biology. 2005; **25**(12):2542-2547

[86] Cheng H, Huang H, Guo Z, Chang Y, Li Z. Role of prostaglandin E2 in tissue repair and regeneration. Theranostics. 2021;**11**(18):8836-8854

[87] Jiang W, Xu J. Immune modulation by mesenchymal stem cells. Cell Proliferation. 2020;**53**(1):e12712

[88] Chen W, Huang Y, Han J, Yu L, Li Y, Lu Z, et al. Immunomodulatory effects of mesenchymal stromal cells-derived exosome. Immunologic Research. 2016; **64**(4):831-840

[89] Krause DS, Theise ND, Collector MI, Henegariu O, Hwang S, Gardner R, et al. Multi-organ, multi-lineage engraftment by a single bone marrow-derived stem cell. Cell. 2001;**105**(3):369-377

[90] Ortiz LA, Gambelli F, McBride C, Gaupp D, Baddoo M, Kaminski N, et al. Mesenchymal stem cell engraftment in lung is enhanced in response to bleomycin exposure and ameliorates its fibrotic effects. Proceedings of the National Academy of Sciences of the United States of America. 2003;**100**(14): 8407-8411

[91] Orozco L, Munar A, Soler R, Alberca M, Soler F, Huguet M, et al. Treatment of knee osteoarthritis with autologous mesenchymal stem cells: two-year follow-up results. Transplantation. 2014;**97**(11):e66-e68

[92] Huskisson EC. Measurement of pain. Lancet. 1974;**2**(7889):1127-1131

[93] Orozco L, Munar A, Soler R, Alberca M, Soler F, Huguet M, et al. Treatment of knee osteoarthritis with autologous mesenchymal stem cells: A pilot study. Transplantation. 2013; **95**(12):1535-1541

[94] Matas J, Orrego M, Amenabar D, Infante C, Tapia-Limonchi R, Cadiz MI, et al. Umbilical cord-derived mesenchymal stromal cells (MSCs) for knee osteoarthritis: Repeated MSC dosing is superior to a single MSC dose and to hyaluronic acid in a controlled randomized phase I/II Trial. Stem Cells Translational Medicine. 2019;**8**(3):215-224

[95] Buzaboon N, Alshammary S. Clinical applicability of adult human mesenchymal stem cell therapy in the treatment of knee osteoarthritis. Stem Cells Cloning. 2020;**13**:117-136

[96] Cui GH, Wang YY, Li CJ, Shi CH, Wang WS. Efficacy of mesenchymal stem cells in treating patients with osteoarthritis of the knee: A meta-analysis. Experimental and Therapeutic Medicine. 2016;**12**(5): 3390-3400

[97] Wu KC, Chang YH, Liu HW, Ding DC. Transplanting human umbilical cord mesenchymal stem cells and hyaluronate hydrogel repairs cartilage of osteoarthritis in the minipig model. Ci Ji Yi Xue Za Zhi. 2019;**31**(1):11-19

[98] Zscharnack M, Hepp P, Richter R, Aigner T, Schulz R, Somerson J, et al. Repair of chronic osteochondral defects using predifferentiated mesenchymal stem cells in an ovine model. The American Journal of Sports Medicine. 2010;**38**(9):1857-1869

Chapter 12

Ayurveda Research on *Agnikarma* in Osteoarthritis of Knee Joint

Tukaram Dudhamal

Abstract

In Ayurveda, treatment with intentional therapeutic heat burns is called *Agnikarma* (thermal cauterization), which is one of the para-surgical procedures. It is also called *Dahan Karma* (thermal cauterization). Various painful conditions like joint pain, sciatica, tendinopathies, headache, abdominal cramps/discomfort, and few convulsive disorders like epilepsy, schizophrenia, psycho-somatic disorders, and some skin diseases can be treated with this intentional heat burn therapy. *Agnikarma* has widely been used in clinical practice since time immemorial and is said to have immediate and long-lasting relief, as mentioned in the Indian traditional therapy. This para-surgical procedure is practiced in all teaching institutes of Ayurveda in India, and many researchers are publishing the research work done on *Agnikarma* in musculo-skeletal disorders. In this chapter, the concept of *Agnikarma* along with a brief procedure and published evidence-based research studies on osteoarthritis (OA) of the knee joint treated with *Agnikarma* are critically analyzed. This chapter contributes the knowledge of the Indian traditional para-surgical procedure in musculoskeletal disorders in general and OA knee joint in particular.

Keywords: *Agnikarma*, ayurveda, OA knee joint

1. Introduction

According to Sushruta, *Agnikarma* (intentional therapeutic heat burns) is a superior *Anu-shastra Karma* (para-surgical procedure), and in patients treated with the *Agnikarma* (cauterization) procedure, the disease usually did not recur [1]. Depending on the disease, different materials heated at different temperatures are used for *Agnikarma*; that is, depending upon the disease and its predominant doshas (body humors), different materials and temperatures are selected for the treatment; for example, in the case of *Agnikarma* on the skin, less hot *shalakas* (probes) are used [2, 3].

Snigdha Agnikarma is cauterization with the help of heated liquids, semi-liquids, or fats, while *Ruksha Agnikarma* is cauterization with the help of heated metal [4]. Local *Agnikarma (sthanika)* is done at the disease site, such as skin disorders, and distant *Agnikarma (sthanantriya)* is done away from the actual diseased area.

Four kinds of shape of the *Agnikarma* are described in Ayurveda classics: *Valay* – circular, *Bindu* – dotted with a pointed object, *Vilekha* – linear, and *Pratisarana* –produced by the rubbing of a heated object upon the site up to the desired extent (Acharya Sushruta) [5]. Three additional shapes of *Agnikarma* are: *Ardhachandra* – semilunar or crescent shaped, *Swastika* – cross shaped, and *Ashtapada* – having eight arms or limbs (Acharya Vagbhata) [6].

According to the depth and tissue involved, four kinds of *Agnikarma* are *Twak Dagdha, Mamsa Dagdha, Sira snayu Dagdha,* and *Sandhi Asthi Dagdha* [7].

1.1 Indications of *Agnikarma*

A number of diseases and conditions belonging to the musculo-skeletal system, eyes, ENT, hernias, sciatica, elephantiasis, hemorrhoids, sinuses and fistulae, headache, and benign neoplasms have been explained in texts where *Agnikarma* is indicated as a therapeutic measure [8].

The above statement is based on the indications mentioned in the Ayurveda text, that is, in *Sushruta Samhita*. On the basis of this concept, some clinical trials are conducted in Ayurveda research institutes and published in the PubMed indexed journals. The clinical pieces of evidence in the context of *Agnikarma* in the management of musculo-skeletal disorders are Tennis elbow [9], lumbar spondylosis [10], osteoarthritis of the knee joint [11, 12], sciatica [13, 14], migraine [15], and benign growths like warts [16, 17].

The clinical pieces of evidence in the context of *Agnikarma* in musculo-skeletal disorders with doi numbers are review articles [18, 19], trigger finger [20], calcaneal spur [21], de Quervain's tenosynovitis [22], plantar fasciitis [23], cervical erosion [24], gynecomastia [25], and mucocele [26].

The clinical pieces of evidences other than PubMed-indexed journals in the context of *Agnikarma* in the management of musculo-skeletal disorders are corn [27, 28], direct inguinal hernia [29], osteoarthritis of the knee joint [30, 31], cervical spondylosis [32, 33], planter fasciitis (calcaneum spur) [34, 35], and sciatica [36].

1.2 Contra-indications of *Agnikarma*

It should not be done in *Pitta Prakriti* (*Pitta*-dominating body constitution), *Bhinna kosthas* (abdominal perforations), *Dourbalya* (general debility), *Vriddha* (old age), *Baala* (children), *Bheeru* (fearful or bogey man), a person afflicted with a large number of *Vrana* (multiple wounds), *Antah shonita* (internal hemorrhage) [37], and a person who is unfit for *svedana* (unfit for hot fomentation) (Anuddhrita Shalya) [38]. According to Acharya Charaka, *Agnikarma* should not be done in the *vrana* of *snayu* (tendon or ligament injuries), *marma* (vital parts), *Netra* (eyes), *kushtha* (leprosy), and *vrana with visha and Shalya* (wounds with poison or retained foreign body) [39].

1.3 Suitable time or *Ritu* (Season) for *Agnikarma*

Agnikarma can be done during all the seasons except *Grishma* (summer) and *Sharad* (extreme winters) [40]. It is because in *Sharad*, there is vitiation of *Pitta* and *Agnikarma* also aggravates *Pitta*, and it may lead to further *Pitta* vitiation. During *Grishma* season, there is increase in environmental temperature and *Bala* (vital force) of the patient remains weak. Even in these seasons, in emergent conditions that are amenable only to *Agnikarma*, it may be used after taking appropriate countermeasures to protect the patients from the complications.

1.4 Methodology of *Agnikarma*

1.4.1 Pre-operative measures

The collection of instruments, other required articles, and assistance should be ready. Diet: All the required *Agnikarma* should be done after feeding the patient with *Pichhila* diet (slimy diet/curd rice).

Examination, investigations, and other precautions: Before going for any surgical or para-surgical procedure, a complete assessment should be carried out regarding all the factors, such as routine blood investigations like CBC, blood sugar, etc. Tetanus prophylaxis is given. Patient's *Bala* (strength), *Marmasthana* (vital parts), *Roga*, and *Ritu* (season) should be properly assessed. Only after that *Agnikarma* should be done [41]. After confirmation of the site of *Agnikarma*, it is marked (maximum tenderness). The selected site is cleaned with *Triphala kwath* or normal saline (in any condition, spirit should not be applied). The area is covered with a sterile holed towel.

1.4.2 Main procedure

After completion of the assessment of the patient and making final diagnosis, *Agnikarma* should be done with a suitable instrument according to the *Dosha* (body humor) and *Dhatu* (body tissue) involved and on the site mentioned for the disease until the *Samyaka Dagdha lakshanas* are produced. Depending on the nature of the disease, the predominance of the *Dosha*, and its site, 10–12 heat burns are made with appropriate *Shalakas* (probes). According to the disease, superficial burns, that is, '*Twaka dagda*', are done for the disease receding superficially, and deep heat burns, that is, *Mamsa Dagda*, are done for deep-seated diseases. During the procedure, the patient may feel pain, so he or she should be taken in confidence and assistance may be required to hold him or her so that the procedure can be performed appropriately. During and after *Agnikarma*, *aloe vera* pulp should be applied to minimize the burning sensation.

1.4.3 Post-operative Measures

After completion of *Agnikarma*, the part where *Agnikarma* has been done should be anointed with *Madhu* (honey) and *Ghrita* (clarified butter) for *Ropana* (healing) of *Dagdha Vrana* (burn wound). Wound should not be made wet to prevent the wound infection.

1.5 Probable complications

1. *Heena Dagdha*: If the *Shalaka* is not properly heated, it will produce this type of *Dagdha*.

2. *Ati-Dagdha*: This complication is produced due to transfer of more heat from the red-hot *Shalaka* to the diseased part.

3. *Marmaghata*: Due to the fear of burn, the patient may go in vasovagal shock. Emergency treatment should be given to the patient.

4. *Daha (burning)*: More or less burning pain is experienced by each and every patient undergoing *Agnikarma Chikitsa*. This may be treated by *Avachurna* (dusting) of *Yashtimadhu* powder or *Lepa* of *Ghritkumari Swarasa*.

5. *Shopha* (odema): Inflammation is one of the complications; it should be treated accordingly with *shothahar* (anti-inflammatory drugs).

6. *Dushta Vranata*: Infection at the burn site is one of the complications, which should be treated accordingly as a superficial burn.

2. Evidence-based research studies

The research studies carried out by researchers of Ayurveda with the help of different sources of *Agnikarma* in the management of OA knee joint has been summarized with a brief methodology and results citing the references of published research studies for further details.

Pragnesh D. Pandya had conducted a study on 18 patients of *Sandhigata Vata* (osteoarthritis) of knee joint with the aim to evaluate the role of *Agnikarma* and internal Ayurveda medicine in the management of OA knee joint [42]. Selected patients were divided into 3 groups. In group A (n = 6), patients were treated with *Binduvata Agnikarma* by boiling *Ghrita* (clarified butter) after local anesthesia (2% lignocaine) in the respective knee joint one time. In group B (n = 6), patients were treated by *Vata Vidhvansadi Yoga* followed by *Shuddha Guggulu Vati* as internal medicines for 12 weeks. In group C (n = 6), patients were treated with both the therapies, that is, *Agnikarma* locally and drugs internally. Those patients who were in group A and B were observed with equally benefited patients who were treated locally as well as with internal medicines, that is, patients in group C, showed comparatively better results than group A and B. The study concluded that *Agnikarma* offers a better and competent solution in the management of *Sandhigata Vata* (OA of knee joint).

Dhiraj D. Chandasna had done further study on 21 patients of *Sandhigata Vata* (OA of knee joint) [43]. All 21 patients were divided in 3 groups. In group A (n = 7), patients were treated with *Binduvata Agnikarma* by boiling *Ghrita* (clarified butter) after local anesthesia on the affected knee joint one time. In group B (n = 7), patients were treated with *Vata Vidhvansadi Yoga* followed by *Shuddha Guggulu Vati* as internal medicines for one month. In group C (n = 7), patients were treated with both the therapies, that is, *Agnikarma* locally and drugs internally. 100% relief in all the symptoms was found in 4 patients out of 7 in group A, 1 patient out of 7 in group B, and all 7 patients in group C. Those patients who were in group C showed comparatively better relief among the 3 groups. The study concluded that *Agnikarma* is effective in the management of *Sandhigata Vata* (osteoarthritis).

Nilesh G. Jethava reported a study on 28 patients of *Janu Sandhigata Vata* to evaluate the efficacy of *Agnikarma* with *Rajata* and *Loha Shalaka* in the management of *Janu Sandhigata Vata* (OA of knee joint) [44]. A study was carried out in two groups, in which patients of group A received *Agnikarma* treatment with *Rajata Shalaka* and patients of group B received *Agnikarma* treatment with *Loha Shalaka* once a week for 4 weeks. Both groups showed statistically insignificant difference in the result. *Loha Shalaka* showed better result for pain relief compared to *Rajata Shalaka*. The study has proven the efficacy of *Agnikarma* in *Janu Sandhigata Vata* (OA of knee joint) for pain management.

Sucheta Ray conducted RCT on *Agnikarma* with two different Shalakas in OA of knee joint [45]. A total of 30 patients were divided into two groups: *Rajat Shalaka* and *Tamra Shalaka*. Assessment was done after the follow-up on 7th and 14th days. In patients treated with *Rajat Shalaka*, complete remission was seen in 3 patients (20%), remarkable improvement in 6 patients (40%), and moderate improvement in 6 patients (40%). In patients treated with *Tamra Shalaka*, complete remission was seen in 2 patients (13.33%), remarkable improvement in 4 patients (26.66%), and moderate improvement in 9 patients (60%). Results in both groups were statistically highly significant with p value of ≤ 0.0001. The study showed that *Agnikarma* with *Rajata Shalaka* was more effective than *Tamra Shalaka* in relieving the pain, tenderness, and other signs and symptoms of *Janu Sandhigata Vata* (OA of knee joint).

Aneesh Sharma carried out RCT on *Agnikarma* and *Panchatikta Guggulu* in the management of *Sandhivata* (OA of knee joint) [11]. A total 33 patients with *Janugata Sandhivata* were divided into 2 groups; in group A ($n = 18$), *Agnikarma* was done with *Panchadhatu Shalaka* once every week for one month, while in group B ($n = 15$), *Agnikarma* was done along with *Panchatikta Guggulu* given orally for one month.

Sandhishula (pain), *Sparshaasahyata* (tenderness), *Sandhisphutana* (crepitus), and *Sandhigraha* (stiffness) were weekly assessed by subjective gradation, and a range of movement (ROM) was recorded in research proforma. In *Sandhishula*, 86% relief was seen in group A, whereas 77.78% relief was seen in group B. *Sparshaasahyata* was reduced by 69% in group A, while 87.78% in Group B. Nearly 39% improvement was seen in *Sandhisphutana* in Group A, while 46.67% in Group B. In *Sandhigraha*, 63% relief was obtained in each of the groups. The patients got relief from the pain after first sitting of *Agnikarma* in both the groups. The relief was sustained for more than 3 months in most of the patients, as noted during follow-up. There was no significant difference in radiological findings before and after treatment in both the groups.

Mohasin Kadegaon et al. conducted a clinical study on 30 patients of *Sandhigata Vata* with special reference to *Janu Sandhi* (OA of knee joint) [46]. The aim of the study was to evaluate the efficacy of *Agnikarma* and *Svedana* in the management of OA of the knee joint. All the selected patients were equally divided into 2 groups. In group A ($n = 15$), patients were treated with *Agnikarma* in the affected knee joint in a single sitting by *Lohadhatu Shalaka*, and in group B ($n = 15$), patients were treated with *Dashamula Nadisveda* for 7 days. Follow-up was done on 7th and 14th days. *Agnikarma* with *Lohashalaka* is more effective in the management of *Vedana* and *Stambha*, whereas *Dashamula Nadisveda* is more effective in treating *Sandhisotha*. The overall result of improvement seen in group A was 74.62%, while in group B it was 70.19%. The study showed better and quick result in *Agnikarma* with *Lohashalaka* as compared to *Dashamula Nadisveda* (OA of knee joint).

Parth Pandya et al. did further study on 30 patients with *Janu Sandhigata Vata* (OA of knee joint) [47]. In group A ($n = 15$), patients were treated with *Agnikarma* by *Panchadhatu Shalaka* once a week for one month. In group B ($n = 15$), patients were treated with *Agnikarma* by *Panchadhatu Shalaka* along with *Panchatikta Guggulu* orally for one month. There was not much difference in the percentage of improvement in both groups. However, the combined effect of *Agnikarma* and oral *Panchatikta Guggulu* showed better results in reference to relief in the complaints of joint pain, joint stiffness, and crepitus.

Anju Lata et al. carried out RCT on a comparative study of conductive and direct method of *Agnikarma* with *Tamra Shalaka* in *Sandhigatvata* [48]. A total of 60 patients with OA of knee joint were divided into two groups. In the conductive method ($n = 30$) and direct method ($n = 30$) of *Agnikarma* with *Tamra Shalaka* at an average temperature of 150°C and 50°C, respectively, it was found that the pain, tenderness, and swelling were significantly reduced after treatment by both methods with a p-value less than 0.05. But in the direct method, more effective and satisfactory result was found than in the conductive, which method might be due to a high temperature of about 150°C. The study concluded that *Agnikarma* shows good results in pain relief when the temperature of the *Shalaka* is 150°C and more in conditions like osteoarthritis of knee joint.

Ruchi Pandey carried out an RCT to evaluate the effect of *Agnikarma* along with *Panchatikta* Guggulu in the management of *Janu Sandhigata Vata* (osteoarthritis of knee joint) [49]. In group A ($n = 21$), 4 sittings of *Agnikarma* were done with *Panchadhatu Shalaka*. In group B ($n = 20$), 4 sittings of *Agnikarma* were done with *Panchadhatu Shalaka* along with *Panchatikta Guggulu* orally for one month. Significant relief was observed in both groups in all subjective parameters. Clinically and percentage wise, group B showed better results. The study concluded that *Agnikarma* alone has a definite role in reducing the knee joint pain and tenderness, but the addition of *Panchatikta Guggulu* showed convincing results in stiffness, swelling, and range of movement of knee joint. The author also demonstrated a video of *Agnikarma* for the same study [50].

Shubham Puri conducted a study on *Agnikarma* and indigenous drugs in the management of *Janu Sandhigata Vata* w.s.r. to OA of knee joint [51]. In this study, in group A, 15 patients received oral indigenous drugs, while in group B, 15 patients received *Agnikarma* with *Rajat Shalaka. Agnikarma* was done in four sittings with a weekly interval. The group of patients who received *Agnikarma* showed better results as compared with the orally treated group of patients. In terms of the two parameters of pain and range of movements, *Agnikarma*-treated patients showed very good result as compared to patients treated with oral medications. The study concluded that *Agnikarma* was found to be very effective in the management of *Janu Sandhigata Vata* (OA knee joint).

Syyed MJ carried out RCT on *Agnikarma* in 60 patients of *Janu Sandhigata Vata* w.s.r to OA of knee joint [52]. Patients were randomly allocated to receive either conservative medicine or *Agnikarma* for a period of 15 days. Clinical efficacy was evaluated on 7th and 14th days on the basis of cardinal symptoms with a visual analogue scale. Treatment with *Agnikarma* produced a significant drop in the severity of pain ($p < 0.001$). Radiological assessment, however, did not show any significant changes in both the groups.

Lobo SJ did a comparative clinical trial on 60 patients with *Janu Sandhigata Vata* (OA of knee joint) [53]. The aim of the study was to evaluate the effect of *Agnikarma* (therapeutic heat burn) by *Suvarna Shalaka* (rod made of gold) and *Panchadhatu Shalaka* (rod made up of five metals). All patients were divided into two groups. In group A ($n = 30$), patients were treated by *Agnikarma* with *Suvarna Shalaka*, and in group B ($n = 30$), patients were treated by *Agnikarma* with *Panchadhatu Shalaka* once a week for four weeks. All patients were followed up after 15th and 30th days. The statistical analysis showed that *Agnikarma* by *Suvarna Shalaka* was statistically more significant in reduction of pain, tenderness, crepitus, swelling, angle of flexion, and extension compared to *Agnikarma* by *Panchadhatu Shalaka.* Thus, the study concluded that *Suvarna Shalaka Agnikarma* is found more beneficial than *Agnikarma* using *Panchadhatu Shalaka* in prime symptoms of *Janu Sandhigata Vata* (OA of knee joint).

Raut SR conducted a case-based study on pain management by the conductive method of *Agnikarma* with *Suvarna Shalaka* in *Janu Sandhigata Vata* [54] in three sittings. On every 7th day, it was observed that the response of the patient was good to conductive *Agnikarma* therapy. The pain is reduced in VAS from 7/10 to 0/10. ROM flexion improved from 110 to 135 with no burn marks.

3. Conclusions

Thus, in conclusion, *Agnikarma* is practiced in India with positive outcomes in the management of OA as a conservative measure, and its effects are sustained for up to 6 months. This procedure needs further evaluation with other parameters like inflammatory markers in a scientific way in more number of cases. Data on more number of cases with specific parameters and multicentric trial are needed for the exact mode of action and scientific validation.

Acknowledgements

The author thanks Prof. Dr. Anup Thakar, Director, ITRA, Jamnagar, Gujarat, India, for providing all facilities at the department for continuous research studies on para-surgical procedures.

Conflict of interest

None declared.

Author details

Tukaram Dudhamal
Department of Shalya Tantra, Institute of Teaching and Research in Ayurveda (institute of National Importance), Ministry of AYUSH, Government of India, Jamnagar, Gujarat, India

*Address all correspondence to: dudhamal@itra.edu.in; drtsdudhamal@gmail.com

References

[1] Shastri AD, editor. Sushruta Samhita, Sutra Sthana 12/3. 1st ed. Varanasi: Chaukhamba Sanskrit Sansthan; 2007. p. 50

[2] Shastri AD, editor. Sushruta Samhita, Sutra Sthana 12/4. 1st ed. Varanasi: Chaukhamba Sanskrit Sansthan; 2007. pp. 51-52

[3] Gupta PD. Agnikarma technological Innovations. 1st ed. Nagpur: Prabha Publication; 1992. pp. 25-26

[4] Shastri AD, editor. Sushruta Samhita, Sutra Sthana 12/4. 1st ed. Varanasi: Chaukhamba Sanskrit Sansthan; 2007. p. 51

[5] Shastri AD, editor. Sushruta Samhita, Sutra Sthana 12/11. 1st ed. Varanasi: Chaukhamba Sanskrit Sansthan; 2007. p. 52

[6] Gupta KA. Ashtang Sangrah, Sutra Stahana 40/4. Varanasi: Chaukhamba Sanskrit Sansthan; 2000. p. 227

[7] Shastri AD, editor. Sushruta Samhita, Sutra Sthana 12/8. 1st ed. Varanasi: Chaukhamba Sanskrit Sansthan; 2007. p. 52

[8] Shastri AD, editor. Sushruta Samhita, Sutra Sthana 12/9-10. 1st ed. Varanasi: Chaukhamba Sanskrit Sansthan; 2007. p. 52

[9] Mahanta V, Dudhamal TS, Gupta SK. Management of tennis elbow by Agnikarma. Journal of Ayurveda Integrative Medicine. 2013;**4**(1):45-47

[10] Joshi F, Mahanta V, Dudhamal TS, Gupta SK. Effect of Agnikarma (therapeutic heat burns) and Raktamokshana (therapeutic bloodletting) in the management of Kati Sandhigata Vata (lumbar spondylosis). Ayurveda. 2019;**40**(2):79-88

[11] Sharma AV, Dudhamal TS, Gupta SK, Mahanta V. Clinical study of Agnikarma and Panchatikta Guggulu in the management of Sandhivata (osteoartheritis of knee joint). Ayurveda. 2016;**37**(1):38-44

[12] Jethava NG, Dudhamal TS. A role of Agnikarma in Sandhigata Vata (osteoarthritis of knee joint). PG research work submitted to Gujarat Ayurveda University, Jamnagar. 2015;**36**(1):23-28. DOI: 10.4103/0974-8520.169017

[13] Bali Y, Vijayasarathi R, Ebnezar J, Venkatesh B. Efficacy of Agnikarma over the padakanistakam (little toe) and Katibasti in Gridhrasi: A comparative study. International Journal of Ayurveda Research. 2010;**1**(4):223-230

[14] Vaneet Kumar J, Dudhamal TS, Gupta SK, Mahanta V. A comparative clinical study of Siravedha and Agnikarma in management of Gridhrasi (sciatica). Ayurveda. 2014;**35**(3):270-276

[15] Kanakhara B, Chaudhari V. A pilot study on clinical efficacy of Agnikarma and Pathyadi decoction (an Ayurvedic formulation) in the management of Ardhavabhedaka (migraine). Ayurveda. 2018;**39**(1):56-61

[16] Sekhar Namburi UR, Omprakash BG. A review on management of warts in Ayurveda. Ayurveda. 2011 Jan;**32**(1):100-102

[17] Shindhe P, Kiran M. Carmakila: An effective management by kshara karma. Journal of Ayurveda Integrative Medicine. 2013;**4**(3):181-183

[18] Singh B, Rajiv Dole R, Deep G, Yogitha Bali MR. Application of Agnikarma with Shalaka Dahana Upakaranas in the Management of Musculoskeletal Disorders – A Comprehensive Review. International Journal of Ayurveda and Pharma Research. 2022;**9**(12):68-72

[19] Badwe Y, Shilvant R, Shinde J. Role of Agnikarma in pain management of various musculoskeletal disorders: A Review Study. International Journal of Ayurveda and Pharma Research. 2021;**9**(8):89-96

[20] Gadve BN, Patil MS. A Clinical Case Study of Agnikarma with Panchadhatu Shalaka in Trigger Finger (Snayugat Vata). World Journal of Pharmaceutical Research. 2021;**10**(12):257-263

[21] Mugilmathi BK, Reddy V, Vipin SG. Role of Bindu Dagdha type of Agnikarma in management of Vatakantaka with Special Reference to Calcaneal Spur: A Case Study. International Journal of Research in Ayurveda and Pharmacy. 2022;**13**(5):43-46

[22] Jeetendra AJ, Santhosh KJ. A Clinical Study on Effect of Agnikarma in Urdwa Shakhagata Kurchasira Marmaghata (De Quervain's Tenosynovitis). IAMJ. 2020

[23] Yadav P, Shukla D. Role of Viddha-Agnikarma in Chronic Plantar Fasciitis-A Case Study. Environment Conservation Journal. 2019;**20**(1):47-50

[24] Tiwari R, Pushpalatha B, Bharathi K. Clinical study to evaluate the efficacy of Agnikarma In Karnini with special reference to cervical erosion. International Journal of Ayurveda and Pharma Research. 2020;**8**(11):53-58

[25] Sharma R, Barahate G, Neralkar U. Case Study of Agni Karma in Stanya Granthi with Special Reference to Gynecomastia. International Journal of Research in Ayurveda and Pharmacy. 2022;**13**(3)

[26] Bharankar SD, Dhakate VG. A Case Study of Agnikarma Procedure in the Management of Mucocele (Jalarbuda). World Journal of Pharmaceutical Research. 2021;**10**(12):1568-1572

[27] Sonam R, Shah B, Sah R. Management of Kadara (Corn) By Agnikarma - A case report. International Journal of AYUSH Case Reports. 2019;**3**(2):188-191

[28] Roy S, Katheeja KM. Agnikarma in the Management of Kadara (Corn) - A Case Report. International Journal of AYUSH Case Reports. 2022;**6**(1):34-38

[29] Shukkoor MA, Subhi N. Improvised Agnikarma with Infrared Photocoagulator in Direct Inguinal hernia –A Single Case Report. International Journal of AYUSH Case Reports. 2022;**6**(1):39-43

[30] Rathod K, Kumar N, Dudhamal T. Management of Janusandhigata Vata w.s.r. to Osteoarthritis of knee joint with modified method of Agnikarma by the use of electrocautery- A Case Report. International Journal of AYUSH Case Reports. 2022;**6**(3):318-324

[31] Lobo S, Bhuyan C, Das A. Agnikarma with Suvarna Shalaka in Janu Sandhigata Vata (Osteoarthritis of Knee Joint) - A Case Report. International Journal of AYUSH Case Reports. 2019;**3**(1):105-111

[32] Daga H, Jethava N, Toshikhane H. Management of Sandhigata Vata (Cervical Spondylosis) by Agnikarma with Lauha Shalaka - An Observational Pilot study. International Journal of AYUSH Case Reports. 2018;**2**(1):36-42

[33] Sehgal U, Rajagopala M, Dwivedi RR, Bavalatti N. Role of Agnikarma and

Ajamodadivati in the management of Sandhigata Vata w.s.r. to Cervical Spondylosis. Ayurveda. 2009;**30**(3):345-349

[34] Ganatra R, Kapadiya M, Dudhamal T. Agnikarma (therapeutic heat burn) an unique approach in the management of vatakantaka w.s.r. to plantar fasciitis- A single Case Report. International Journal of AYUSH Case Reports. 2021;**5**(1):30-35

[35] Kusuma A, Mitra VC, Deep P, Kutty M, Nair PKS, Prabhakaran VA, et al. A preliminary study on evaluation of clinical effect of Agnikarma Chikitsa on Parsnisula (Plantar Fascitis). Journal of Research in Ayurveda and Siddha. 2009;**30**(2):57-70

[36] Lohith BA, Prasad BS. Effect of Bindu Agnikarma (Cauterisation) in Grdhrasi (Sciatica) - A Clinical Study. Aryavaidyan. 2010;**23**(4):226-230

[37] Shastri AD, editor. Sushruta Samhita, Sutra Sthana 12/14. 1st ed. Varanasi: Chaukhamba Sanskrit Sansthan; 2007. p. 53

[38] Shastri AD, editor. Sushruta Samhita, Chikitsa Sthana 32/25. 1st ed. Varanasi: Chaukhamba Sanskrit Sansthan; 2007. p. 176

[39] Shastri KN, Chaturvedi GN. Sushruta Samhita, Chikitsa Sthana 25/105, 106. 17th ed. Varanasi: Chaukhamba Sanskrit Sansthan; 2007. p. 176

[40] Shastri AD, editor. Sushruta Samhita, Sutra Sthana 12/5. 1st ed. Varanasi: Chaukhamba Sanskrit Sansthan; 2007. p. 51

[41] Shastri AD, editor. Sushruta Samhita, Sutra Sthana 12/12. 1st ed. Varanasi: Chaukhamba Sanskrit Sansthan; 2007. p. 52

[42] Pandya PD, Singh K. Role of Agnikarma in the management of Sandhigata Vata. Jamnagar, India: Gujarat Ayurveda University; 1990

[43] Chandasna DD, Singh K. Further Studies on Agnikarma in Sandhigata Vata. Jamnagar, India: Gujarat Ayurveda University; 1991

[44] Jethava NG, Dudhamal TS. Role of agnikrma in management of sandhigatavata. Jamnagar: PG Research Work Submitted to Gujarat Ayurveda University; July 2012

[45] Ray S. A Comparative Study on Efficacy of Agnikarma by Rajat and Tamra shalaka in sandhigata vata which Special Reference to janu sandhi. Bangalore India: Rajeev Gandhi University of Health Sciences (RGUHS); 2012

[46] Mohasin K, Udayashankar H, Yunus M. Management of Sandhigatavata w.s.r to Janusandhi by Agnikarma and Svedana - A comparative clinical study. Aryavaidyan. 2014;**27**(1):52-56

[47] Pandya P, Gupta SK, et al. A Further Study on Agnikarma with Panchatikta Guggulu in the Management of Sandhigatavata w.s.r. to Knee Joint Osteoarthritis. Jamnagar, India: Gujarat Ayurveda University; 2015

[48] Lata A, Badwe Y, Vaidya U. A Comparative Study of Conductive and Direct Method of Agnikarma with Tamra Shalaka in Sandhigatvata with Special Reference to Osteoarthritis of Knee Joint. International Journal of Ayurveda and Pharma Research. 2015;**3**(10):1-6

[49] Ruchi P. Dudhamal TS Effect of Agnikarma along with Panchatikta Guggulu in the management of Janusandhigatavata (Osteoarthritis of Knee Joint). Journal of Ayurved Campus (JAC). 2020;**1**(1):1-6

[50] Pandey R. Agnikarma (therapeutic heat application) in Osteoarthritis of Knee joint- A video demonstration. International Journal of AYUSH Case Reports. 2017;**1**(1):36-37

[51] Puri S, Savadi BS. A comparative study on agnikarma and indigenous drugs in the management of Janu sandhigata vata w.s.r. to osteoarthritis of knee joint. International Journal of Ayurveda and Pharma Research. 2019;**7**(1):39-44

[52] Syyed MJ. Clinical study on efficacy of agnikarma in the management janu sandhigata vata w.s.r to knee joint osteoarthritis. PIJAR. 2019;**3**(4):1-15

[53] Lobo SJ, Bhuyan C, Das AK, Shukla A. A comparative clinical study of Agnikarma (Therapeutic heat burn) with Suvarna Shalaka (Rod of gold) and Panchadhatu Shalaka (Rod made up of five metals) in Janusandhigata Vata w.s.r. to Osteoarthritis of Knee Joint. Journal of Natural Remedies. 2021;**21**(4):303-316

[54] Raut SR, Badole S. Pain Management by Conductive Method of Agnikarma with Suvarna Shalaka in Janusandhigata Vata W.S.R. Knee OA: A Case Report. International Journal of Ayurveda. 2021;**6**(2):42-46